GW01279760

Variability in Drug Therapy
Description, Estimation, and Control

A Sandoz Workshop

Variability in Drug Therapy
Description, Estimation, and Control

A Sandoz Workshop

Editors

Malcolm Rowland, Ph.D.
Professor of Pharmacy
Department of Pharmacy
University of Manchester
Manchester, United Kingdom

Lewis B. Sheiner, M.D.
Professor of Laboratory Medicine and
of Medicine
Departments of Laboratory Medicine
and of Medicine
School of Medicine
University of California
San Francisco, California

Jean-Louis Steimer, Ph.D.
Chargé de Recherches
Institut National de la Santé et de la Recherche Médicale
Unité 194
CHU Pitié-Salpêtrière
Paris, France

Raven Press ● New York

Raven Press, 1185 Avenue of the Americas, New York, New York 10036

© 1985 by Raven Press Books, Ltd. All rights reserved. This book is protected by copyright. No part of it may be reproduced, stored in a retrieval system, or transmitted, in any form or by any means, electronic, mechanical, photocopying, recording, or otherwise, without the prior written permission of the publisher.

Made in the United States of America

Library of Congress Cataloging in Publication Data
Main entry under title:

Variability in drug therapy.

 Based on a meeting held in Rome in May 1984.
 Includes bibliographies and index.
 1. Drugs—Dose-response relationship—Congresses.
2. Pharmacokinetics—Congresses. 3. Biochemical
variation—Congresses. 4. Chemotherapy—Congresses.
I. Rowland, Malcolm. II. Sheiner, Lewis B. III. Steimer,
Jean-Louis. IV. Sandoz AG. [DNLM: 1. Dose-Response
Relationship, Drug—congresses. 2. Drugs—administration
& dosage—congresses. 3. Drugs—metabolism—congresses.
4. Drug Therapy—congresses. QV 38 V299 1984]
RM301.8.V37   1985   615'.7   85-1888
ISBN 0-88167-080-4

The material contained in this volume was submitted as previously unpublished material, except in the instances in which credit has been given to the source from which some of the illustrative material was derived.

Great care has been taken to maintain the accuracy of the information contained in the volume. However, Raven Press cannot be held responsible for errors or for any consequences arising from the use of the information contained herein.

Materials appearing in this book prepared by individuals as part of their official duties as U.S. Government employees are not covered by the above-mentioned copyright.

0   9   8   7   6   5   4   3   2

To Dawn, Lisa, and Michelle
To Michael, Amanda, and Tim
To Elise and Charles

Preface

Even if we try to forget, we are constantly reminded, by one experience or another, that patients differ in their responses to drugs. Manifestations of such variability are seen in differences in the doses of drugs required to produce the same therapeutic end point, and in differences in responses to the same doses or dosage regimens of a drug. Sometimes differences in responses are so small, or the therapeutic index of the drug is so large, that variability is of little therapeutic concern. But, all too often, the degree of variability is too large, and adjustment of dosage in the individual is needed, if ineffective therapy or excessive toxicity, with occasional fatality, is to be avoided. Here variability both between and within individuals needs to be considered. Also to be considered are the sources of variability, which can broadly be divided into pharmacokinetics and pharmacodynamics. Pharmacokinetics relates dosage to concentration achieved and includes absorption, distribution, and elimination; pharmacodynamics relates concentration to response. Among the causes of variability are genetics, disease, age, drugs, and a variety of environmental factors.

Although the subject of variability is old, the development of new insights into the way that the body handles and responds to drugs, as well as the development of new statistical approaches to the question of variability, prompted this volume, *Variability in Drug Therapy: Description, Estimation, and Control.* The authors are from a wide spectrum of specialties, including clinical pharmacology, pharmacokinetics, analytical chemistry, biomathematics, and statistics.

The book is divided into four sections, each with several chapters. The first section, entitled Basics in Variability, deals with evidence of variability in response of patients to drugs, models used to describe pharmacokinetic variability, and chemical assay variability. The second section, entitled Modeling and Estimation of Pharmacokinetic Variability, deals with modeling of variability on both the molecular level and macroscopic level, a comparison of methods used to estimate interindividual pharmacokinetic variability, and statistical considerations of issues in population pharmacokinetics. The third section, entitled Variability in Dose–Effect Relationships, considers evidence for variability in animal and human pharmacodynamics, modeling of the concentration–effect relationship, and integration of pharmacokinetic and pharmacodynamic data. The fourth section, Management of the Individual: Forecasting and Control, directs its attention to the question of optimal design for individual parameter estimation, application of control theory to drug therapy, and clinical application of bayesian feedback to dosage adjustment. Specific discussions follow the majority of chapters, and the book closes with a general discussion.

We, the editors, hope that through the book, we have advanced understanding of variability in drug therapy. Because of the broad impact of variability, the contents of this book should be of interest to all those involved in the development, production, prescribing, and optimal use of medicines for the well-being of patients.

Malcolm Rowland
Lewis B. Sheiner
Jean-Louis Steimer

Acknowledgments

This volume is based on the workshop entitled "Variability in Drug Therapy: Description, Estimation, and Control" held in Rome, in May 1984.

The editors acknowledge Sandoz Ltd., Basle, Switzerland, for sponsorship of the workshop and the Swiss Gerontological Society for support. We are especially indebted to Dr. Leo Abisch, Marketing, and Dr. Werner Niederberger, Biopharmaceutical Department, from Sandoz Ltd., Basle, Switzerland, and to Dr. Helmut Eckert, head of Sandoz Forschungsinstitut, Vienna, Austria, for advice and dedicated assistance in the planning and organization of the workshop. We are also grateful to Mrs. Verena Ceresoli and to Messrs. Fritz Baldus and Guido Nussbaumer, all from Convention Services, Sandoz Ltd., Basle, Switzerland, for technical assistance of the highest level. We also thank Dr. R. Temple, of the U.S. Food and Drug Administration for allowing us to reproduce his discussion paper on testing of drugs in the elderly. Last, but not least, we would like to thank Mrs. Sandra Carozzi, Antonella Fantuzzi, Martine Fréchelin, Anne Maurer, and Albine Stalder for excellent secretarial help.

Contents

Basics in Variability

Interindividual Differences in Drug Responses: An Overview 1
Folke Sjöqvist

Models to Identify Sources of Pharmacokinetic Variability 11
Malcolm Rowland

Accounting for Assay Variability 29
Leon Aarons

Modeling and Estimation of Pharmacokinetic Variability

Modeling Pharmacokinetic Variability on the Molecular Level
  with Stochastic Compartmental Systems 31
James H. Matis and Thomas E. Wehrly

Modeling Pharmacokinetic/Pharmacodynamic Variability 51
Lewis B. Sheiner

Estimating Interindividual Pharmacokinetic Variability 65
Jean-Louis Steimer, Alain Mallet, and France Mentré

Models, Formulations, and Statistics 113
David J. Finney

Variability in Dose-Effect Relationships

Variability in Animal and Human Pharmacodynamic Studies .. 125
Gerhard Levy

Modeling Pharmacodynamics: Parametric and Nonparametric
  Approaches 139
Lewis B. Sheiner

Integrating Pharmacokinetics and Dynamics: Variability in
  Thiopental's Dose Requirement, Pharmacokinetics, and
  Pharmacodynamics 153
Donald R. Stanski and Jo Hermans

Variability in Bioavailability: Concentration Versus Effect 167
Lennart K. Paalzow, Gudrun H. M. Paalzow, and Peer Tfelt-Hansen

Management of the Individual: Forecasting and Control

Optimal Design for Individual Parameter Estimation in
    Pharmacokinetics 187
Elliot M. Landaw

Control of Uncertain Dynamic Systems: Methods,
    Implementation, and Application to Drug Therapy 201
Darryl Katz

Clinical Application of Bayesian Feedback for Dosage
    Adjustment: Rationale and Experience 211
Samuel Vožeh, Toshihiko Uematsu, and Ferenc Follath

Discussion: Principles and Evaluation of Variability in
    Drug Therapy 219
Laszlo Endrenyi (Editor)

Concluding Remarks: Respective Roles of Pharmacokinetics
    and Pharmacodynamics in Drug Development 235
Giorgio Segre

Subject Index 239

Contributors and Discussants

Leon Aarons
Department of Pharmacy
University of Manchester
Oxford Road
Manchester M13 9PL, United Kingdom

Leo Abisch
Marketing
Sandoz AG
CH-4002 Basel, Switzerland

Helmut Eckert
Sandoz Forschungsinstitut
Brunnerstrasse 59
A-1235 Wien, Austria

Laszlo Endrenyi
Department of Pharmacology
University of Toronto
Toronto, Ontario M5S 1A8, Canada

David J. Finney
Department of Statistics
University of Edinburgh
James Clerk Maxwell Building
Mayfield Road
Edinburgh EH9 3JZ, United Kingdom

Ferenc Follath
Division of Clinical Pharmacology
Department of Research and Internal
  Medicine
University Hospital
CH-4031 Basel, Switzerland

U. Gundert-Remy
Institut für Arzneimittelforschung
des Bundesgesundheitsamtes
Seestrasse 10
D-1000 Berlin 65, Federal Republic
  of Germany

Jo Hermans
Department of Medical Statistics
Leiden University School of Medicine
NL-2333 AA Leiden, The Netherlands

Darryl Katz
Department of Mathematics
California State University
Fullerton, California 92634

Jean-René Kiechel
Centre de Recherche
  Pharmacocinétique
Laboratories Sandoz SA
14, Bd Richelieu
Boîte postale
F-92506 Rueil-Malmaison, France

Thomas Kissel
Pharma Development
Sandoz AG
CH-4002 Basel, Switzerland

Klaus Kutz
Clinical Research
Sandoz AG
CH-4002 Basel, Switzerland

Elliot M. Landaw
Department of Biomathematics
University of California at
  Los Angeles School of Medicine
Los Angeles, California 90024

Gerhard Levy
Department of Pharmaceutics
School of Pharmacy
State University of New York at Buffalo
H547 Cooke-Hochstetter Complex
Amherst, New York 14260

Ray Lipicki
Division of Cardiorenal Drug Products
Food and Drug Administration
5600 Fishers Lane
Rockville, Maryland 20857

Contributors

Alain Mallet
INSERM U194
Départment de Biomathématiques
91, Bd de l'Hôpital
F-75634 Paris Cedex 13, France

James H. Matis
Department of Statistics
Texas A&M University
College Station, Texas 77843

Wolfgang Meister
Medizinische Klinik Innenstadt
der Universität München
Ziemssenstrasse 1
D-8000 München 2, Federal
Republic of Germany

France Mentré
INSERM U194
Départment de Biomathématiques
91, Bd de l'Hôpital
F-75634 Paris Cedex 13, France

Werner Niederberger
Pharma Development
Sandoz AG
CH-4002 Basel, Switzerland

Erich Nüesch
Clinical Research
Sandoz AG
CH-4002 Basel, Switzerland

Gudrun H. M. Paalzow
Department of Pharmacology
Faculty of Pharmacy
University of Uppsala, BMC
Box 580
S-751 23 Uppsala, Sweden

Lennart K. Paalzow
Department of Biopharmaceutics and
  Pharmacokinetics
Faculty of Pharmacy
University of Uppsala, BMC
Box 580
S-751 23 Uppsala, Sweden

William T. Robinson
Drug Metabolism
Sandoz Inc.
P.O. Box 11
East Hanover, New Jersey 07936

Malcolm Rowland
Department of Pharmacy
University of Manchester
Oxford Road
Manchester M13 9PL, United Kingdom

Peter C. Rüegg
Clinical Research
Sandoz AG
CH-4002 Basel, Switzerland

Wilfried Schiess
Sandoz AG
Deutschherrnstrasse 15
D-8500 Nürnberg, Federal Republic
  of Germany

Hans J. Schwarz
Drug Metabolism
Sandoz Inc.
P.O. Box 11
East Hanover, New Jersey 07936

Giorgio Segre
Istituto di Farmacologia
Università di Siena
I-53100 Siena, Italy

Lewis B. Sheiner
Clinics—255
Department of Laboratory Medicine and
  Division of Clinical Pharmacology
University of California
San Francisco, California 94143

Pierre Simon
Départment de Médecine
Faculté de Médecine
Pitié-Salpétrière
91, Bd de l'Hôpital
F-75634 Paris Cedex 13, France

Folke Sjöqvist
Department of Clinical Pharmacology
Karolinska Institute
Huddinge Hospital
S-1411 86 Huddinge, Sweden

CONTRIBUTORS

Donald Stanski
Departments of Anesthesia and Medicine
 (Clinical Pharmacology)
Stanford University Medical School
Stanford, California 94305;
 and
Anesthesia
Academisch Ziekenhuis Leiden
Rijnsburgerweg 10
Department of NL-2333 AA Leiden,
 The Netherlands

Jean-Louis Steimer
INSERM U194
Départment de Biomathématiques
91, Bd de l'Hôpital
F-75634 Paris Cedex 13, France;
 and
Biopharmaceutical Department
Sandoz Ltd.
CH-4002 Basel, Switzerland

Egon Stürmer
Marketing
Sandoz AG
CH-4002 Basel, Switzerland

Heinz Sucker
Pharma Development
Sandoz AG
CH-4002 Basel, Switzerland

Peer Tfelt-Hansen
Department of Neurology
Rigshospitalet
DK-2100 Copenhagen Ø, Denmark

Toshihiko Uematsu
Division of Clinical Pharmacology
Department of Research and Internal
 Medicine
University Hospital
CH-4031 Basel, Switzerland

Samuel Vožeh
Division of Clinical Pharmacology
Department of Research and Internal
 Medicine
University Hospital
CH-4031 Basel, Switzerland

Thomas E. Wehrly
Department of Statistics
Texas A&M University
College Station, Texas 77843

Alan Wood
Clinical Research
Sandoz AG
CH-4002 Basel, Switzerland

Foreword

The primary purpose of the research-based pharmaceutical industry always has been to provide patients and physicians with safe and effective drugs. Recently, however, the industry's self-assessment of its role in the health arena has propelled it a step farther. To provide society with useful and sometimes even novel drugs is no longer enough; we also must deliver ideas and concepts of how we envisage those drugs to be used. This broader role comprises therapy rather than only therapeutics. Therapy must be based on knowledge of a drug's absorption, metabolism, distribution, and excretion, and of its half-life and its availability. Perhaps even more important, it must, if possible, be based on an ability to measure the effects of a drug in humans reliably and also to determine those pharmacodynamic and pharmacokinetic parameters that forebode toxicity and that indicate to the physician that the patient is moving beyond the therapeutic range of a drug and that, therefore, the dosage will have to be reduced.

In providing drugs that are meant to be useful for the treatment of a large number of people, we must generalize. In our clinical trials we try to determine the dose and the dosage regimen of a new drug that will work in most patients without exposing them to the hazards or inconveniences of side effects. Of course, these recommendations are generalizations—which will work in most cases but not in all. Although they work in the majority, these generalizations may not provide the achievable therapeutic optimum to each single patient. The necessity to generalize also leads to standardization. The chemical identity of the active principle, its purity, the particle size of the active substance, and many galenical parameters like the stability and the dissolution rate of a particular preparation are kept constant within very narrow limits. With many important drugs this is done on a worldwide scale, so that a doctor working in Honolulu is able to give the patient exactly the same preparation that colleagues in Central Europe or South Africa are using.

Our ability to generalize and to standardize provides the therapist with the possibility to individualize. If absolutely equivalent preparations work to different extents in different individuals, then obviously the source of variability must be in the patient, not in the drug preparation. The objective common to both the pharmaceutical industry and the physician is to deliver effective concentrations of drugs to the biological targets for adequate periods of time in order to achieve therapeutic effects. At the same time, toxic reactions must be avoided. If the effects to be achieved and the side effects to be avoided are easily observable, variations in dose and dosing interval can be oriented toward these effects alone. Where this is not the case, a "target concentration strategy" may be appropriate. In these cases the dosage is adapted to provide a certain concentration of the drug at the target for an adequate time.

Drug variability can result from a large number of parameters: absorption, metabolism, distribution, protein binding, and excretion being the dominant ones. Especially in the presence of other drugs and during diseases, there is also the possibility that the interactions of drugs and their targets will be altered, e.g., through the up- or down-regulation of receptors.

This volume contains chapters written by distinguished specialists and attempts to find answers to questions that have practical relevance to the issue of variability in drug therapy:

1. What are the reasons for interindividual and intraindividual variability?
2. Is variability merely a nuisance, or can it become a serious therapeutic problem?
3. Are interindividual and/or intraindividual variabilities commonly seen with all drugs, or is there a chemical proneness to variability seen only with some drugs and not with others?
4. Does variability in kinetic parameters always indicate variability of efficacy? Are there exceptions?
5. What strategies are available to the physician in dealing with drug variability?
6. What can be done in drug research and development to avoid variability, if anything?

These represent only a few questions. However, we hope to learn more about the phenomenon of variability in drug therapy and hope to find new methods to deal with it more effectively.

Jürgen Drews
Pharmaceutical Research and Development
Sandoz Ltd.
Basel, Switzerland

Symbols and Abbreviations

SYMBOLS

Pharmacokinetics and Pharmacodynamics

A .... coefficient of the exponential model
C .... concentration
C_e .... concentration in effect compartment
C_{e50} .. C_e eliciting half-maximum effect
CL ... clearance
C_p ... plasma concentration
C_{p50}, C_{pss50} . steady-state C_p eliciting half-maximum effect
E .... effect
E_{max} .. maximum effect
k, k_e .. first-order rate constant for drug elimination
k_{eo} ... first-order rate constant for equilibration between effect compartment and plasma
k_{ij} .... first-order rate constant for movement of drug from compartment i to compartment j
K_m ... Michaelis-Menten constant
R .... dosing rate
t ..... time
$T_{½}$ ... half-life of drug
V .... volume of distribution
V_m ... maximum velocity for saturable drug elimination
γ ..... Hill coefficient
λ ..... exponent of the exponential model

Modeling, Estimation, Statistics

$E(\cdot)$ .. expected value of a random variable
$f(\cdot)$ ... a mathematical (e.g., pharmacokinetic) model
$F(\cdot), F$ a probability distribution (e.g., of pharmacokinetic parameters in a population of individuals)
M .... (asymptotic) variance–covariance matrix of the estimates of an individual's parameters
n ..... number of measurements from an individual (e.g., number of blood samples)
N .... number of individuals in a study (i.e., sample size)
p ..... dimension of the parameter vector (number of parameters in model f)
$\text{Var}(\cdot)$. variance of a scalar random variable
y ..... experimental data
ϵ ..... residual error (between experimental data and model predictions)
ζ ..... exponent of the power variance model
η ..... (random) shift (of the pa-

SYMBOLS AND ABBREVIATIONS

θ ..... rameters for an individual) from the mean value
parameters describing the population probability distribution ("population characteristics")
μ ..... expected value of the parameters in the population
σ^2 .... variance of a random variable (e.g., σ_ϵ^2 for ϵ)
ϕ ..... parameters (e.g., pharmacokinetic) describing an individual
Φ .... random-variable "parameters" whose distribution is F
Ψ .... expected value of a response (e.g., a serum-level profile)
Ω .... variance–covariance matrix of the parameters in the population
$\hat{\phi}, \hat{\mu}, \hat{\Omega}$ estimates of ϕ, μ, Ω
IR ... set of real numbers

Remarks: In several chapters, individuals as well as data for a single individual had to be indexed. Subscripts i (for the data) and j (for the individuals) have been used consistently for that purpose. Accordingly:

n_j .... number of measurements for individual j
y_{ij} .... ith data with the jth individual
$y_{ij}; i = 1, \ldots, n_j$ .. data from individual j (n_j values)
y_j .... data from individual j (vector notation)
$y_j; j = 1, \ldots, N$ .. all data from the N individuals of the sample

Note: These symbols have been chosen for unifying the notation across chapters when the same concepts are extensively used and discussed by several authors in different chapters. One or another symbol in this list might appear at some place in a given chapter with another meaning. Such occurrences are rare and are stated.

ABBREVIATIONS

APTT	activated partial thromboplastin time
AUC	area under the curve
CNS	central nervous system
ED_{50}	effective dose fifty
EEG	electroencephalogram
ELS	extended least squares
EP	experimental pharmacokinetics
GFR	glomerular filtration rate
GTS	global two-stage (method)
HPLC	high-performance liquid chromatography
ITS	iterated two-stage (method)
LD_{50}	lethal dose fifty
MAE	maximum average efficiency
MAP	maximum a posteriori
MRT	mean residence time
NAD	naive averaging of data
NLME	nonlinear mixed-effect (model)
NONMEM	nonlinear mixed-effect model with first-order approximation
NPD	naive pooled data
NPML	nonparametric maximum likelihood
PP	population pharmacokinetics
QF	rapid intercompartmental clearance
QS	slow intercompartmental clearance
SEM	standard error of the mean
STS	standard two-stage (method)
TCA	tricyclic antidepressants
VRT	variance of residence time

Variability
in Drug Therapy
Description, Estimation, and Control

A Sandoz Workshop

Interindividual Differences in Drug Responses: An Overview

Folke Sjöqvist

Department of Clinical Pharmacology, Karolinska Institute, Huddinge Hospital, S-1411 86 Huddinge, Sweden

Both irrational and rational factors contribute to the well-known variability among patients in their responses to a fixed dosage schedule of a drug (Table 1). To the former belong variable compliance with the drug regimen and placebo effects. Spontaneous fluctuations in symptoms and thereby in apparent drug effects are exceedingly difficult to evaluate in the individual case. Another irrational factor is the presence of drugs on the market with poor and variable absorption. The latter problem is of decreasing importance in many countries because of more rigorous drug regulation.

Poor drug compliance as a source of variability in drug responses cannot be neglected. Unfortunately, most studies of compliance have been performed with questionable methods such as pill counts and interviews with patients. Using an electronic device, Norell (11) was able to record when patients with glaucoma actually opened their eye-drop bottles (pilocarpine). Thereby, medication records were obtained that amply illustrated the fundamental differences among patients in their attitudes to drug therapy prescribed thrice daily (Fig. 1). A frequency-distribution histogram of the dosage intervals practiced by 82 patients showed a peak at 8 hr, but with variations from a few to 160 hr. It appeared possible to affect the medication behavior toward the prescribed regimen by educating the patients about the purpose and long-term benefits of using pilocarpine regularly (Fig. 2). This method is presently being developed in our hospital for recording tablet medication. It should be mentioned that the clinical importance of poor compliance entirely depends on the precision with which drug therapy has been prescribed. As an example, many elderly patients may be saved from digoxin intoxication simply by not complying with a dosage schedule that would better fit a middle-aged individual with normal kidney function (3).

There is no doubt that the *psychological individuality* of patients has important implications for the outcome of drug therapy. Pharmacologists, however, prefer to stress the importance of *biochemical individuality,* which is easier to

TABLE 1. *Interindividual differences in drug responses*

Contributing factors	Comments
Psychological individuality	
Poor compliance with drug therapy	Tailoring of the dosage schedule, drug education
Placebo effects	
Biochemical individuality	
True interindividual differences in:	Genetic and environmental factors contribute to the variability
First-pass metabolism	
Systemic clearance	
Renal excretion	
Spontaneous fluctuation in symptoms and disease	Difficult to predict and evaluate in the individual case
Receptor variability	Must be explored under controlled kinetic conditions
Pathophysiological individuality	
Disease-mediated changes in pharmacokinetics:	
Kidney disease	Impaired renal excretion of drugs and metabolites; the creatinine clearance satisfactorily predicts this impairment
Cardiovascular disease	
Age-dependent individuality	Impaired renal excretion of drugs in the elderly is well documented

evaluate in well-designed experiments producing hard data. Ideally, such studies should focus on interindividual differences in drug responses, but in practice most of them concern variability in pharmacokinetic parameters taken out of clinical context. Thus, data supporting the clinical value of measuring plasma drug levels are still limited, and it is not uncommon that therapeutic drug monitoring leads to "treatment" of the plasma level rather than the patient.

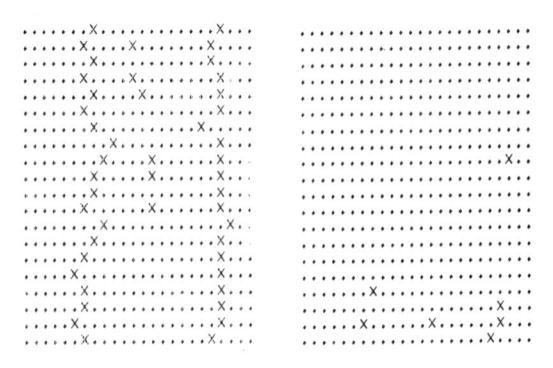

FIG. 1. Monitor records from 2 patients who had been prescribed pilocarpine eye drops thrice daily. One patient was compliant **(left)**, and one started dropping shortly before revisiting the eye clinic **(right)**. (From Norell et al., ref. 12, with permission.)

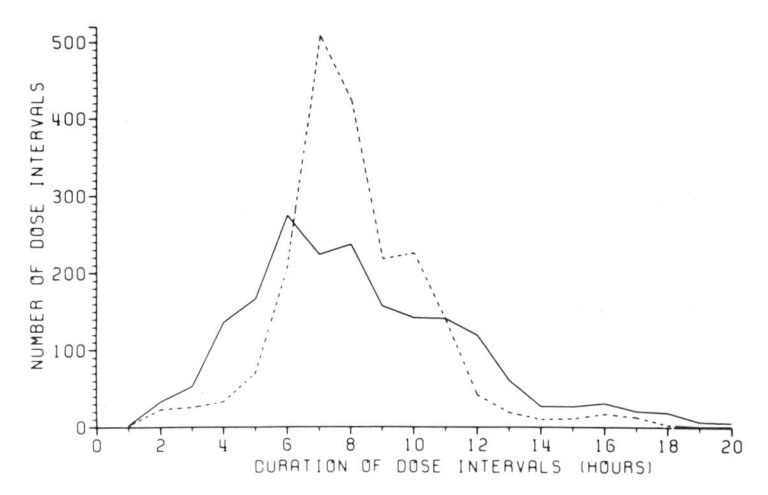

FIG. 2. Frequency distributions of dose intervals for pilocarpine during the first (*solid line*) and second (*dotted line*) 20-day periods. Before the second period the patients underwent a 30-min drug education and tailoring program. The patients were not aware of the recordings. (From Norell, ref. 11, with permission.)

In order to explore the clinical significance of interindividual differences in drug kinetics it is necessary to use an interdisciplinary research strategy. Accurate bioanalysis and elegant kinetics are not sufficient. Equally important are pharmacodynamic measurements and reproducible assessment of clinical drug effects. Many controversies in the literature regarding the clinical use of pharmacokinetics are due to the fact that one or several of these aspects have been neglected. During our interdisciplinary work on the role of kinetic variability in clinical responses to tricyclic antidepressants (TCA) we have had to continuously reevaluate the bioanalytic, pharmacodynamic, and clinical methods used (Table 2). The modest efficacy of these drugs has been a major complication in these studies. In spite of this, there is now a consensus (6,13) that plasma levels of some TCAs are important determinants for their effects in patients with endogenous depression (Fig. 3). The many studies that have failed to demonstrate concentration–effect relationships for TCAs support the notion that these drugs are prescribed on ill-defined indications, where there is little reason to expect a response beyond the placebo effect. Extrapolating the therapeutic range of plasma concentrations established in patients with endogenous depression to all patients with depression or to all patients being prescribed these drugs would result in abuse of clinical pharmacokinetic concepts. The commercialization of drug analyses that is now taking place must therefore be balanced by proper education of physicians (and laboratory people, for that matter) in clinical pharmacology.

An important aim of clinical pharmacokinetic research is to find easily measurable *predictors of drug response.* It would be particularly valuable to have access to methods that would distinguish responders from nonresponders and

TABLE 2. *Sequence of events in our attempts to explore the clinical significance of interindividual variability in the kinetics of TCAs*

Bioanalysis and pharmacokinetics
- 1 Sensitive method for analysis of TCA
- 2 Exploring the kinetics, binding, and metabolism of TCA: role of genetic and environmental factors
- 8 Refined analytical methods for TCA and metabolites (mass fragmentography, high-performance liquid chromatography)
- 9 Mass fragmentographic methods for monoamine metabolites in cerebrospinal fluid (CSF)
- 14 Reevaluation of the role of genetic factors in the oxidation of TCA (relationship to debrisoquine hydroxylation phenotype)
- 16 Imipramine receptor binding assay
- 17 Methods for peptides in CSF

Pharmacodynamics
- 3 Inhibition of monoamine uptake in neurons incubated in plasma drawn from patients
- 4 Blockade of tyramine pressor effects in patients
- 10 Effects of TCA on monoamine metabolites in CSF
- 13 Reevaluation of the effects of drug metabolites on noradrenaline (NA), serotonin (5-HT), and acetylcholine neurons; importance of stereoisomers
- 15 Differential effects of TCA in subgroups of depression

Clinical outcome (psychiatry)
- 5 Rating scale for adverse effect
- 6 Application of depression rating scales
- 7 Interrater reliability assessed
- 11 A comprehensive psychiatric rating scale (CPRS) being developed
- 12 Clinical outcomes in biochemical subgroups [low and high 5-hydroxyindolacetic acid (5-HIAA) in CSF] of depressives (relationship to suicidal behavior)

that would predict patients at risk to develop adverse drug reactions on standard doses. Receptor binding techniques have so far failed to provide such means. Pharmacogenetic research seems to be more promising. It has been known for 20 years that a small proportion of patients are slow in oxidizing certain drugs, such as phenytoin (8) and TCAs (7). The possibility of phenotyping slow drug oxidizers (Fig. 4) with sparteine (5) or debrisoquine (10) is of great interest for both pharmacotherapy and early drug evaluation. Knowing the individual's hydroxylation phenotype may help the investigator to understand mechanisms involved in variability in drug responses. Two examples from our own work may illustrate this point.

While studying the kinetics of various beta-blockers (alprenolol, timolol, metoprolol) we found 4 patients with significantly higher steady-state plasma concentrations than the remainder. All 4 patients turned out to be slow hydroxylators of debrisoquine (Fig. 5). Subsequent studies showed that metoprolol seems to be dependent on the debrisoquine hydroxylase for its metabolism (9). Fortunately, beta-blockers have a broad margin of safety. The situation is quite different for TCAs, whose metabolism also co-varies with the debrisoquine hydroxylation phenotype (15). Thus, it is permitted to hypothesize that

INDIVIDUALITY IN DRUG RESPONSES

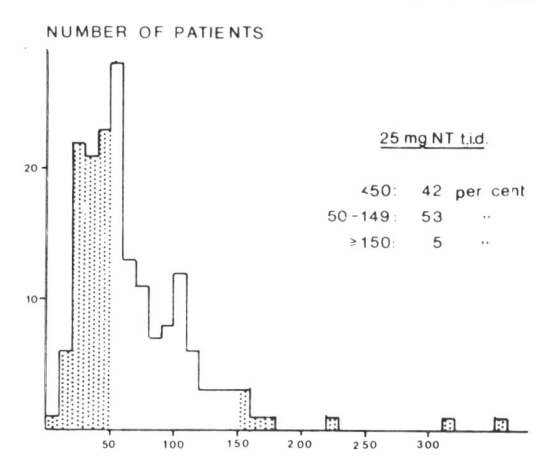

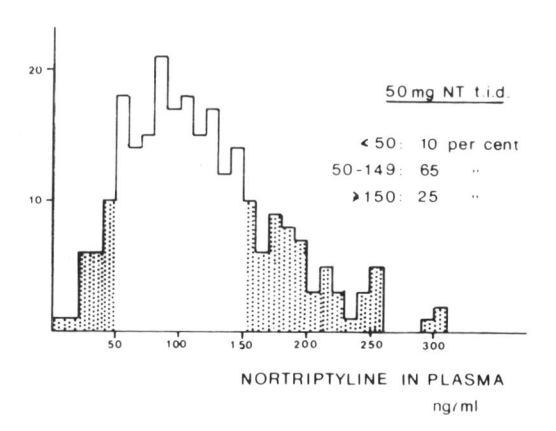

FIG. 3. Frequency distributions of plasma levels of nortriptyline (NT) on two dosage regimens. The therapeutic range of plasma levels (50–150 ng/ml) is indicated for endogenously depressed patients. On a standard dosage of 50 mg t.i.d., 65% of Swedish patients achieved these concentrations. On the basis of such population kinetics a rational dosage strategy can be developed. Slow hydroxylators develop high plasma levels and may get adverse drug reactions as well as poor antidepressant effect. Slow hydroxylators of NT (and other tricyclics) are also slow hydroxylators of debrisoquine.

patients who develop severe side effects on standard dosages of TCAs are slow hydroxylators. The hypothesis can be verified in the individual case by monitoring the plasma concentration of TCA or phenotyping the individual with debrisoquine (14).

The other example stems from a phase-I study of the new selective monoamine oxidase (MAO) inhibitor amiflamine (2). Volunteers taking this drug showed remarkably different renal excretions of the demethylated metabolites, but two distinct patterns emerged when the subjects were grouped according to their hydroxylation phenotypes (Table 3). It might thus be of value to perform

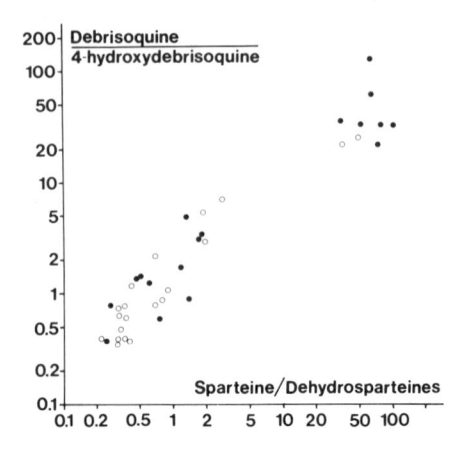

FIG. 4. Relationship between the metabolic ratios of debrisoquine and sparteine in 18 healthy German (*filled circles*) and 30 healthy Swedish (*open circles*) subjects ($r_S = 0.91$; $p < 0.001$). Both drugs can be used to phenotype individuals into rapid and slow hydroxylators. This phenotypic classification is also relevant for the oxidation of some other drugs such as certain beta-blockers and TCAs. (From Eichelbaum et al., ref. 4, with permission.)

phase-I studies of new drugs in volunteers whose biochemical individualities with respect to the cytochrome P-450 isozymes have been assessed.

Pharmacogenetic variability occurs with both high- and low-clearance drugs. Nortriptyline is usually classified as a high-clearance drug, but it must be emphasized that the clearance values in the population vary 10-fold and that there are individuals who show low clearance of this drug. It is the variability rather

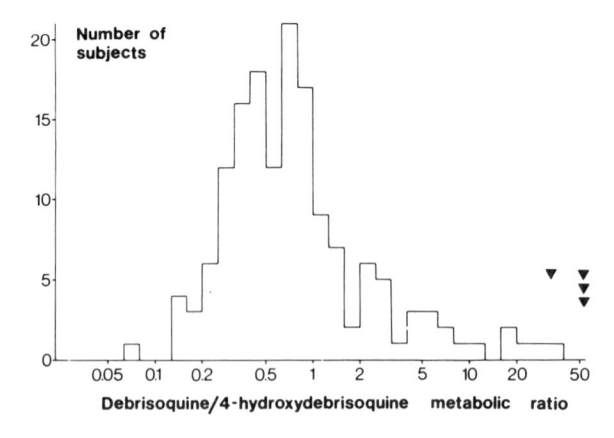

FIG. 5. Debrisoquine metabolic ratios in 4 outliers (*filled triangles*) with unusually high plasma concentrations of the beta-blockers metoprolol (2 subjects), alprenolol, and timolol. Ratios in 155 healthy Swedish volunteers are shown for comparison; individuals with ratios above 12.6 are poor hydroxylators. (From Alván et al., ref. 1, with permission.)

TABLE 3. Urinary recovery of amiflamine and its metabolites in rapid and slow hydroxylators of debrisoquine

Subject	Debrisoquine ratio	Percentage of dose recovered as				Ratios between products		
		Parent compound	Desmethyl metabolite	Didesmethyl metabolite	Parent drug/ desmethyl	Desmethyl/ disdesmethyl	Parent drug didesmethyl
G.A.	0.18	0.05	2.37	43.40	0.02	0.05	0.001
L.G.	0.50	0.26	12.08	39.50	0.02	0.31	0.007
O.W.	0.72	0.29	14.11	53.32	0.02	0.26	0.005
B.E.W.	21.6	15.27	33.87	7.30	0.45	4.64	2.09
A.B.	39	17.67	17.40	2.51	1.02	6.93	7.04

than the magnitude of clearance that matters clinically. Another important aspect is the stability (reproducibility) of the kinetics of a drug. It appears that some drugs have rather consistent kinetics over time within the individual, whereas others may show marked intraindividual variability. The latter may be a clinical disadvantage. A new classification of drugs being metabolized might be of interest for drug selection. The first class would be those with stable metabolism, which mainly is governed by genetic factors, and the second class would be those with unstable kinetics due to the influence of a variety of environmental factors.

Finally, *pathophysiological individuality* and *age-dependent individuality* contribute to the variability in drug responses. Pharmacokinetic studies in the elderly are now commonly performed as part of the documentation of new drugs. The premises for some of these studies are not clear. As an example, it is questionable whether or not there are clinically important differences between elderly and other patients in the metabolism of drugs.

ACKNOWLEDGMENT

Supported by grants from the Swedish Medical Research Council (04X-3902).

REFERENCES

1. Alván, G., von Bahr, C., Seideman, P., and Sjöqvist, F. (1982): High plasma concentrations of beta-receptor blocking drugs and deficient debrisoquine hydroxylation. *Lancet*, 1:333–334.
2. Alván, G., Grind, M., Graffner, C., and Sjöqvist, F. (1984): Relationship of N-demethylations of amiflamine and its metabolite to debrisoquine hydroxylation polymorphism. *Clin. Pharmacol. Ther.*, 36:515–519.
3. Boethius, G., and Sjöqvist, F. (1978): Doses and dosage intervals of drugs—clinical practice versus pharmacokinetic principles. *Clin. Pharmacol. Ther.*, 24:255–263.
4. Eichelbaum, M., Bertilsson, L., Säwe, J., and Zekorn, C. (1982): Polymorphic oxidation of sparteine and debrisoquine: Related pharmacogenetic entities. *Clin. Pharmacol. Ther.*, 31:184–186.
5. Eichelbaum, M., Spannbrucker, N., Steinecke, B., and Dengler, H. (1979): Defective N-oxidation of sparteine in man: A new pharmacogenetic defect. *Eur. J. Clin. Pharmacol.*, 16:183–187.
6. Gram, L., Kragh-Sørensen, P., Kristensen, C., Møller, M., Pedersen, O., and Thayssen, P. (1984): Plasma level monitoring of antidepressants: Theoretical basis and clinical application. In: *Frontiers in Biochemical and Pharmacological Research in Depression*, edited by E. Usdin, M. Åsberg, L. Bertilsson, and F. Sjöqvist, pp. 399–412. Raven Press, New York.
7. Hammer, W., and Sjöqvist, F. (1967): Plasma levels of monomethylated tricyclic antidepressants during treatment with imipramine-like compounds. *Life Sci.*, 6:1895–1903.
8. Kutt, H., Wolk, M., Scherman, R., and McDowell, F. (1964): Insufficient parahydroxylation as a cause of diphenylhydantoin toxicity. *Neurology (Minneap.)*, 14:542–548.
9. Lennard, M., Silas, J., Freestone, S., Ramsay, L., Tucker, G., and Woods, H. (1982): Oxidation phenotype—a major determinant of metoprolol metabolism and response. *N. Engl. J. Med.*, 307:1558–1560.
10. Mahgoub, A., Idle, J.R., Pring, L.G., Lancaster, R., and Smith, R.C. (1977): Polymorphic hydroxylation of debrisoquine in man. *Lancet*, 2:584–586.

11. Norell, S.E. (1979): Improving medication compliance: A randomised clinical trial. *Br. Med. J.,* 2:1031–1033.
12. Norell, S.E., Granström, P.A., and Wassén, R. (1980): A medication monitor and fluorescein technique designed to study medication behaviour. *Acta Ophtalmol.* 58:459–567.
13. Potter, W.Z., Bertilsson, L., and Sjöqvist, F. (1981): Clinical pharmacokinetics of psychotropic drugs: Fundamental and practical aspects. In: *Handbook of Biological Psychiatry. Part VI. Practical Applications of Psychotropic Drugs and Other Biological Treatments,* edited by H.M. van Praag, M.H. Lader, O.J. Rafaelsen, and E.J. Sachar, pp. 71–134. Marcel Dekker, New York.
14. Sjöqvist, F. (1984): Polymorphisms in drug metabolism: Implications for drug utilization. *Biochemical Society Transactions,* 12:101–103.
15. Sjöqvist, F., and Bertilsson, L. (1984): Clinical pharmacology of antidepressant drugs: Pharmacogenetics. In: *Frontiers in Biochemical and Pharmacological Research in Depression,* edited by E. Usdin, M. Åsberg, L. Bertilsson, and F. Sjöqvist, pp. 359–372. Raven Press, New York.

DISCUSSION

Discussant 1 (D1): I would like to comment on the idea of a dichotomy between intraindividual variability and interindividual variability. Perhaps neither is that stable. Perhaps I differ from myself 20 years ago more than I did then from another 25-year-old.

Speaker (S): That may be so for certain characteristics, but not for others. I was just throwing out this idea for further discussion. I am fully prepared to drop the concept, but I don't think that we can generalize from studies of a few probe drugs such as antipyrine. Investigators working with different drugs have different experiences regarding intraindividual reproducibility, which has rarely been investigated in longitudinal pharmacokinetic studies. It would have been nice, for example, to have determined your kinetics for several drugs 20 years ago and have repeated the determination now.

We found, in a collaborative study with Dr. Woolhouse in Ghana (2), that the clearance of nortriptyline and the debrisoquine index come out very similar in the two different places. We have also found that nortriptyline kinetics are amazingly reproducible within an individual. On the other hand, one is reminded of the observation by Conney and associates (1), many years ago, that after only a few days' diet with charcoal-broiled beefsteak, the kinetics of phenacetine changed drastically. Clearly, it is an advantage in clinical medicine to have a drug that shows only small intraindividual variability in its pharmacokinetics.

D2: You mentioned the establishment of concentration–response relationships. Do you think that psychometric testing involving the subjective response from a psychiatric patient is sensitive and reproducible and reliable enough over a population to be useful for defining a concentration–response relationship to such drugs as the antidepressants?

S: Yes. Reliability studies have been done with psychiatric rating scales used in depression. In the hands of academically trained psychiatrists, good correlations come out, both within and between departments.

REFERENCES

1. Conney, A.G., Pantuck, E.J., Hsiao, K.C., Garland, W.A., Anderson, K.E., Alvares, A.P., and Kappas, A. (1976): Enhanced phenacetine metabolism in humans fed charcoal broiled beef. *Clin. Pharmacol. Ther.,* 20:633–642.
2. Woolhouse, N., Adjepon-Yamoah, K.K., Mellström, B., Hedman, A., Bertilsson, L., and Sjöqvist, F. (1984): Nortriptypline and debrisoquine hydroxylations in Ghanaian and Swedish subjects. *Clin Pharmacol. Ther.,* 36:374–378.

*Variability in Drug Therapy:
Description, Estimation, and Control,*
edited by M. Rowland et al.
Raven Press, New York © 1985.

Models to Identify Sources of Pharmacokinetic Variability

Malcolm Rowland

*Department of Pharmacy, University of Manchester,
Manchester M13 9PL, United Kingdom*

Mathematical models serve to summarize a large collection of data, to make predictions, and to gain insight into the underlying processes responsible for the observations. Such models vary in complexity depending on the amount and quality of information available and on the intended use of the model. These general comments apply, of course, to models used in pharmacokinetics, where measurements are often limited in number and in kind.

In the past, pharmacokinetic models were little more than extensions of those used to describe simple reaction-beaker kinetics. However, in recent years the trend has been to place pharmacokinetic models in a physiological context, with considerable benefit to our understanding of the factors controlling the fate of administered drugs.

Specifically, in this chapter, I should like to illustrate how physiologically-based models can help both to identify sources of pharmacokinetic variability and to predict how such variability is expressed in terms of commonly estimated parameters. Inferences are generally based on measurements of drug or metabolite or both in plasma (blood) and urine that reflect a balance between input (absorption) and disposition. To fully appreciate the overall situation, it is appropriate to separate these processes, starting first with disposition.

DISPOSITION

Distribution and elimination both cause the concentration of drug in plasma to decline. Although variable, distribution kinetics are generally rapid compared with those of elimination, and consequently in many applications of pharmacokinetics, distribution is assumed to occur spontaneously, with the extent of distribution outside of plasma being characterized by the volume of distribution V. Exceptions arise, particularly when there is a therapeutic interest in the early non-steady-state situation, e.g., anesthesia, and when distribution into effector-site tissues is very slow relative to elimination, usually because of a membrane permeability limitation, e.g., aminoglycoside distribution (38). Besides membrane permeability, other factors controlling the rate of drug distribution are vascular perfusion rate and the relative distribution of drug between blood and tissues.

An elimination half-life ($T_{1/2}$) or an elimination rate constant (k) is frequently used to characterize the disposition kinetics of a drug. For many purposes, including identification of sources of variability, it is best, however, to characterize disposition by volume of distribution and clearance, CL, which is a measure of the efficiency of organs for drug elimination. This is so because clearance and volume of distribution are the independent parameters that control half-life ($T_{1/2} = 0.693 V/\text{CL}$). Both volume of distribution and clearance, and hence half-life, vary widely between drugs and for a given drug can vary widely between individuals. Reasons for the observed differences in degree of variability in volume of distribution and clearance among drugs become apparent when these pharmacokinetic parameters are interpreted in the context of physiologic models.

Distribution

The major determinants of volume of distribution are body composition, binding of drug in blood and in tissues, and, for sufficiently lipophilic drugs, partitioning into adipose tissue. The fraction of drug unbound in plasma (f_u) varies widely among drugs, and often (for highly bound drugs) among individuals. Differences in binding among drugs arise primarily from differences in affinity of drug for the binding protein, which may be albumin (especially for acids), α_1 acidic glycoprotein (especially for many amines), or specific proteins (such as cortisol-binding globulin and sex-hormone-binding globulin). Differences in binding protein concentrations, differences in concentrations of drug (if it approaches the molar concentration of binding protein), and the presence or absence of displacers are primary sources of variability among individuals in the degree of plasma binding of a drug (15,31). Whether or not changes in plasma binding alter the volume of distribution of a drug depends on its basic distributional pattern. This is illustrated in Fig. 1. Only for drugs with relatively large volumes of distribution (> 30 liters / 70 kg) that are bound substantially to plasma proteins will variations in plasma binding produce corresponding changes in volume of distribution. The unbound volume of distribution, V_u ($= V/f_u$), which relates the amount of drug in the body to the concentration of the important unbound (pharmacologically active) drug, does not change in this instance, however. With a large volume of distribution, the percentage of drug in plasma is too small for changes in the amount of drug on the plasma protein to materially affect the unbound pool, which reflects the total amount of drug in the body. The opposite is true for a drug with a small volume of distribution (~ 10 liters/70 kg), because of predominant binding

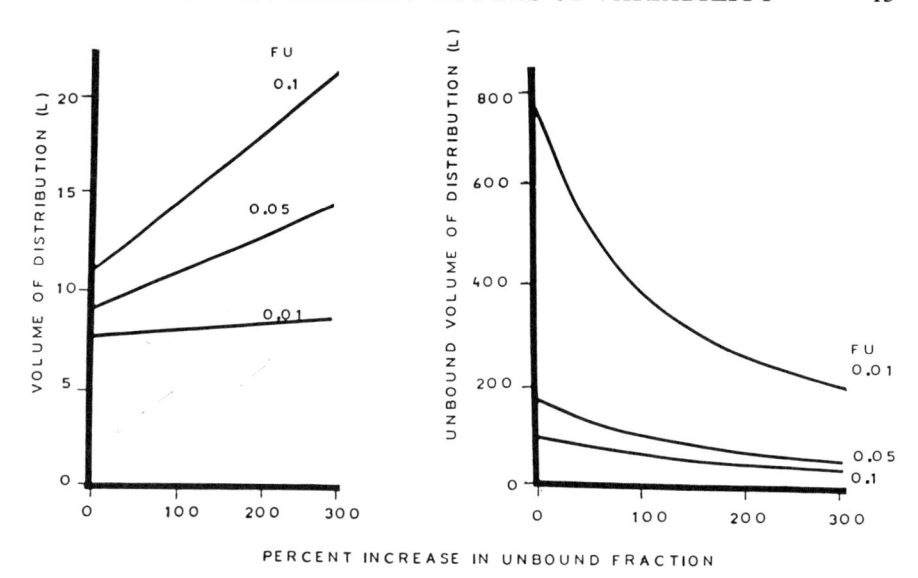

FIG. 1. Changes in the volume of distribution **(left)** and unbound volume of distribution **(right)** with increases in the fraction of drug unbound in plasma (f_u) for a drug bound only to albumin and distributing into total-body water space (42 liters). (Adapted from Tozer, ref. 41.)

within the body to plasma proteins (usually albumin). Here variations in plasma binding produce little change in V but a relatively large change in V_u (Fig. 1). The reason lies in the distribution of plasma protein between the plasma and the remaining extracellular fluid (27); any change in plasma binding is reflected by a proportional change in tissue binding, with little change in distribution of total drug within the body. However, with most of the drug in the body bound initially, then as drug binding both within and outside the plasma changes, so does the unbound pool. Models that include this distribution of plasma proteins have done much to help explain drug distribution under a variety of conditions (22,42).

Clearance

The concept of clearance has received wide application in pharmacokinetics (30,33,35,41,46). Organ clearance is the product of organ blood flow (Q) and extraction ratio (E). The primary determinants of clearance are organ blood flow, binding of drug within blood, membrane permeability, and intrinsic cellular activity, frequently referred to as the intrinsic clearance of the system, CL_{int}. The meaning of intrinsic clearance depends on the organ and the nature of the elimination process. Often elimination is via metabolism, in which case intrinsic clearance is a function of the maximum velocity and Michaelis-Menten constant for each of the enzymes involved. When dealing with transport systems, as occurs in biliary and renal secretion, the corresponding parameters of interest are the maximum transport rate and the affinity constant of the drug for the system(s).

When attempting to identify sources of variability in clearance, it is extremely important, whenever possible, to partition intrinsic clearance into its component parts. This often means identifying and measuring metabolites in plasma and urine and determining the metabolic sequences involved. Interpretation of the data is based on the use of the same pharmacokinetic models as are applied to drugs themselves (13,32). Despite the many difficulties involved in such partitioning of intrinsic clearance, the rewards are many. Those metabolic pathways showing greatest interindividual variability are beginning to be characterized, and through correlation studies involving the administration of several extensively oxidized drugs to the same individuals, common oxidative metabolic pathways for different drugs have been identified (6).

To help predict the influences of the factors affecting clearance, drugs have been classified according to the magnitude of the extraction ratio. For drugs of high extraction ($E > 0.7$), clearance approaches and is limited by blood flow; it is relatively insensitive to changes in binding or cellular activity. At the other extreme are drugs of low extraction ($E < 0.2$). For these, theory predicts that clearance should be sensitive to changes in binding and cellular activity and relatively insensitive to changes in perfusion. That is,

$$\mathrm{CL} = f_\mathrm{u} \cdot \mathrm{CL}_\mathrm{u} \qquad (1)$$

where CL_u is the clearance based on unbound drug, which, when the limitation lies at the enzymatic level, is equal to the intrinsic clearance CL_int. An increasing body of experimental evidence (12,19,37) supports equation (1). Between the extremes are drugs of intermediate extraction ratio, for which all determinants of clearance must be considered.

The foregoing classification of drugs in terms of extraction-ratio values is somewhat arbitrary, as it is possible to change a high-extraction drug to a low-extraction drug by changing sufficiently, for example, the degree of binding within plasma (34). In practice, however, a parameter rarely varies by more than 5- to 10-fold within the population, and often may vary much less, so that the foregoing statements are reasonable approximations. Notwithstanding, prediction and interpretation of the exact relationships between the determinants of clearance and clearance itself require the formulation of a model.

Although the concept of clearance is applicable to any eliminating organ, most work in this area has been concerned with hepatic elimination. Several models of hepatic clearance have been prosposed, and experimental data supporting one or another of them have been forthcoming (3,9,17,24,25,47). When interpreting sources of variation in clearance, it is therefore important to realize that there is some uncertainty in the model used, and this applies especially to drugs of high extraction ratio; at low extraction, all models collapse to a similar form, and in essence the prediction is independent of the model chosen (37).

With regard to the other major process, renal excretion, all drugs are filtered at the renal glomeruli. Some are also actively secreted into the lumen of the nephron, and others are reabsorbed from the lumen, predominantly by passive diffusion. If only filtration occurs, renal clearance is given by equation (1), where CL_u is the glomerular filtration rate (GFR). For such drugs, renal clearance varies with binding of drug within plasma and probably to some extent with renal perfusion, which affects GFR. Reabsorption occurs principally with lipophilic drugs, and for these, renal clearance can vary with urine flow and (if weak electrolytes) with urine pH. Physiologic models have been developed that successfully accommodate and predict the influences of variations in protein binding and urine flow rate on renal clearance, based on the differential permeability characteristics of the luminal epithelium to drug and water (12,39).

Total clearance is the net result of clearances by different organs, usually the liver and kidneys, but it can include clearances by the lungs, the blood, and other tissues. When attempting to predict or to interpret the influences of variations in factors on total clearance, it is important to recognize the anatomic relationships among different organs (e.g., gut, liver, and lungs are in series; liver and kidneys are in parallel). Also, separation into clearances by the individual organs is desirable, particularly if the drug is extracted well by one organ but not by another and if the processes involved in elimination of drug from the organs differ (36).

Disposition Kinetics

Variability in Intrinsic Clearance

Combining models of drug distribution and clearance allows prediction and interpretation of variability in drug disposition data. The large interindividual variability in the half-life of antipyrine (45) is explained primarily by variations in intrinsic hepatic clearance, probably associated with variations in the amounts of the mixed-function oxidase enzymes responsible for the metabolism of this compound; antipyrine is predominantly metabolized, has a low hepatic extraction ratio, is negligibly bound to plasma or tissue components, and is sufficiently lipophilic to pass membranes to occupy total-body water space. A similar explanation probably applies to theophylline, which also exhibits large variability in disposition kinetics, has low clearance, and is only moderately bound (16). Such a high degree of variability in intrinsic clearance will be masked by the perfusion limitation for a drug of high hepatic clearance, and because hepatic blood flow rate is relatively constant among normal individuals, at around 90 liters/hr, little variation in clearance between them is expected. Moreover, unless plasma binding and tissue binding are very variable,

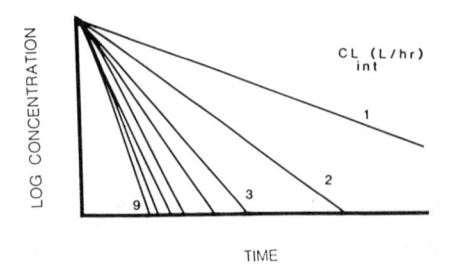

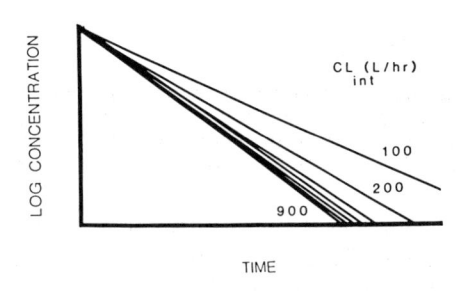

FIG. 2. Expected plasma drug concentration–time profiles following an intravenous bolus dose with changes in intrinsic clearance for drugs of low extraction ratio **(top)** and high extraction ratio **(bottom)**. Intrinsic clearance was varied over a ninefold range in both cases, from 1 to 9 liters/hr for the poorly extracted drug and from 100 to 900 liters/hr for the highly extracted drug. Simulation based on the well-stirred model of hepatic elimination (24), assuming hepatic elimination, only, a hepatic blood flow of 90 liters/hr, and a volume of distribution greater than 30 liters.

the volume of distribution and hence the disposition kinetics for such a drug will be much the same for all normal individuals (Fig. 2). This, indeed, has been found true for lidocaine (29,36), propranolol (18), and alprenolol (1), all drugs of high hepatic clearance.

Variability in Plasma Binding

Any variability in plasma protein binding will manifest itself in disposition kinetics differently for drugs of low and high extraction ratios. The situation is illustrated in Fig. 3 for a drug with a moderately large volume of distribution (that is, one in which V_u is unaffected by changes in plasma binding, *vide supra*). For a drug of low extraction ratio, because neither CL_u nor V_u has changed, neither will the half-life. All that happens is that with increased binding, and hence smaller V, a higher total (but not unbound) plasma concentration is seen. In contrast, for a drug of high extraction ratio, a change in binding produces little change in clearance. But with V varying so does the half-life, becoming shorter the greater the degree of binding of the drug to plasma pro-

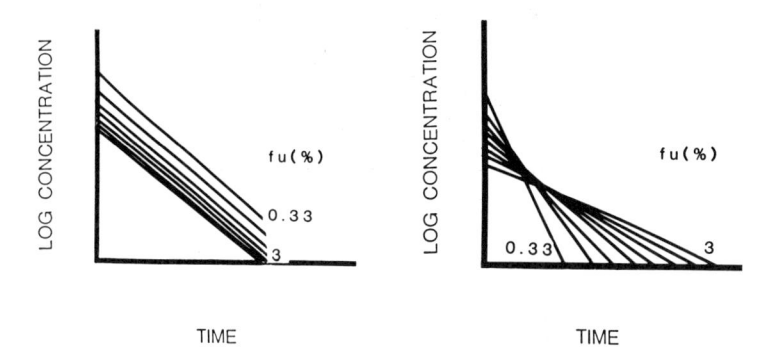

FIG. 3. Expected plasma drug concentration–time profiles following an intravenous bolus dose with changes in plasma protein binding for drugs of low intrinsic clearance (**left**) and high intrinsic clearance (**right**). In each case the fraction of drug unbound (f_u) was varied ninefold, from 0.33 to 3%. See Fig. 2 for assumptions.

teins. The situation is somewhat different for those drugs that are predominantly bound to albumin. Then the half-life tends to be most sensitive to variations in plasma binding for drugs of low intrinsic clearance (23).

The impact of variability in plasma binding on the events at steady state, following a constant-rate intravenous infusion, is worth noting. At plateau,

$$\frac{\text{concentration}}{\text{at plateau}} = \frac{\text{infusion rate}}{\text{clearance}} \tag{2}$$

With a drug of low clearance ($CL = f_u \cdot CL_u$), altered binding (f_u) affects clearance but not unbound clearance, so that the plateau plasma concentration varies, but not the concentration of unbound (pharmacologically active) drug. This situation is nicely illustrated with phenytoin, a drug of low clearance. Although plasma protein binding is less in uremic patients and in patients with the nephrotic syndrome than in normals, no adjustment in the usual daily dosing rate of this antiepileptic drug is required (11). Variation in plasma binding has more profound consequences for drugs of high clearance. For them, although clearance and hence total plasma plateau concentration will vary little, the unbound concentration at plateau must inversely reflect any variation in the fraction of drug unbound.

ABSORPTION AND DISPOSITION

Hepatic First Pass

With all orally administered drugs having to pass through the liver, some will be lost before entering the general circulation; the higher the hepatic extraction ratio the greater is the loss (and the lower is the oral bioavailability, F)

due to this *first-pass* effect. Analysis shows that when the hepatic extraction ratio is high, bioavailability reflects variation in intrinsic clearance (CL_{int}). Accordingly, with subsequent disposition being controlled by hepatic perfusion, a series of similarly shaped plasma drug concentration–time curves, but reaching different peak concentrations, should be seen among individuals receiving the same oral dosage of drug (Fig. 4). Such has been observed with high-clearance drugs, including propranolol (18) and lidocaine (4). In contrast, for drugs of low hepatic extraction ratio, variation in intrinsic clearance is reflected by variance in clearance (and half-life) rather than in bioavailability (and maximum plasma concentration), that is always high (Fig. 4).

An impression prevails that variability in bioavailability, because of the high first-pass effect, imposes an inherent limitation on a drug. This expression of variability in hepatic intrinsic clearance may result in subjects needing different single oral doses of drug to produce the same effect, but on chronic dosing the degree of variability in the plateau concentration for such a drug is inherently no different than exists for a drug of low hepatic clearance, with the same degree of variability in intrinsic clearance (Fig. 5). At plateau, the time-average concentration (C_{av}) is given by

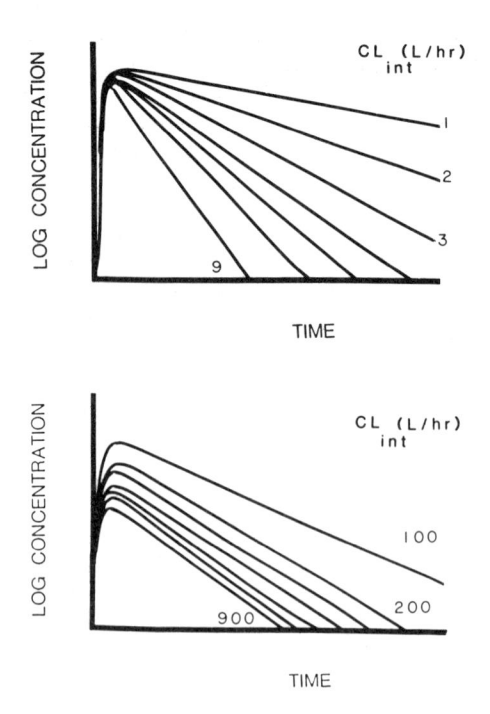

FIG. 4. Expected plasma drug concentration–time profiles following a single oral dose of drug with changes in intrinsic clearance for drugs of low extraction ratio **(top)** and high extraction ratio **(bottom)**. See Fig. 2 for assumptions and conditions.

$$C_{av} = \frac{F \cdot \text{dose}}{CL \cdot \tau} \qquad (3)$$

where τ is the dosing interval. For drugs of high hepatic clearance, variability in C_{av} reflects variability in intrinsic clearance through F, whereas with drugs of low hepatic clearance the variability in C_{av} reflects variability in intrinsic clearance through CL (with $F \simeq 1$). In both cases the dosing rate (dose/τ) would need to be adjusted to maintain a common C_{av} within subjects, this being achieved by simply adjusting the dose for the high-clearance drug (as half-life is relatively constant) and perhaps by a mixture of adjusting dose and dosing interval (given that half-life varies) for the low-clearance drug. Of major importance is the underlying variation in enzymatic activities, which differ from one enzyme system to another. Obviously, to minimize variation in pharmacokinetics, molecules should be selected that, if metabolized, are substrates of enzymatic systems that show the least variability among subjects.

Considering the individual, it follows from the foregoing that there is no inherent reason to believe that there should be any greater intraindividual variation in pharmacokinetic parameters or in C_{av} for drugs of high hepatic extraction than for drugs of low hepatic extraction, caused by a set variation in intrinsic clearance due to variations in enzyme levels, inhibitors, or inducers and so forth. The lack of obvious difference in the degree of intraindividual variability in pharmacokinetics between lidocaine (Fig. 6), a drug of high hepatic clearance, and theophylline (43), a drug of low hepatic clearance, would support this hypothesis. If substantiated, it follows that there should be nothing to choose between high- and low-clearance drugs with regard to maintaining a desired plasma drug concentration within an individual patient receiving chronic therapy.

In patients with normal kidney function, interindividual differences in renal clearance of drugs are often considerably smaller than those for hepatic clearance. Accordingly, whereas variability in bioavailability for drugs of high hepatic extraction will persist, variability in total clearance for all drugs will

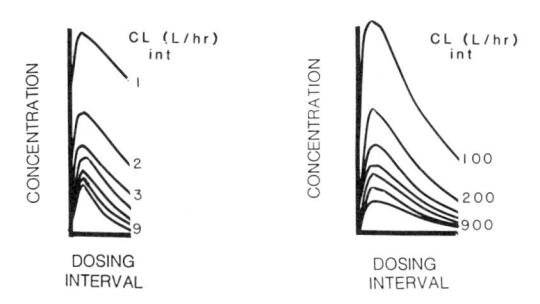

FIG. 5. Expected plasma drug concentration–time profiles at steady state following chronic oral administration of a drug with changes in intrinsic clearance for drugs of low extraction ratio **(left)** and high extraction ratio **(right)**. See Fig. 2 for assumptions and conditions.

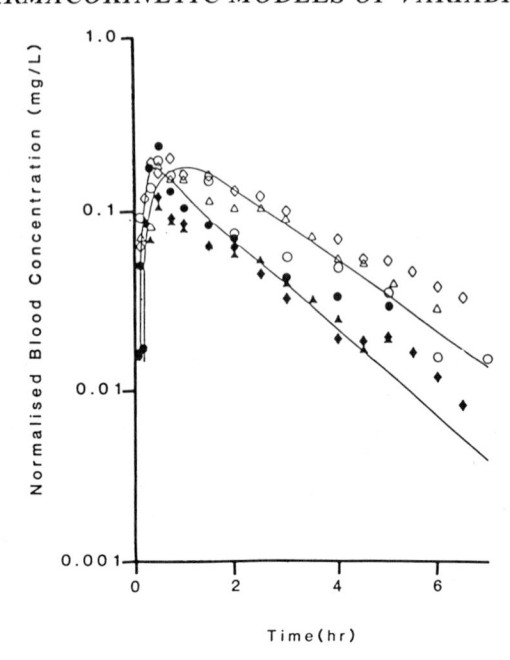

FIG. 6. The virtual superimposition of the plasma concentrations of lidocaine and its de-ethylated metabolite, MEGX, when a subject received different oral doses (100, 300, 500 mg) of lidocaine implies that intraindividual variability in the disposition kinetics of lidocaine and its metabolite must be small. (From Bennett et al., ref. 4, with permission.)

diminish with a greater contribution of renal excretion to overall drug elimination.

In terms of total drug in plasma (or blood), the effect of variation in plasma binding on C_{av} should be similar to that seen with variation in intrinsic hepatocellular activity. The contribution of differences in binding should, however, be minimal or absent when considering unbound drug at steady state (Fig. 7).

Prehepatic Metabolism

Metabolite data can provide support for any suggestion that low oral bioavailability of a drug is solely due to hepatic first-pass loss. For this suggestion to hold, the fraction of the dose of drug converted to metabolite [reflected by its corresponding total area under the concentration–time curve (AUC) or cumulative excretion] should be the same, independent of route of drug administration. This follows because under these circumstances the amount of drug reaching the liver, whether given orally or parenterally, is the same (provided that the liver is the primary organ of elimination). This is indeed seen with MEGX, a primary metabolite of lidocaine (Fig. 8), and with 10-hydroxynortriptyline, a primary metabolite of nortriptyline (39); both lidocaine and nor

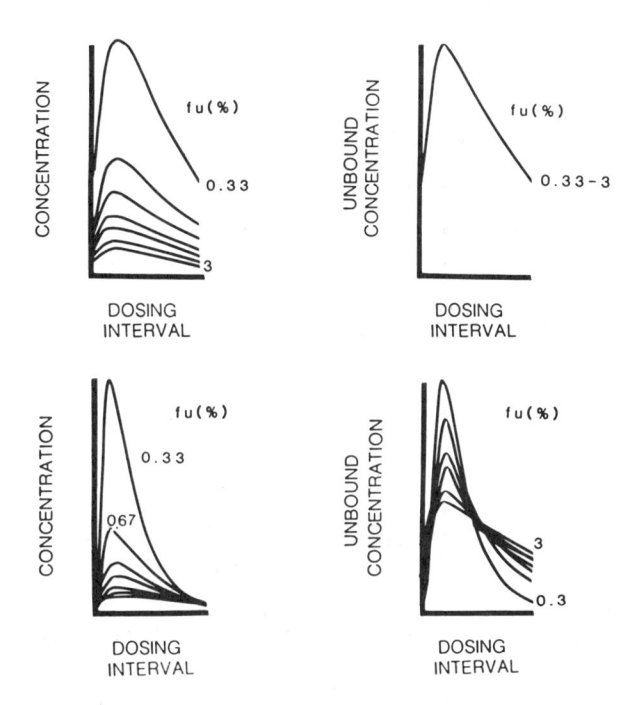

FIG. 7. Expected total **(left)** and unbound **(right)** plateau drug concentrations with a ninefold variation in the fraction of drug unbound in plasma (0.33–3%) for drugs of low extraction ratio **(top)** and high extraction ratio **(bottom)** when given as a chronic oral dosage regimen. Note that for the drug of high clearance, variation in f_u causes the shape of the curve, but not necessarily the area under the unbound curve, to change; no change in unbound drug concentration is expected for the drug of low clearance. See Fig. 2 for assumptions and conditions.

triptyline show low oral bioavailability due to a high hepatic first-pass loss.

Prehepatic metabolism is an additional cause for a decrease in oral bioavailability. It can also be a source of pronounced interindividual and intraindividual variability in absorption of drug. Possible sites of prehepatic metabolism are the gastrointestinal epithelium (10) and the intestinal microflora (14). Given the heterogeneous distribution of enzymes along the gut wall and the fluctuations in populations of intestinal microflora of interest, which reside primarily in the lower part of the small intestine and large bowel, both the rate and extent of intestinal metabolism may vary from one occasion to another. A clue to the occurrence of prehepatic metabolism is a greater AUC for a metabolite (or greater amount excreted in urine) when drug is given orally than when given parenterally. Such is the case for isoproterenol (with respect to sulfate conjugation) (8) and for L-DOPA (with respect to decarboxylation) (5). Giving a peripheral decarboxylase inhibitor improves the situation for L-DOPA by increasing the extent of, and decreasing the variability in, its absorption (5).

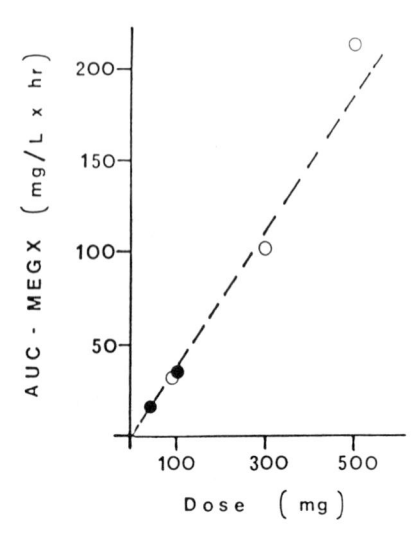

FIG. 8. Because the AUC for the de-ethylated metabolite of lidocaine, MEGX, is the same for a given dose of lidocaine whether given orally (*open circles*) or intravenously (*filled circles*), the low oral bioavailability of lidocaine (~ 30%) is probably due to hepatic first-pass elimination. The direct proportionality between the AUC for MEGX and the dose of lidocaine indicates that the system is linear. (From Bennett et al., ref. 4, with permission.)

Incomplete Dissolution

Most drugs are administered orally in solid dosage forms, and dissolution must proceed for absorption to occur. Generally, incomplete dissolution of solid drug not only lowers the amount absorbed but also increases the variability in absorption, and as such is a cause for concern in drug therapy. This source of variability can often be identified by comparing the bioavailability performance between a solution of drug (if sufficiently soluble) and the solid dosage form, or between two solid dosage forms with widely differing dissolution profiles. Metabolite data can provide supportive information. Thus, if incomplete dissolution has occurred, then although the amount of drug absorbed is lower, the ratio of areas between drug and metabolite (or ratio of cumulative amounts excreted) should be unchanged. This approach assumes that the extent of metabolism during the absorption process is unaffected by differences in rates of drug dissolution, a reasonable assumption in many, but not all, cases.

Gastric Emptying

Being absorbed primarily from the intestine rather than from the stomach, it is not surprising that gastrointestinal absorption of drugs is often affected by the stomach emptying rate, which varies between and within individuals (21).

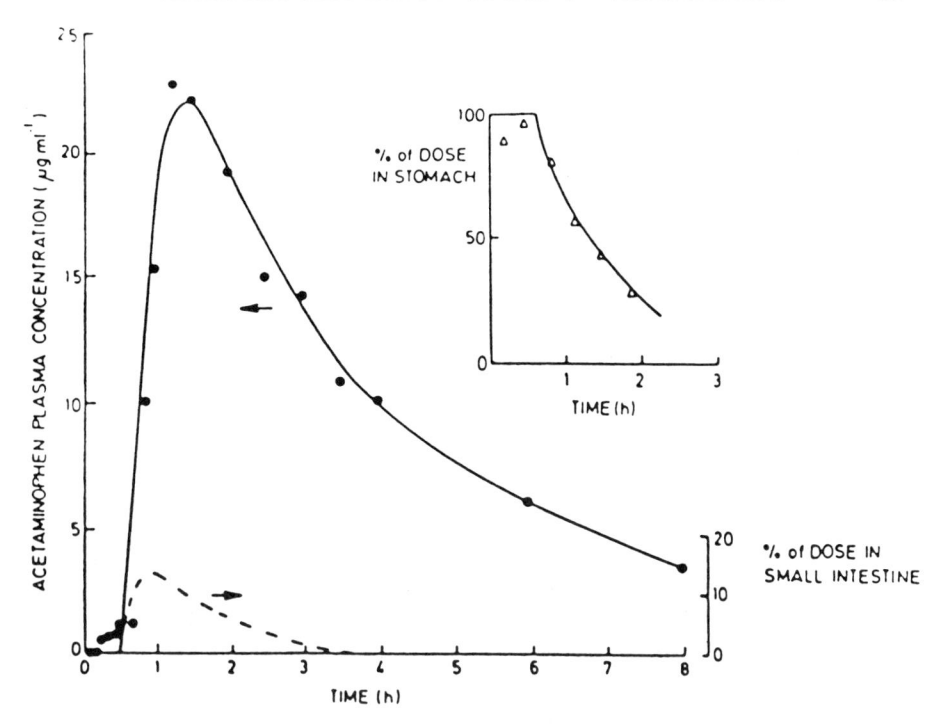

FIG. 9. By incorporating independent data on the percentage of acetaminophen remaining in the stomach **(inset)**, the plasma acetaminophen concentration–time profile following an oral dose of drug can be adequately described. (From Clements et al., ref. 7, with permission.)

This source of variability in drug absorption can be identified and accounted for by independently measuring gastric emptying and using that as the input function for drug entering the intestine. This approach was successfully used to model the kinetics of absorption for acetaminophen in humans (Fig. 9).

Saturable Elimination

So far, saturation of metabolic pathways and transport systems has been ignored, but this occurs frequently in practice (26,44). Its occurrence complicates interpretation, particularly when there is a multiplicity of enzymes involved, as often occurs, and when a drug has to pass through several metabolic organs (gut wall, liver, lung) before reaching the site of measurement. The time dependence in pharmacokinetic parameters (20), due, for example, to autoinduction, further complicates the situation. Without detailed modeling of the entire system, which at best is usually limited to animal studies, it is impossible to make precise quantitative estimates of the contributions of individual metabolic enzyme systems to overall variability in a drug's pharmacokinetics.

A possible consequence of saturable metabolism is amplification in the expression of variability. One striking example is the profound (100–200-fold) increase in the AUC when the oral dose of salicylamide is raised from 1 to 2 g (2). Following an oral dose, the AUC is given by

$$\text{AUC} = \frac{F \cdot \text{dose}}{\text{CL}} \quad (4)$$

At low doses, salicylamide exhibits a high first-pass loss due to presystemic metabolism. With saturation, bioavailability is increased and clearance decreased, both effects increasing the AUC. Under these circumstances the AUC is particularly sensitive to the rate of absorption, as well as to the dose (28).

Another example is seen in the steady-state plasma concentration (C_{ss}) of a drug like phenytoin, which undergoes elimination almost entirely via a saturable metabolic pathway. At steady state,

$$C_{ss} = \frac{F \cdot R_0 K_m}{V_m - F \cdot R_0} \quad (5)$$

where K_m is the Michaelis-Menten constant, V_m is maximum velocity, F is bioavailability, and R_0 is the rate of drug administration. From equation (5) it is clear that for a given steady-state concentration, the greater the degree of saturation (the closer FR_0 is to V_m) the greater is the sensitivity of C_{ss} to a change in either F or V_m, occurring within or between individuals. This explains why the plateau phenytoin concentration can be so sensitive to relatively minor differences in bioavailability performances of drug products, which may be difficult to detect from *in vitro* dissolution studies, and why minor changes in dosages in some individuals have such marked effects on plateau concentrations (40).

CONCLUDING REMARKS

Much progress has been made in developing models that allow insight into the processes controlling drug absorption and disposition. They vary in complexity depending on the intended application. Used sensibly, these models do help to identify sources of pharmacokinetic variability. Once identified, however, it still remains for us to assess their significance in regard to overall variability in drug therapy.

REFERENCES

1. Alvan, G., Piasky, K., Lind, M., and von Bahr, C. (1977): Effect of pentobarbital on the disposition of alprenolol. *Clin. Pharmacol. Ther.*, 22:316–321.
2. Barr, W.H. (1969): Factors involved in the assessment of systemic or biological availability of drug products. *Drug Information Bulletin*, 3:27–69.
3. Bass, L., Robinson, P., and Bracken, A.J. (1978): Hepatic elimination of flowing substances: The distributed model. *J. Theor. Biol.*, 72:161–184.

4. Bennett, P.N., Aarons, L.J., Bending, M.R., Steiner, J.A., and Rowland, M. (1982): Pharmacokinetics of lidocaine and its de-ethylated metabolite: Dose and time dependency studies in man. *J. Pharmacokinet. Biopharm.*, 10:265–281.
5. Bianchine, J.R., and Shaw, G.M. (1976): Clinical pharmacokinetics of levodopa in Parkinson's disease. *Clin. Pharmacokinet.*, 1:313–358.
6. Breimer, D.D. (1983): Interindividual variations in drug disposition: Clinical implications and methods of investigation. *Clin. Pharmacokinet.*, 8:371–377.
7. Clements, J.A., Heading, R.C., Nimmo, W.S., and Prescott, M.D. (1978): Kinetics of acetaminophen-absorption and gastric emptying in man. *Clin. Pharmacol. Ther.*, 24:420–431.
8. Conolly, M.E., Davies, D.S., Dollery, C.T., Morgan, C.D., Paterson, J.W., and Sandler, M.L. (1972): Metabolism of isoprenaline in dog and man. *Br. J. Pharmacol.*, 46:458–472.
9. Forker, E.K., and Luxon, B. (1978): Hepatic transport kinetics and plasma disappearance curves: Distributed modelling versus conventional approach. *Am. J. Physiol.*, 235:E648–660.
10. George, C.F. (1981): Drug metabolism by the gastrointestinal mucosa. *Clin. Pharmacokinet.*, 6:259–274.
11. Gugler, R., and Azarnoff, D.L. (1976): Drug protein binding and the nephrotic syndrome. *Clin. Pharmacokinet.*, 1:25–35.
12. Hall, S., and Rowland, M. (1984): Relationship between renal clearance, protein binding and urine flow for digitoxin, a compound of low clearance in the isolated perfused rat kidney. *J. Pharmacol. Exp. Ther.*, 227:174–179.
13. Houston, J.B. (1981): Drug metabolite kinetics. *Pharmacol. Ther.*, 15:521–552.
14. Illing, H.P.A. (1981): Techniques for microfloral and associated metabolic studies in relation to the absorption and entero-hepatic circulation of drugs. *Xenobiotica*, 11:815–830.
15. Jusko, W.J., and Gretch, M. (1976): Plasma and tissue protein binding of drugs in pharmacokinetics. *Drug Metab. Rev.*, 5:43–140.
16. Jusko, W.J., Schentag, J.J., Clark, J.H., Gardner, M., and Yurchak, A.M. (1978): Enhanced biotransformation of theophylline in marijuana and tobacco smokers. *Clin. Pharmacol. Ther.*, 24:406–410.
17. Kieding, S., and Chiarantini, E. (1978): Effect of sinusoidal perfusion on galactose elimination kinetics in the perfused rat liver. *J. Pharmacol. Exp. Ther.*, 205:465–470.
18. Kornhauser, D.M., Wood, J.J., Vestal, R.E., Wilkinson, G.R., Branch, R.A., and Shand, D.G. (1978): Biological determinants of propranolol disposition in man. *Clin. Pharmacol. Ther.*, 23:165–174.
19. Levy, G., and Yacobi, A. (1974): Effect of protein binding on the elimination of warfarin. *J. Pharm. Sci.*, 63:805–806.
20. Levy, R.H. (1982): Time dependent kinetics. *Pharmacol. Ther.*, 17:383–399.
21. Nimmo, W.S. (1976): Drugs, disease and gastric emptying. *Clin. Pharmacokinet.*, 1:109–203.
22. Øie, S., and Tozer, T.N. (1979): Effect of altered plasma protein binding on apparent volume of distribution. *J. Pharm. Sci.*, 68:1203–1205.
23. Øie, S., Guentert, T.W., and Tozer, T.N. (1980): Effect of saturable binding on the pharmacokinetics of drugs: A simulation. *J. Pharm. Pharmacol.*, 32:471–477.
24. Pang, K.S., and Rowland, M. (1978): Hepatic clearance of drugs. I. Theoretical considerations of a "well-stirred" model and a "parallel tube" model. Influence of hepatic blood flow, plasma and blood cell binding, and the hepatocellular enzymatic activity on hepatic drug clearance. *J. Pharmacokinet. Biopharm.*, 5:625–653.
25. Pang, K.S., and Rowland, M. (1978): Hepatic clearance of drugs. II. Experimental evidence for acceptance of the "well-stirred" model over the "parallel tube" model using lidocaine in the perfused rat liver *in situ* preparation. *J. Pharmacokinet. Biopharm.*, 5:655–680.
26. Pond, S.M., and Tozer, T.N. (1984): First-pass elimination: Basic concepts and clinical consequences. *Clin. Pharmacokinet.*, 9:1–25.
27. Rothschild, M.A., Bauman, A., Yalow, R.S., and Benson, S.A. (1955): Tissue distribution of I^{131} labelled human serum albumin following intravenous administration. *J. Clin. Invest.*, 34:1354–1358.
28. Rowland, M. (1971): Effect of some physiologic factors on the bioavailability of oral

dosage forms. In: *Current Concepts in the Pharmaceutical Sciences, Vol. 2,* edited by J. Swarbrick, pp. 182–222. Lea & Febiger, Philadelphia.
29. Rowland, M., Thompson, P.D., Guichard, A., and Melmon, K.L. (1971): Disposition kinetics of lidocaine in normal subjects. *Ann. N.Y. Acad. Sci.,* 179:383–398.
30. Rowland, M., Benet, L.Z., and Graham, G.G. (1973): Clearance concepts in pharmacokinetics. *J. Pharmacokinet. Biopharm.,* 1:123–136.
31. Rowland, M. (1980): Plasma protein binding and therapeutic drug monitoring. *Therap. Drug Monitor.,* 2:29–37.
32. Rowland, M., and Tozer, T.N. (1980): *Clinical Pharmacokinetics: Concepts and Applications,* pp. 124–137. Lea & Febiger, Philadelphia.
33. Rowland, M., and Tozer, T.N. (1980): *Clinical Pharmacokinetics: Concepts and Applications,* pp. 49–76. Lea & Febiger, Philadelphia.
34. Rowland, M., Leitch, D., Fleming, G., and Smith, B. (1983): Protein binding and hepatic extraction of diazepam across the rat liver. *J. Pharm. Pharmacol.,* 35:383–384.
35. Rowland, M. (1984): Protein binding and drug clearance. *Clin. Parmacokinet.* [*Suppl. 1*], 9:10–17.
36. Rowland, M. (1981): Clearance: Models, validation and implications. In: *Pharmacokinetics: A Modern View, Vol. 6,* edited by L.Z. Benet, pp. 259–274. Plenum Press, New York.
37. Schary, W.L., and Rowland, M. (1983): Protein binding and hepatic clearance: Studies with tolbutamide, a drug of low intrinsic clearance, in the isolated perfused rat liver preparation. *J. Pharmacokinet. Biopharm.,* 11:225–243.
38. Schentag, J.J., Jusko, W.J., Vance, J.W., Cumbo, T.J., Abrutyn, E., Delattre, M., and Gerbracht, L.M. (1977): Gentamicin disposition and tissue accumulation on multiple dosing. *J. Pharmacokinet. Biopharm.,* 5:559–577.
39. Tang-Lin, D.D., Tozer, T.N., and Riegelman, S. (1983): Dependence of renal clearance on urine flow—a mathematical model and its applications. *J. Pharm. Sci.,* 72:154–158.
40. Tozer, T.N., and Winter, M.E. (1980): Phenytoin. In: *Applied Pharmacokinetics,* edited by W.E. Evans, J.J. Schentag, and W.J. Jusko, pp. 275–314. Applied Therapeutics, San Francisco.
41. Tozer, T.N. (1981): Concepts basic to pharmacokinetics. *Pharmacol, Ther.,* 12:109–132.
42. Tozer, T.N. (1984): Implications of altered plasma protein binding in disease states. In: *Pharmacokinetic Basis for Drug Treatment,* edited by L.Z. Benet, N. Massoud, and J.G. Gambertoglio, pp. 173–194. Raven Press, New York.
43. Upton, R.A., Thiercelin, J.F., Guentert, T.W., Wallace, S.M., Powell, J.R., Sansom, L., and Riegelman, S. (1982): Intraindividual variability in theophylline pharmacokinetics: Statistical verification in 39 of 60 healthy young volunteers. *J. Pharmacokinet. Biopharm.,* 10:123–134.
44. Van Rossum, J.M., Van Lingen, G., and Burgess, J.P.T. (1983): Dose dependent kinetics. *Pharmacol. Ther.,* 21:77–100.
45. Vestal, R.B., Norris, A.H., Robin, J.D., Cohen, B.H., Shock, N.W., and Anches, R. (1975): Antipyrine metabolism in man: Influence of age, alcohol, caffeine and smoking. *Clin. Pharmacol. Ther.,* 18:425–432.
46. Wilkinson, G.R., and Shand, D.G. (1975): Commentary: A physiological approach to hepatic drug clearance. *Clin. Pharmacol. Ther.,* 18:377–390.
47. Winkler, K., Bass, L., Kieding, S., and Tygstrup, M. (1974): The effect of hepatic perfusion on assessment of kinetic constants. In: *Regulation of Hepatic Metabolism,* edited by L. Lundqvist, and N. Tygstrup, pp. 797–807. Munksgaard, Copenhagen.

DISCUSSION

Discussant 1 (D1): I would like to question an assumption of yours: the relatively low variability in liver blood flow. This may be true in normal volunteers; it may not be true in patients. We have data on theophylline and lidocaine in patients, both given intravenously. The interpatient variabilities in total body clearance are about the same. According to your simulation, however, it should be much lower for lidocaine. The patients receiving lidocaine were patients with myocardial infarction, so that they may have had hemodynamic problems that caused large variability in liver blood flow. Perhaps this occurs under other circumstances. If so, would not the variability in clearance be higher for drugs of high hepatic clearance when given orally?

Speaker (S): That may be so. Within the patient population there are many sources of, and contributions to, variability. However, one problem facing a pharmaceutical company is to try to develop a drug that exhibits minimal variability when used clinically. Obviously, one cannot be sure of the magnitude of variability until the drug is used widely. What concerns me is that drugs that exhibit a variable first-pass effect are automatically damned. If you want to damn anything, it is large interindividual variability in amounts of those enzymes responsible for certain metabolic transformations. It might be nice to know those enzymes that show the least variability among patients and target the drug for such enzymes. Making a drug that is not metabolized may sound attractive. But it may then need to be so polar, or possess such a long half-life, that it displays poor and large variability in absorption or becomes too difficult to use in practice.

D2: Under normal circumstances, hepatic blood flow varies relatively little, but enzymatic activity can vary very widely.

D3: If I understood you correctly, knowing that a drug has a high clearance or low clearance has no special predictive value with respect to predicting variability at steady state during a multiple-dose regimen.

S: That's correct. A drug, whether of high or low hepatic clearance, simply manifests the variability in the responsible enzyme(s). The fact that one drug happens to be a good substrate and another not so is incidental.

D3: What, then, has predictive value?

S: The magnitude of the extraction ratio, as it allows one to predict the likely influence of changing blood flow or changing binding, and so forth, on clearance and steady-state concentrations, when drugs are given parenterally.

D4: I would like to illustrate some of the concepts raised in your talk by reference to results of kinetic studies we have performed in many healthy subjects over the years with three drugs: caffeine, guanfacine, and dihydroergotamine. The first two are well absorbed, with high bioavailability and low clearance, caffeine being almost exclusively metabolized, whereas much of guanfacine is cleared renally unchanged. In contrast, dihydroergotamine is a high-clearance drug characterized by incomplete absorption, a high first-pass loss, and extensive metabolism and biliary excretion. For caffeine and guanfacine, given orally, bioavailability varied little, but clearance varied considerably, with coefficients of variation of 62 and 40% respectively. In contrast, the oral bioavailability of dihydroergotamine varied considerably (coefficient of variability of 30–40%), but the AUC (and hence the predicted average steady-state concentration) for dihydroergotamine was not more variable than that for either caffeine or guanfacine.

D5: I think your work raises a methodological issue for those of us who think about analyzing data. The question is, What kind of tools ought we to be giving the experimentalist to allow him to simulate a distribution of inputs and a distribution of parameters and look at the resulting distribution of outputs?

S: I do see another kind of methodological problem; that is, attempts to compare differences in the degree of variability between drugs that have differences in half-life. Often, but not always, a drug with a high clearance has a shorter half-life than one with a low clearance. This may mean that within a dosing interval at steady state there may well be a much lower degree of fluctuation in the plasma concentration for the low-clearance drug, so that the time of sampling to assess variability in the average plateau concentration (which depends on availability and clearance) will not be anywhere near so critical as that for a high-clearance drug. The net effect may be the claim that the short-half-life drug exhibits more variability in its pharmacokinetics than that of the longer-half-life drug, when the real issue is methodology.

D6: You assumed passive absorption in your models. What happens if active transport occurs?

S: Several things occur. One is dose dependence, and, more specifically, a concentration dependence in the absorption of the drug. The second is that probably the distribution of the transport system along the gastrointestinal tract is heterogeneous, in which case absorption will be highly variable and sensitive to pharmaceutical formulation, in that the formulation can influence the time (and hence the site) at which dissolution of drugs occurs.

D7: Assessment of the sources of variability is really a matter of knowing what the potential rate-limiting steps are. One has to know a lot about the drug. One has to know what the biotransformation pathways are. This and other basic knowledge is unfortunately not available until and unless the drug is successful and justifies the necessary research investment. Moreover, different patient populations can exhibit different rate-limiting steps.

D5: I think you can do a sort of sensitivity analysis to determine the influence of the major factors on the output you are interested in.

D8: You can actually use these sensitivity tests to see whether or not blood flow is important. Start with a very complex physiological model, and it's amazing how much can be thrown out because it turns out to be irrelevant or not rate-limiting.

*Variability in Drug Therapy:
Description, Estimation, and Control,*
edited by M. Rowland et al.
Raven Press, New York © 1985.

Accounting for Assay Variability

Leon Aarons

*Department of Pharmacy, University of Manchester,
Manchester M13 9PL, United Kingdom*

Variability in drug therapy arises from many sources. In particular, one can identify variability due to biopharmaceutics, pharmacokinetics, and pharmacodynamics. Therefore, one of the objectives of therapeutic drug monitoring is, by measuring plasma or blood concentrations, to account for some of the biopharmaceutical and pharmacokinetic variability. However, it is often forgotten that determination of plasma or blood concentrations is subject to errors that can contribute significantly to the overall variability. The magnitude of assay error depends on the drug, the assay, and the dose, or, more specifically, the plasma or blood concentration. In this contribution I want to briefly discuss the various sources of assay error and how they can be reduced. An assay can be divided into four stages:

1. Sampling
2. Workup
3. End point determination
4. Calibration

Sampling times are an avoidable source of variability. All too often the sampling times that are submitted are the nominal times rather than the actual times. Although sampling times are not normally the province of the analyst, error in sampling time is lumped into the analytical error.

The workup can involve aliquoting, extraction, evaporation, and/or derivatization. All of these procedures can introduce errors and losses. Careful management is required to minimize error at this stage. In modern times, end point determination is either spectrophotometric or chromatographic, with emphasis shifting toward high-pressure liquid chromatography. Again, careful and skilled operation is needed to get the best out of these techniques.

An assessment of assay error is provided at the calibration stage and should be part of the assay validation. The validation procedure should include a test for linearity, assessment of variability and bias, and some statement about sensitivity. A correlation coefficient is not a sufficient measure of linearity, and a lack-of-fit statistic should be employed. Intra-day variability should be determined over a range of concentrations, but particularly at the low and high ends of the calibration. Inter-day variability really has no meaning for assays that are calibrated every day. Bias is very difficult to estimate for assays in biological fluids, as no absolute standard exists. There are many definitions of sensitivity, but the most practical definition is one that gives some estimate of the confidence with which the lowest concentration can be measured. The composition of the calibrators needs to be looked at carefully. It is often more convenient to use aqueous calibrators, but equivalence with standards made up in plasma or blood needs to be established. Finally, interference from endogenous and exogenous substances needs to be eliminated.

The vast majority of calibrations are linear, and the method of ordinary unweighted least squares is often employed to find the line of best fit. However, in the author's experience, the variance associated with assay data is commonly heteroscedastic, usually increasing with concentration. Unweighted least squares, although on average producing unbiased parameter estimates, gives rise to imprecise parameter estimates and poor estimates of confidence associated with the predictions based on the calibration. Weighted least squares should be used, with weights being chosen to be proportional to the reciprocal of the variance. However, variances obtained from calibration data (if this is done at all) are not good estimates, and the variances associated with concentrations between calibrators have to be obtained by interpolation. A method like extended least squares (2) that attempts to define a variance model as well as a structural model overcomes these difficulties at the expense of computational complexity. However, with the proliferation of microcomputers, this is ceasing to be a problem.

The analyst has one other choice to make as far as the calibration is concerned: which concentrations to choose. Obviously the concentrations should span the region of interest, but it is more efficient to divide the calibrators into two groups, replicating half at the lowest concentration and the other half at the highest concentration (1). The advantage of this design over the conventional design of uniformly spacing the calibrators throughout the concentration range is greatest for a small number of calibrators. The danger of the two-point design is that it will not detect departure from linearity. However, by the time the assay goes into routine use, linearity should not be a question.

In conclusion, I would like to emphasize that good pharmacokinetics relies on good assay methodology. Assay error may contribute significantly to overall variability, but at least by careful design and management it can be minimized.

REFERENCES

1. Aarons, L. (1981): Effect of experimental design on assay calibration. *Analyst*, 106:1249–1256.
2. Sheiner, L.B., and Beal, S.L. (1980): Evaluation of methods for estimating population pharmacokinetic parameters. I. Michaelis-Menten model. *J. Pharmacokinet. Biopharm.*, 8:553–571.

Variability in Drug Therapy:
Description, Estimation, and Control,
edited by M. Rowland et al.
Raven Press, New York © 1985.

Modeling Pharmacokinetic Variability on the Molecular Level with Stochastic Compartmental Systems

James H. Matis and Thomas E. Wehrly

Department of Statistics, Texas A&M University, College Station, Texas 77843

Linear compartmental models have been widely used to model pharmacokinetic systems. Most of the previous modeling theory and virtually all of the previous applications have been based on a deterministic formulation of a compartmental system (6,7,17). In the deterministic formulation, a compartment can be defined as a mass or concentration $X(t)$ that is governed by the differential equation

$$dX(t)/dt = -KX(t) + f(t) \tag{1}$$

where K is the relative rate of elimination from and $f(t)$ is the rate of entry into the compartment (4,18).

This chapter reviews an alternative, stochastic formulation of a compartmental model. The existence of variability, hence stochasticity, on the molecular level has long been recognized by writers describing the foundations of compartmental modeling. However rigorous, detailed stochastic formulations of such variability are usually not presented, being regarded either as unimportant or as intuitive from the deterministic model. However, in our opinion, a rigorous formulation for such stochastic models is needed for three reasons: (a) to clarify the theoretical foundations of compartmental theory, (b) to generate many statistical moments that are of practical interest, and (c) to derive new, generalized stochastic models that will be useful in data analysis. All of these points will be illustrated subsequently.

This chapter is an extension of earlier work by Matis, Wehrly, and Metzler (13), henceforth denoted MWM. The second section reviews the matrix formulation of a deterministic model and illustrates its use with several simple two-compartment models. The third section presents a stochastic model for particle location in the system. This model is slightly different from that in MWM and is a closer analogue to the deterministic formulation. The fourth

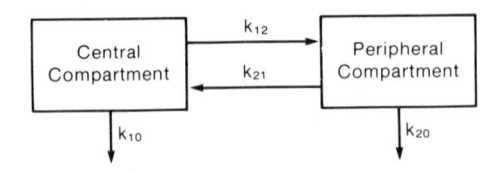

[FIGURE: The general two-compartment model showing Central Compartment and Peripheral Compartment with rates k_{12}, k_{21}, k_{10}, k_{20}]

FIG. 1. The general two-compartment model.

section extends the statistical moments presented in MWM to include other random variables related to residence times. The statistical moments from the compartmental approach are then compared to those from the noncompartmental approach. The fifth section generalizes the stochastic models for location and residence time to include systems whose transition rates are functions of the particle retention times. Such "age-dependent" models are illustrated with simple examples.

DETERMINISTIC FORMULATION

General Theory

For the purposes of this chapter we shall consider only models with two compartments. However, the formulation is extended to n compartments in MWM. The general two-compartment model is given in Fig. 1 and requires the following definitions:

1. Let $X_{ij}(t)$, with $i, j = 1, 2$, denote the amount of a drug that originated in i at time 0 and that is in j at time t.
2. Let $\dot{X}_{ij}(t)$ denote the time derivative if $X_{ij}(t)$.
3. Let k_{ij}, with $i = 1, 2, j = 0, 1, 2, i \neq j$, denote the constant transfer rate from i to j, where 0 denotes the system exterior.

One set of linear differential equations describing the deterministic compartmental model in Fig. 1 is

$$\dot{X}_{i1}(t) = -(k_{10} + k_{12})X_{i1}(t) + k_{21}X_{i2}(t)$$
$$\dot{X}_{i2}(t) = k_{12}X_{i1}(t) - (k_{20} + k_{21})X_{i2}(t) \quad \text{for } i = 1, 2 \quad (2)$$

These equations are of the form in equation (1) and usually appear without the designation of the compartment of origin, i. This designation is added here for subsequent convenience. The following matrix definitions are also helpful:

4. Let

$$X(t) = \begin{bmatrix} X_{11}(t) & X_{12}(t) \\ X_{21}(t) & X_{22}(t) \end{bmatrix}$$

denote the matrix of amounts and $\dot{X}(t)$ the matrix of derivatives.

5. Let
$$K = \begin{bmatrix} -(k_{10} + k_{12}) & k_{12} \\ k_{21} & -(k_{20} + k_{21}) \end{bmatrix}$$
be the coefficient matrix.

6. Let
$$\Lambda = \begin{bmatrix} \lambda_1 & 0 \\ 0 & \lambda_2 \end{bmatrix} \quad \text{and} \quad T = [T_1, T_2]$$
be matrices of eigenvalues, λ_i, and corresponding eigenvectors, T_i, of K. Equation (2) can now be written in matrix form as
$$\dot{X}(t) = X(t)K \tag{3}$$
which generalizes equation (1). The general matrix solution is
$$X(t) = X(0)e^{Kt} \tag{4}$$
which for distinct eigenvalues can be written as
$$X(t) = X(0)Te^{\Lambda t}T^{-1} \tag{5}$$
where $e^{\Lambda t}$ is a diagonal matrix with elements $e^{\lambda_i t}$. Equation (5) implies that the solutions for $X_{ij}(t)$ are sums of exponentials.

These equations can be solved explicitly as functions of the k_{ij} parameters for many simply two- and three-compartment models, as will be illustrated subsequently. Often one measures concentrations, defined as $C_{ij}(t) = X_{ij}(t)/V_j$, where V_j is the apparent volume of the compartment j. The transformation to $C_{ij}(t)$ is easy to implement in equation (5).

Numerical Examples

There are three characteristic structures of the two-compartment model based on the source(s) of elimination. As simple examples, consider the specific numerical examples given in Fig. 2 illustrating each of the structures. For simplicity, we assume a unit initial dose into compartment 1, i.e., $X_{11}(0) = 1$. The numerical solutions for $X_{11}(t)$ and $X_{12}(t)$ are available from formulas given on pages 85 and 90 of Gilbaldi and Perrier (6) for the first two models or on page 28 of Rescigno and Segre (17) for all three models. These solutions are listed in Table 1. Table 1 also contains the intermediate matrix results that when substituted into equation (5) yield the numerical solutions. Solutions for $X_{21}(t)$ and $X_{22}(t)$ are easy to find from equation (5) for any initial amount $X_{22}(0)$.

STOCHASTIC FORMULATION FOR PARTICLE LOCATION

The description and solution of the stochastic particle model for particle location are similar to those for the previous deterministic model. Conceptually,

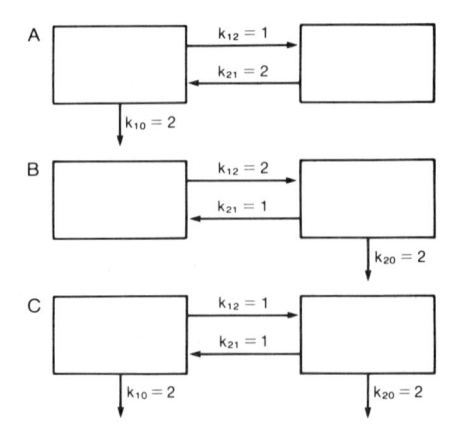

FIG. 2. A specific illustration of each two-compartment model structure based on the source(s) of elimination. **A:** Elimination central. **B:** Elimination peripheral. **C:** Elimination central and peripheral.

TABLE 1. *Solution for drug distribution over time for selected two-compartment models*

Model A: Elimination central, with $k_{10} = 2$, $k_{12} = 1$, $k_{21} = 2$

$X_{11}(t) = (e^{-t} + 2e^{-4t})/3$, $\quad X_{12}(t) = (e^{-t} - e^{-4t})/3$

$$K = \begin{bmatrix} -3 & 1 \\ 2 & -2 \end{bmatrix}, \quad e^{\Lambda t} = \begin{bmatrix} e^{-t} & 0 \\ 0 & e^{-4t} \end{bmatrix}, \quad T = \begin{bmatrix} 1 & 1 \\ 2 & -1 \end{bmatrix}, \quad T^{-1} = \begin{bmatrix} 1/3 & 1/3 \\ 2/3 & -1/3 \end{bmatrix}$$

Model B: Elimination peripheral, with $k_{12} = 2$, $k_{20} = 2$, $k_{21} = 1$

$X_{11}(t) = (2e^{-t} + e^{-4t})/3$, $\quad X_{12}(t) = 2(e^{-t} - e^{-4t})/3$

$$K = \begin{bmatrix} -2 & 2 \\ 1 & -3 \end{bmatrix}, \quad e^{\Lambda t} = \begin{bmatrix} e^{-t} & 0 \\ 0 & e^{-4t} \end{bmatrix}, \quad T = \begin{bmatrix} 1 & 1 \\ 1/2 & -1 \end{bmatrix}, \quad T^{-1} = \begin{bmatrix} 2/3 & 2/3 \\ 1/3 & -2/3 \end{bmatrix}$$

Model C: Elimination central and peripheral, with $k_{10} = k_{20} = 2$ and $k_{12} = k_{21} = 1$

$X_{11}(t) = (e^{-2t} + e^{-4t})/2$, $\quad X_{12}(t) = (e^{-2t} - e^{-4t})/2$

$$K = \begin{bmatrix} -3 & 1 \\ 1 & -3 \end{bmatrix}, \quad e^{\Lambda t} = \begin{bmatrix} e^{-2t} & 0 \\ 0 & e^{-4t} \end{bmatrix}, \quad T = \begin{bmatrix} 1 & 1 \\ 1 & -1 \end{bmatrix}, \quad T^{-1} = \begin{bmatrix} 1/2 & 1/2 \\ 1/2 & -1/2 \end{bmatrix}$$

---

the stochastic model is based on *probabilities* of particle transfers in given time increments, whereas the deterministic model is based on *proportional* flows of material. Figure 1 also represents the general two-compartment stochastic model with the following redefinitions:

1'. Let $p_{ij}(t)$, with $i, j = 1, 2$, denote the probability that a particle originating in i at time 0 is in j at time t.

2'. Let $\dot{p}_{ij}(t)$ denote the time derivative of $p_{ij}(t)$.

3'. Let k_{ij}, with $i = 1, 2$ and $j = 0, 1, 2$, $i \neq j$, denote the probability intensity coefficient in units of time^{-1}. When multiplied by a small time increment, it yields a transfer probability. It can be defined more rigorously by the following probability statement:

$$\text{Prob\{a given particle in } i \text{ at time } t \text{ is in } j \text{ at } t + \Delta t\} = k_{ij}\Delta t + o(\Delta t) \quad (6)$$

where $o(\Delta t)$ denotes all terms $(\Delta t)^2, (\Delta t)^3, \ldots$.

From this chance mechanism one can construct the following set of differential equations describing the stochastic compartmental model:

$$\dot{p}_{i1}(t) = -(k_{10} + k_{12})p_{i1}(t) + k_{21}p_{i2}(t)$$
$$\dot{p}_{i2}(t) = k_{12}p_{i1}(t) - (k_{20} + k_{21})p_{i2}(t) \quad \text{for } i = 1, 2 \quad (7)$$

These equations are often called the Kolmogorov forward equations; see page 417 of Chiang (1). Letting $P(t) = [p_{ij}(t)]$ denote the matrix of probabilities, with $\dot{P}(t)$ denoting the matrix of derivatives, one can rewrite equation (7) as

$$\dot{P}(t) = P(t)K \quad (8)$$

which has the same form as equation (3). Therefore, for distinct eigenvalues, its solution is

$$P(t) = Te^{\Lambda t}T^{-1} \quad (9)$$

because $P(0)$ is the identity matrix.

As numerical examples, consider the previous solutions of the models in Fig. 2 as given in Table 1. Because the deterministic model assumed a unit initial dose, $X_{11}(0) = 1$, the solutions in Table 1 hold for the stochastic particle model with $p_{1j}(t)$ replacing $X_{1j}(t)$ for $j = 1, 2$. In general, the *proportional* dose solutions in the deterministic model will equal the corresponding solutions for the absolute *probabilities* in the stochastic model.

The preceding formulation holds for single particles originating in any given compartment. The results can be extended to yield the probability distribution of initial populations of X_{11} and/or X_{22} particles. The means, variances, and other moments of such counts are also available. In particular, it is shown in MWM that the means of the X_{ii} particles remaining in the compartments have solutions of the same form as equations (5) and (9).

STOCHASTIC FORMULATION FOR PARTICLE RESIDENCE TIMES AND RELATED VARIABLES

Theoretical Results for the Compartmental Approach

The mean and variance of the residence times were given in MWM for a structured compartmental model. These considerations can be extended to include other useful time-related variables. The following definitions are helpful:

7. Let R_{ij}, with $i, j = 1, 2$, denote the random "lifetime" during the current visit of a particle in i whose next transfer will be to j.

8. Let R_i, with $i = 1, 2$, denote the random *retention time* (also called *transit time*) during the current visit of a particle in i prior to its next transfer out of i (to any other compartment or to the exterior). Clearly, $R_i \leq R_{ij}$.

9. Let V_{ij}, with $i, j = 1, 2$, denote the random number of *visitations* that a particle originating in i, say at $t = 0$, will make to j prior to its departure from the system.

10. Let S_{ij}, with $i, j = 1, 2$, denote the total *residence* (or sojourn) time that a particle originating in i will accumulate in j during its V_{ij} visits. Thus, S_{ij} is the sum of V_{ij} independent and identically distributed R_j random variables.

11. Let $S_{i.} = \sum_j S_{ij}$, with $i = 1, 2$, denote the total *residence* time that a particle originating in i will accumulate in the system prior to its departure.

One very fundamental result is the implication of equation (6) for the distribution of retention times. Note that equation (6) implies that the event of a transfer is independent of the retention time that the given particle has spent in compartment i. This is often termed the lack-of-memory property (or the Markov property), and it can be shown that the only retention-time distribution with such property is the exponential distribution. It follows, therefore, that R_{ij} is distributed as an exponential random variable with parameter k_{ij}. Therefore, the density function of R_{ij} can be written as

$$f_{R_{ij}}(a; k_{ij}) = k_{ij} \exp(-k_{ij}a) \quad (a \geq 0, k_{ij} \geq 0) \tag{10}$$

where a is the measure of "age" (12). The mean and variance of R_{ij} follow as

$$E(R_{ij}) = (k_{ij})^{-1} \tag{11}$$

$$\text{Var}(R_{ij}) = (k_{ij})^{-2} \tag{12}$$

Using a statement analogous to equation (6), it can be shown that the R_i retention time is distributed as an exponential random variable with parameter

$$k_i = \sum_{\substack{j=0 \\ j \neq i}}^{2} k_{ij}$$

For example, the mean and variance of R_1 are

$$E(R_1) = (k_{10} + k_{12})^{-1} \tag{13}$$

$$\text{Var}(R_1) = (k_{10} + k_{12})^{-2} \tag{14}$$

Simple formulas exist also for the moments of the numbers of visitations and the residence times describing particle kinetics. The following definitions are helpful:

12. Let τ_{ij} and γ_{ij} denote the mean and variance of the residence time S_{ij}.
13. Let τ'_{ij} and γ'_{ij} denote the mean and variance of the number of visitations V_{ij}.
14. Let $\tau_{i.}$ and $\gamma_{i.}$ denote the mean and variance of the total residence time $S_{i.}$. These are often denoted as MRT and VRT, respectively.
15. Let $\tau = (\tau_{ij})$, $\tau' = (\tau'_{ij})$, $\gamma = (\gamma_{ij})$, and $\gamma' = (\gamma'_{ij})$ be matrices of means and variances.

The following results have been proved:

$$\text{(i)} \quad \tau = -K^{-1} \tag{15}$$

$$\text{(ii)} \quad \gamma = 2\tau\tau_D - \tau_{(2)} \tag{16}$$

where τ_D is the diagonal matrix $(\tau_{11}, \tau_{22}, \ldots)$ and $\tau_{(2)}$ is the matrix of squared elements of τ,

$$\text{(iii)} \quad \tau' = (I - K^*)^{-1} \tag{17}$$

where K^* is the normalized K matrix such that $k^*_{ii} = 0$ and $k^*_{ij} = -k_{ij}/k_{ii}$ for $i \neq j$, and

$$\text{(iv)} \quad \gamma' = 2\tau'\tau'_D - \tau'_{(2)} \tag{18}$$

where τ'_D and $\tau'_{(2)}$ are defined as in equation (16).

Equations (15) and (16) are given in MWM and equations (17) and (18) in Matis et al. (12). Note that all of these moments calculations are based on relatively simple mathematical operations, namely matrix multiplication and inversion of the K matrix. Higher-order moments, e.g., for skewness and kurtosis, and cross-moments can be found from formulas in Olson and Matis (14). In particular, the covariance between two residence times is shown to be

$$\text{(v)} \quad \text{Cov}[S_{ij}, S_{ik}] = \tau_{ij}\tau_{jk} + \tau_{ik}\tau_{kj} - \tau_{ij}\tau_{ik} \tag{19}$$

Numerical Illustration of Results for Compartmental Approach

Table 2 contains the results when the previous formulas based on the compartmental approach are implemented for the three models given previously. For model A, note that the expected retention times per visit are $E(R_1) = 1/3$ in 1 and $E(R_2) = 1/2$ in 2. A particle introduced into 1 is expected to make $\tau'_{11} = 3/2$ visits to 1 and $\tau'_{12} = 1/2$ visit to 2. The expected residence times of the particle are $\tau_{11} = 1/2$ in 1 and $\tau_{12} = 1/4$ in 2. The total expected residence time in the system, i.e., the mean residence time, is the sum of the residence times in the individual compartments. Therefore, for the present particle one has

$$\text{MRT} = \tau_{1.} = \tau_{11} + \tau_{12} = \frac{3}{4}$$

TABLE 2. *Solution for statistical moments based on compartmental approach for selected two-compartment models*

Model A: Elimination central, with $k_{10} = 2$, $k_{12} = 1$, $k_{21} = 2$

$E(R_1) = 1/3$, $E(R_2) = 1/2$

$$K = \begin{bmatrix} -3 & 1 \\ 2 & -2 \end{bmatrix}, \quad \tau = \begin{bmatrix} 1/2 & 1/4 \\ 1/2 & 3/4 \end{bmatrix}, \quad \gamma = \begin{bmatrix} 1/4 & 5/16 \\ 1/4 & 9/16 \end{bmatrix}$$

$$K^* = \begin{bmatrix} 0 & 1/3 \\ 1 & 0 \end{bmatrix}, \quad \tau' = \begin{bmatrix} 3/2 & 1/2 \\ 3/2 & 3/2 \end{bmatrix}, \quad \gamma' = \begin{bmatrix} 9/4 & 5/4 \\ 9/4 & 9/4 \end{bmatrix}$$

Model B: Elimination peripheral, with $k_{12} = 2$, $k_{20} = 2$, $k_{21} = 1$

$E(R_1) = 1/2$, $E(R_2) = 1/3$

$$K = \begin{bmatrix} -2 & 2 \\ 1 & -3 \end{bmatrix}, \quad \tau = \begin{bmatrix} 3/4 & 1/2 \\ 1/4 & 1/2 \end{bmatrix}, \quad \gamma = \begin{bmatrix} 9/16 & 1/4 \\ 5/16 & 1/4 \end{bmatrix}$$

$$K^* = \begin{bmatrix} 0 & 1 \\ 1/3 & 0 \end{bmatrix}, \quad \tau' = \begin{bmatrix} 3/2 & 3/2 \\ 1/2 & 3/2 \end{bmatrix}, \quad \gamma' = \begin{bmatrix} 9/4 & 9/4 \\ 5/4 & 9/4 \end{bmatrix}$$

Model C: Elimination central and peripheral, with $k_{10} = k_{20} = 2$ and $k_{12} = k_{21} = 1$

$E(R_1) = 1/3$, $E(R_2) = 1/3$

$$K = \begin{bmatrix} -3 & 1 \\ 1 & -3 \end{bmatrix}, \quad \tau = \begin{bmatrix} 3/8 & 1/8 \\ 1/8 & 3/8 \end{bmatrix}, \quad \gamma = \begin{bmatrix} 9/64 & 5/64 \\ 5/64 & 9/64 \end{bmatrix}$$

$$K^* = \begin{bmatrix} 0 & 1/3 \\ 1/3 & 0 \end{bmatrix}, \quad \tau' = \begin{bmatrix} 9/8 & 3/8 \\ 3/8 & 9/8 \end{bmatrix}, \quad \gamma' = \begin{bmatrix} 81/64 & 45/64 \\ 45/64 & 81/64 \end{bmatrix}$$

The variance of the total residence time, or VRT, is the sum of the individual variances in the compartments plus twice the covariance. The covariance between S_{11} and S_{12} is found from equation (19) to be 1/8; therefore, for the present particle, one has

$$\text{VRT} = \gamma_{1.} = \gamma_{11} + \gamma_{12} + 2 \text{ Cov} = 13/16$$

Clearly, many other moments are available to describe the kinetics of particles in model A. For example, a particle initially in compartment 2 has a MRT of $\tau_{2.} = 5/4$ and a VRT of $\gamma_{2.} = 17/16$. Also, a particle originating in 1 is expected to visit a compartment $\tau'_{1.} = 2$ times. These and many other moments, including higher-order moments, are useful in developing monitoring tests for the basic assumptions, e.g., of constant rates. Such tests are under current investigation.

The particle kinetics of models B and C can also be described in detail from the solutions given in Table 2. However, they may be summarized by noting only two moments of great interest in the subsequent development; namely, for model B, one has MRT $= \tau_1 = 5/4$ and VRT $= \gamma_1 = 17/16$, and for model C one has MRT $= \tau_1 = 1/2$ and VRT $= \gamma_1 = 1/4$.

Theoretical Results for the Noncompartmental Approach

A new, noncompartmental approach of finding statistical moments of residence times directly from concentration–time curves [or $X_{11}(t)$] has received wide attention in pharmacokinetic data analysis. The approach was developed originally in chemical engineering (8) and was applied to pharmacokinetics principally by Yamaoka et al. (20) and Riegelman and Collier (19). Because the theory is "noncompartmental," it has led to assertions such as (a) these statistical-moment methods "do not require the assumption of a specific compartmental model," and therefore (b) "there is [now] very much less interest in characterizing the pharmacokinetics of a drug in terms of model-dependent constants" (6). The new approach is very useful when correctly applied; however, the lack of a rigorous stochastic foundation has led to considerable confusion in its implementation.

Consider a particle that is introduced, say, into compartment 1. *If the particle can leave the system only through compartment 1*, then the noncompartmental approach may be very useful in finding certain moments. Of course, of the three models given previously, only model A satisfies the necessary assumptions for the use of the noncompartmental approach.

The basic noncompartmental results relating to residence times are

(i) $\quad \text{AUC} = \int_0^\infty X_{11}(t)\, dt \quad$ (20)

(ii) $\quad \text{MRT} = \int_0^\infty t X_{11}(t)\, dt / \text{AUC} \quad$ (21)

(iii) $\quad \text{VRT} = \int_0^\infty (t - \text{MRT})^2 X_{11}(t)\, dt / \text{AUC} \quad$ (22)

Rescigno et al. (15,16,18) have developed other measures, one of which is

(iv) $\quad \tau_{11} = \text{AUC}/X_{11}(0) \quad$ (23)

Note that all of these results are calculated directly from $X_{11}(t)$, which is often interpreted as the drug level in the plasma and hence is usually observable. Therefore, these measures have the advantage of being estimable directly by numerical integration of $X_{11}(t)$ without assuming a specific compartmental structure and without estimating intermediate k_{ij} rate coefficients, as required in the methods involving equations (10)–(19). However, they are very sensitive to the assumption that the particle can leave only through compartment 1. Cobelli et al. (2) and DiStefano (3) have shown that serious errors in estimation may result when they are applied incorrectly.

Numerical Illustration of Results for Noncompartmental Approach

Consider finding the foregoing measures for model A where $X_{11}(t) = (e^{-t} + 2e^{-4t})/3$. It is easy to show from equations (20)–(23) that AUC = 1/2, MRT = 3/4, and VRT = 13/16. Because $X_{11}(0) = 1$, one has $\tau_{11} = 1/2$. All of these agree with the results found earlier for the compartmental approach.

The assumptions underlying these formulas are not satisfied by either model B or C, and hence improper use of the formulas with these models would be expected to yield incorrect results. To illustrate this point, note that applying equations (20)–(23) to model B would give AUC = 3/4, MRT = 11/12, VRT = 137/144, and $\tau_{11} = 3/4$. Note that the purported MRT and VRT do not agree with the earlier results and hence are incorrect. Similarly, for model C, one would find AUC = 3/8, MRT = 5/12, VRT = 29/144, and $\tau_{11} = 3/8$, where again the purported MRT and VRT are incorrect.

In practice, experimenters have used equations (21) and (22) for general systems of two or more compartments in which leakage occurs from compartments other than the compartment in which the drug is introduced and measured. The simple examples in this chapter demonstrate clearly the error of such procedures. Of course, if the MRT and VRT are in error, it follows that all subsequent calculations based on them, such as the volumes of distribution and the clearances, are also suspect.

As an aside, not that τ_{11} calculated from equation (23) is correct for all models. This follows because $X_{11}(t)$ for any model is proportional to the survivorship function, the integral of which yields the mean or τ_{11}. Unfortunately, τ_{11} alone is not of great interest in subsequent analysis.

Usefulness of Statistical Moments

One objective of a compartmental model is to provide useful measures for subsequent statistical analysis of pharmacokinetic data. The statistical moments of the variables relating to particle age constitute such useful response variables. As an illustration, an example is given in MWM, where data on cholesterol kinetics were analyzed to test for possible differences between drug treatments. It is shown for that example that the estimated mean residence times, τ_{ij}'s, are more sensitive response variables than the estimated rate coefficients, k_{ij}'s; hence, the test is more powerful when analyzed via compartmental residence times. This research was followed by a simulation study (12) of one particular model (model A) to compare under carefully controlled conditions the powers of estimated rate coefficients, mean residence times, and many other response variables, such as half-lives, found in the literature. It was found that the estimated τ_{12}, the mean residence time in the tissue, was the most powerful single variable to detect a wide variety of treatment effects. This variable, also called the mean permanence time by Rescigno (15,16), has intuitive biological appeal as well.

Although τ_{12}, or, in general, τ_{ij} for $j \neq 1$, appears very sensitive in general, it fails completely to detect certain treatment effects, such as increases of similar proportions in both k_{12} and k_{21} of model A. However, in this particular case both γ_{12} and τ'_{12} are sensitive to the change, and, in general, other statistical moments would detect specialized cases. The main point here is that a variety of statistical moments, in addition to simple compartmental residence times, are useful in practical data analysis. Further research is in progress to delineate the conditions under which particular moments would be preferable. We are not aware of similar studies that would determine the power of the MRT and VRT given by the noncompartmental approach, but because of their composite nature, we would expect them, in general, to be less powerful than the more focused τ_{ij}'s, τ''_{ij}'s, γ_{ij}'s, and γ''_{ij}'s.

In summary, we claim that application of the statistical moments from the noncompartmental approach requires the assumption of a particular *class* of compartmental models, and we recommend that the assumption be carefully tested by fitting alternative models to data. Moreover, in our opinion, the demonstrated utility of the statistical moments from the compartmental approach should lead to more, rather than less, interest in characterizing the pharmacokinetics of a drug in terms of model-dependent k_{ij} parameters. In light of these facts, we recommend (a) finding the "best" structured compartmental model for a particular data set through theoretical considerations and statistical analysis, (b) estimating the k_{ij} rate coefficients and thereby the K matrix of the model, and (c) transforming the K matrix to yield estimated statistical moments for further understanding and analysis.

STOCHASTIC FORMULATION WITH AGE-VARYING TRANSFER RATES

Compartment Model with Gamma Retention Times

As noted previously, a compartment can be defined in the deterministic formulation as a mass or concentration governed by linear differential equations of the form of equation (1). The analogous definition in the stochastic formulation is a set of particles whose location probabilities are governed by linear differential equations of the form of equation (7), which in turn are direct consequences of the constant instantaneous flow probabilities of the form of equation (6). An alternative definition in the stochastic formulation is a set of particles whose R_{ij} lifetimes, which govern transfers in the system, are distributed as exponential random variables with parameters k_{ij}, as given in equation (10).

The conceptual implication of the present stochastic (and deterministic) formulation is that the transfer mechanism cannot discriminate on the basis of accumulated retention time. In order to simplify the semantics, we have defined particle "age" as its present retention time in the compartment of interest. In these terms, the present stochastic formulation assumes that the system selects particles at random for transfer without respect to their age.

However, this assumption is questionable in many systems. As a specific example, in physiological modeling, Ellis et al. (5) examined passage through the gastrointestinal tract of ruminants. They noted that the assumed compartments are not homogeneous but rather are subject to imperfect mixing, which results in age discrimination in the passage mechanism. Moreover, particles undergo digestive breakdown in the tract, with the effect that the older particles, which tend to be smaller, are more likely to transfer than the newer particles, which tend to be larger. In general, the heterogeneity inherent in dividing a body into "central" and "peripheral" compartments is widely recognized. One might argue, in fact, that there are few, if any, real biological systems that can be divided into homogeneous compartments with exponential lifetimes.

Of course, the theoretical question whether or not a perfect "exponential" compartment exists in nature does not diminish the practical utility of compartmental modeling and analysis based on exponential compartments. However, it does raise the question whether or not practical alternatives exist that might be useful in the analysis of pharmacokinetic data. One such alternative is the "gamma" compartment model, i.e., a model whose compartments have gamma-distributed retention times.

The assumed gamma distribution, denoted $\Gamma(n, \lambda)$, for a particular retention time is perhaps most readily justified by examining its corresponding probability intensity rate function. This rate function, also called a hazard rate, can be denoted as $k_i(a)$ and defined as

$$\text{Prob}\{\text{a given particle of age } a \text{ in compartment } i \text{ at time } t \text{ is no longer in } i \text{ at time } t + \Delta t\} = k_i(a)\Delta t + o(\Delta t) \quad (24)$$

which is analogous to equation (6). As noted earlier, the exponential distribution of R_i has a constant rate function $k_i(a) = k_i$. Let this exponential distribution be denoted as $\text{Exp}(k_i)$. For the gamma distribution, $\Gamma(n, \lambda)$, the age-varying rate function when n is an integer is (11)

$$k_i(a) = \frac{\lambda^n a^{n-1}/(n-1)!}{\sum_{l=0}^{n-1} (\lambda a)^l / l!} \quad \text{for } a \geq 0 \text{ and } \lambda > 0 \quad (25)$$

Three useful characteristics of this gamma rate function are the following:

1. For $n = 1$, the rate is $k_i(a) = \lambda$. This follows directly from substitution into equation (25), and also from the fact that the exponential is a special case of the gamma, i.e., $\Gamma(1, \lambda) = \text{Exp}(\lambda)$.

2. For $n > 1$, the rate at $a = 0$ is $k_i(0) = 0$, after which it increases. Therefore, equation (25) implies that for $n > 1$ the transfer of newly introduced particles is initially retarded.
3. The rate $k_i(a)$ asymptotes to λ as a becomes large. Hence, equation (25) implies a mechanism by which the age discrimination gradually diminishes as the retention time increases.

Thus, the form of equation (25) is useful in describing transfer of a substance that, perhaps because of incomplete mixing, is initially retarded but that equilibrates with other material over time. Of course, the hypothesis of perfect mixing would be given by the special case $n = 1$.

The parameter n is called the shape parameter and λ the scale parameter. Figure 3 shows some characteristic forms for the age-dependent rate function for several small integers n on a scale where λ is standardized to $\lambda = 1$. The distribution of the R_i retention times corresponding to equation (25) is

$$f_{R_i}(a; n, \lambda_i) = \lambda_i^n \, a^{n-1} \, \exp[-\lambda_i a]/(n-1)! \quad (a > 0) \tag{26}$$

which can be compared to equation (10).

In addition to the retention-time distributions within each compartment, the gamma compartmental model requires the specification of conditional probabilities, denoted α_{ij}, of transfer among the compartments. These α_{ij}'s, assumed time-invariant, give the probabilities of transfer from a donor compartment, i, to each possible recipient compartment, j. It follows that $\alpha_{10} + \alpha_{12} = 1$ and $\alpha_{20} + \alpha_{21} = 1$.

Note that the implementation of the model is nonmechanistic insofar as retention times are concerned. An experimenter might first divide the system into compartments based on known theory. The retention-time distributions within each compartment are specified either through expert knowledge from hazard rates, such as in Fig. 3, or by fitting alternative models to data. The α_{ij} transfer probabilities are then determined. One advantage of using these nonmechanis-

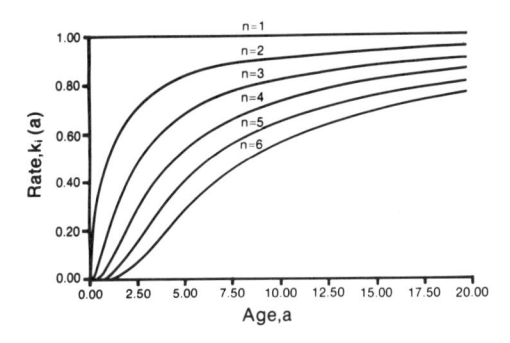

FIG. 3. Age-dependent rate functions for gamma $\Gamma(n, \lambda)$ retention-time distributions for several small integers n and for $\lambda = 1$.

tic retention times is the incorporation of nonhomogeneous compartments and consequential particle age discrimination with a minimum number of additional parameters. This will be illustrated subsequently.

Stochastic Solution for Particle Location in Gamma Compartment Models

Gamma retention times, in addition to their empirical appeal, have benign mathematical properties that make the gamma models tractable. In particular, it can be shown that a $\Gamma(n, \lambda)$ variable can be generated as the sum of n independent $\text{Exp}(\lambda)$ variables. This relationship can be utilized to solve models with gamma retention times through the analysis of equivalent but expanded compartmental models with exponential "pseudocompartments."

To illustrate this, consider the following two examples. As one example (11), consider the generalization of model A to a gamma model with $\Gamma(n_1, \lambda_1)$ and $\Gamma(n_2, \lambda_2)$ retention times and with $\alpha_{12} = p$ as the probability of a transfer from 1 to 2. The equivalent representation of this model with $n_1 + n_2$ exponential compartments is given in Fig. 4. The individual exponential compartments are not intended to be interpreted mechanistically; they exist merely as a mathematical artifice to generate the gamma retention times. As another example (9), consider an irreversible gamma model in which the retention times are $\Gamma(n_1, \lambda_1)$ and $\Gamma(n_2, \lambda_2)$ and the transfer probability is $\alpha_{12} = 1$. This can be regarded as a possible simplification of model B. The equivalent exponential model representation has $n_1 + n_2$ compartments, with n_1 rates equal to λ_1 and n_2 rates equal to λ_2.

As numerical illustrations, consider first the irreversible model that has been applied to passage data by Matis (10). As a simple example, let the retention times be $\Gamma(2, 2)$ and $\text{Exp}(1)$, which gives three pseudocompartments. Letting $\Pi_{ij}(t)$ denote the probability that a particle originating in pseudocompartment i at 0 will be in j at time t, the set of Kolmogorov equations describing the stochastic model for this expanded system is

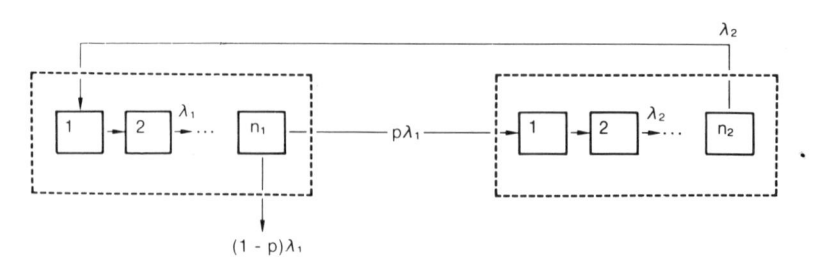

FIG. 4. Representation of model A (elimination central) with gamma $\Gamma(n_i, \lambda_i)$ retention-time distributions as an equivalent system of pseudocompartments with exponential $\text{Exp}(\lambda_i)$ retention-time distributions.

STOCHASTIC COMPARTMENTAL SYSTEMS

$$\dot{\Pi}_{11}(t) = -2\Pi_{11}(t)$$
$$\dot{\Pi}_{12}(t) = 2\Pi_{11}(t) - 2\Pi_{12}(t)$$
$$\dot{\Pi}_{13}(t) = 2\Pi_{12}(t) - \Pi_{13}(t)$$

with coefficient matrix

$$K = \begin{bmatrix} -2 & 2 & 0 \\ 0 & -2 & 2 \\ 1 & 0 & -1 \end{bmatrix} \quad (27)$$

The solution to the expanded system is

$$\Pi_{11}(t) = e^{-2t}$$
$$\Pi_{12}(t) = 2te^{-2t}$$
$$\Pi_{13}(t) = 4e^{-t} - 4(t+1)e^{-2t}$$

which is relatively easy to derive recursively and to verify by substitution. When the pseudocompartments are grouped, the solution for the probabilities of particle location in terms of the original gamma compartments is

$$p_{11}(t) = \Pi_{11}(t) + \Pi_{12}(t) = (1 + 2t)e^{-2t}$$
$$p_{12}(t) = \Pi_{13}(t) = 4e^{-t} - 4(t+1)e^{-2t}$$

Note that the irreversible gamma model leads to equal eigenvalues in the exponential system, and thus to powers of time in the solution.

As a second numerical illustration, consider the reversible model in Fig. 4 with $\Gamma(2, 2)$ and $\text{Exp}(1)$ retention times and with $p = 1/2$. The set of differential equations for the expanded model is

$$\dot{\Pi}_{11}(t) = -2\Pi_{11}(t) + \Pi_{13}(t)$$
$$\dot{\Pi}_{12}(t) = 2\Pi_{11}(t) - 2\Pi_{12}(t)$$
$$\dot{\Pi}_{13}(t) = \Pi_{12}(t) - \Pi_{13}(t)$$

with coefficient matrix

$$K = \begin{bmatrix} -2 & 2 & 0 \\ 0 & -2 & 1 \\ 1 & 0 & -1 \end{bmatrix} \quad (28)$$

It is shown in Matis and Wehrly (11) that such expanded systems that involve cycling almost always have complex eigenvalues, and the solution for this particular model is given as

$$\Pi_{11}(t) = 0.225e^{-0.304t} + e^{-2.35t}[0.775 \cos(1.03t) - 0.110 \sin(1.03t)]$$
$$\Pi_{12}(t) = 0.266e^{-0.304t} + e^{-2.35t}[-0.266 \cos(1.03t) + 1.416 \sin(1.03t)]$$
$$\Pi_{13}(t) = 0.382e^{-0.304t} + e^{-2.35t}[-0.382 \cos(1.03t) - 0.759 \sin(1.03t)]$$

In terms of the original gamma compartments, the solutions are

$$p_{11}(t) = \Pi_{11}(t) + \Pi_{12}(t)$$
$$p_{12}(t) = \Pi_{13}(t)$$

These examples illustrate the point that gamma compartment models are tractable mathematically and can be solved using the previous theory. One qualitative difference is that equal eigenvalues are assumed in irreversible gamma models, giving a solution involving powers of time, and complex eigenvalues arise in almost all reversible gamma models, yielding solutions that contain damped oscillations.

Solution for Statistical Moments in Gamma Compartment Models

The statistical moments of the residence times and related variables for gamma compartment models are easily solved through the foregoing equivalence relationship between gamma compartments and exponential pseudocompartments. To illustrate this, consider first the irreversible gamma model example with expanded K matrix as given in equation (27). The matrices of means and variances for the pseudocompartments are

$$\tau = \begin{bmatrix} \tfrac{1}{2} & \tfrac{1}{2} & 1 \\ 0 & \tfrac{1}{2} & 1 \\ 0 & 0 & 1 \end{bmatrix}, \quad \gamma = \begin{bmatrix} \tfrac{1}{4} & \tfrac{1}{4} & 1 \\ 0 & \tfrac{1}{4} & 1 \\ 0 & 0 & 1 \end{bmatrix}$$

Note that for a particle entering compartment 1, the MRT is

$$\text{MRT} = \tau_{11} + \tau_{12} + \tau_{13} = 2$$

and the VRT is

$$\text{VRT} = \gamma_{11} + \gamma_{12} + \gamma_{13} + 2[\text{Cov}(S_{11}, S_{12}) + \text{Cov}(S_{11}, S_{13}) + \text{Cov}(S_{12}, S_{13})]$$
$$= 3/2$$

The second example with the reversible gamma system is similar. The K matrix in equation (28) gives the following moment matrices for the pseudocompartments:

$$\tau = \begin{bmatrix} 1 & 1 & 1 \\ \tfrac{1}{2} & 1 & 1 \\ 1 & 1 & 2 \end{bmatrix}, \quad \gamma = \begin{bmatrix} 1 & 1 & 3 \\ \tfrac{3}{4} & 1 & 3 \\ 1 & 1 & 4 \end{bmatrix}$$

These also can be combined to give many moments of interest. A particle starting in 1 would have a MRT of

$$\text{MRT} = \tau_{11} + \tau_{12} + \tau_{13} = 3$$

and the VRT of

$$\text{VRT} = \gamma_{11} + \gamma_{12} + \gamma_{13} + 2[\text{Cov}(S_{11}, S_{12}) + \text{Cov}(S_{11}, S_{13}) + \text{Cov}(S_{12}, S_{13})]$$
$$= 18\tfrac{1}{2}$$

Clearly, the statistical moments for the gamma compartment models are easy to determine once the transition rates, on their estimates, are known. If the rates must be estimated from data, one must solve for the models of particle location such as those given in the preceding section. Note also that the noncompartmental methods are not applicable if the compartment of origin has gamma retention times with $n > 1$.

In summary, a generalized approach to compartmental modeling based on gamma retention times has been developed. This formulation incorporates particle age discrimination in the transfer mechanism such as that due to initial incomplete mixing. The models are tractable mathematically, and solutions are available to describe particle location over time and the statistical moments of residence times and related variables. It is recommended that such models be considered routinely to model the molecular variability in pharmacokinetic systems and to analyze pharmacokinetic data.

REFERENCES

1. Chiang, C.L. (1980): *An Introduction to Stochastic Processes and Their Applications.* R.E. Krieger, Huntington, N.Y.
2. Cobelli, C., Nosadini, R., Toffolo, G., McCullogh, A., Avogare, A., Tiengo, A., and Alberti, K.G.M.M. (1982): A model of the kinetics of ketone bodies in humans. *Am. J. Physiol.,* 243(*Regulatory Integrative Comp. Physiol.* 12):R7–R17.
3. DiStefano, J.J., III (1982): Noncompartmental vs. compartmental analysis: Some bases for choice. *Am J. Physiol.,* 243(*Regulatory Integrative Comp. Physiol.* 12):R1–R6.
4. Eisenfeld, J. (1979): Relationship between stochastic and differential models of compartmental system. *Math. Biosci.,* 43:289–305.
5. Ellis, W.C., Matis, J.H., Pond, K.R., Lascano, C.E., and Telford, J.P. (1984): Dietary influences in flow rate and digestive capacity. In: *Herbivore Nutrition in the Subtropics and Tropics,* edited by F.M.C. Gilchrist and R.I. Mackie, 269–293. Science Press, Craighall, South Africa.
6. Gibaldi, M., and Perrier, D. (1982): *Pharmacokinetics,* ed. 2, pp. 409, 475. Marcel Dekker, New York.
7. Godfrey, K., (1983): *Compartmental Models and Their Application.* Academic Press, New York.
8. Himmelblau, D.M., and Bischoff, K.B. (1968): *Process Analysis and Simulation: Deterministic Systems.* Wiley, New York.
9. Hughes, T.H., and Matis, J.H. (1984): An irreversible two-compartment model with age-dependent turnover rates. *Biometrics,* 40:501–505.
10. Matis, J.H. (1972): Gamma time-dependency in Blaxter's compartmental model. *Biometrics,* 28:597–602.
11. Matis, J.H., and Wehrly, T.E. (1984): On the use of residence time moments in the statistical analysis of age-dependent stochastic compartmental systems. In: *Mathematics in Biology and Medicine,* edited by S.L. Paveri-Fontana and V. Capasso, (*in press*). Springer-Verlag, New York.
12. Matis, J.H., Wehrly, T.E., and Gerald, K.B. (1983): The statistical analysis of pharmacokinetic data. In: *Tracer Kinetics and Physiologic Modeling,* edited by R.M. Lambrecht and A. Rescigno, pp. 1–58. Springer-Verlag, New York.
13. Matis, J.H., Wehrly, T.E., and Metzler, C.M. (1983): On some stochastic formulations and related statistical moments of pharmacokinetic models. *J. Pharmacokinet. Biopharm.,* 11:77–92.
14. Olson, D.R., and Matis, J.H. (1984): Residence time moments in compartmental models with age-dependent or time-dependent rates. In: *Mathematics and Computers in Biomedi-*

cal Applications, edited by J. Eisenfeld and C. DeLisi, pp. 237–242. Elsevier, New York.
15. Rescigno, A. (1973): On transfer times in tracer experiments. *J. Theor. Biol.* 39:9–27.
16. Rescigno, A., and Gurpide, E. (1973): Estimation of average times of residence, recycle and interconversion of blood-borne compounds using tracer methods. *J. Clin. Endocrinol. Metab.,* 36:263–276.
17. Rescigno, A., and Segre, G. (1966): *Drug and Tracer Kinetics.* Blaisdell, Waltham, Mass.
18. Rescigno, A., Lambrecht, R.M., and Duncan, C.C. (1983): Mathematical methods in the formulation of pharmacokinetic models. In: *Tracer Kinetics and Physiologic Modeling,* edited by R.M. Lambrecht and A. Rescigno, pp. 59–119. Springer-Verlag, New York.
19. Riegelman, S., and Collier, P. (1980): The application of statistical moment theory to the evaluation of *in vivo* dissolution time and absorption time. *J. Pharmacokinet. Biopharm.,* 8:509–534.
20. Yamaoko, K., Nakagawa, T., and Uno, T. (1978): Statistical moments in pharmacokinetics. *J. Pharmacokinet. Biopharm.,* 6:547–558.

DISCUSSION

Discussant 1 (D1): At the intuitive level, I am intrigued by the idea of factoring the model into two parts: the part that describes the age-dependent transfer and the more mechanical part that sends the particles here and there in the system. Do you really have a general tool for this, or must one use some trick, like the gamma function, to obtain a solution?

Speaker (S): The use of gamma retention times provide a rich system with initial retardation. With such systems, one can solve for the probabilities of particle location at any given time in closed form. One can also find the moments. If any other retention-time distribution is used, it may be very difficult to solve the system in closed form for the probabilities of particle location. But it is easy to solve for the moments of other retention-time distributions, and from these one can find the expected residence time in any particular state. Then one can use the method-of-moments procedure to estimate system parameters.

D1: Would you suggest that we now try to think about models as having two parts: first, the retention-time distribution, and, separately, the connection pattern of the compartments?

S: Yes, it seems to me as though this is a useful approach. If one adopts this general approach and finds that one has homogeneous compartments with exponential retention times, then one is back to the classical system. But it is helpful to have this more general "semi-Markov" formalism. Its implementation is still in a formative stage. At present there is no problem with gamma retention times, which may be as useful for other systems as they are now for gastrointestinal passage models. So I think that is the way the field should be moving. It provides a simple way to describe the variability, or heterogeneity, within the compartments with only a few parameters.

D2: I would like to stress one important aspect of your presentation: There is a big difference between mean residence time and the sojourn time. The mean residence time is the mean time a molecule stays in the system after injection, whereas the sojourn time is the time the particle remains in a given compartment. I would like, moreover, to stress to the pharmacologists here that sojourn time is of interest. Drug effect may, in some way, be connected to it when the integral of the drug level in a compartment over time is important. The sojourn time can be calculated easily through the transfer matrix K, because it is calculated from the value of the AUC in each compartment. This is probably highly correlated with the effect of a drug. For instance, a drug that remains a long time in the body, like the antibiotic cefotriaxone, is much more effective.

D3: Can the "age" dependence of transfer constants be considered to be equivalent to time dependence of the constants?

S: They are really two distinct phenomena. In time-dependent transfer, the transfer rate varies as a function of time, whereas for age-dependent transfer it varies as a function of the age of the particle within the compartment, an endogenous effect rather than an exogenous one. The use of time-varying coefficients is quite different mathematically from the use of age-varying coefficients.

D4: To what kind of biological data have you tried to apply these concepts?

S: We use age-varying models routinely now for any passage data in animal nutrition. In fact, we find that almost without exception, a gamma compartment model provides a better fit to the data than the usual exponential compartment model. The gamma model describes all of the mixing very conveniently with just one additional parameter.

D5: In pharmacokinetics, one of the problems is identifiability; that is, a data set can be described by several possible compartmental models. You seem to imply that you know the compartment model that should be used.

S: In using an age-varying model one can often simplify the system description. Biological considerations will define the compartmental structure, and then we use a very robust way of describing the retention-time distributions within that structure. One can often, therefore, simplify a previous compartmental model that used many compartments.

D6: Does your approach yield any more insight into the system, or are you just finding the most tractable form of describing what you see?

S: We have a simpler, more tractable way of describing what we see. What that means in practice is that we can estimate the model coefficients better and make sharper inferences on some questions of real importance. Part of our task is to find a model that describes the data well with as few parameters as possible and that therefore does not have as many identifiability problems.

D7: I can understand that, for any individual data set, the same information is extracted whether one estimates compartmental microparameters or residence times. Is your implication that in comparing two populations it might be more sensitive to see if there were treatment differences by looking at mean residence times?

S: Yes. In our simulation studies we have a known size of treatment effect. We then find the precision with which we can estimate an individual residence time. Because this "within" variability is less than for microconstants, we can detect a treatment effect with more power.

D7: However, it might be that the population variability for the mean residence times is greater than the population variability for the original compartmental constants. In that case the advantage of being able to estimate an individual residence time with good precision would be negated by the larger interindividual variability.

S: We have not yet simulated tests with interindividual variability. However, empirical results indicate that the estimated mean residence times usually perform very well even with interindividual differences (1).

D8: I am worried by your introduction of the gamma distribution, insofar as it is statistically so convenient. Statisticians often introduce distributions because they like to work with them, rather than because they are the scientific truth. I can see the exponential distribution in the simpler models as having an absolute position. Are you satisfied that by introducing the gamma distribution you are in fact making a closer approach to reality, or are you simply adopting something that is convenient and easily handled mathematically? More than once you referred to particle breakdown. It is not clear to me how a particle remains a particle in your formulation if it breaks down. Ought you really to be saying that there were, for example, five particles originally that were in some way combined, and at a certain age they assumed their separate personalities? Another point that worried me was your emphasis that the parametrization you adopt is more powerful in finding significant differences between treatments. But surely what matters is finding *relevant* differences between the effects of treatments. If one applies any two treatments to replicate materials, one will always find statistically significant differences if one looks hard enough at enough measurements or derived variables. Statistical significance in itself is not the primary purpose of the experiment; rather, it is to find whether or not there are differences in manifestations that are relevant to the output of the system.

S: You are right about the importance of having a relevant transformation. Fortunately, ours are all biologically motivated. The mean residence time, for example, has meaning to biologists. I believe we have found a more powerful parametrization that is biologically interesting; the transformation is suggested by biology, not by some mathematical optimization. We encourage the biologist to have a look at the hazard rates. He does not even have to worry about whether it is a gamma or some other distribution. We can take a look at a catalogue of hazard rates and find one that has a mixing pattern like his. Once he identifies the shape, we have a nonmechanistic description of the mixing and other age-dependent phenomena. Once the particular gamma is identified, the solution follows. Regarding particle breakdown, in forage-passage modeling, a hay particle can be reduced in size and changes in chemical structure due to digestive breakdown. Other particles are indigestible and do not change size. They all are subject to incomplete mixing, however, and so all may be regarded as subject to age-dependent transfer.

REFERENCES

1. Matis, J.M., Wehrly, T.E., and Metzler, C.M. (1983): On some stochastic formulations and related statistical moments of pharmacokinetic models. *J. Pharmacokinet. Biopharm.*, 11:77–92.

Variability in Drug Therapy:
Description, Estimation, and Control,
edited by M. Rowland et al.
Raven Press, New York © 1985.

Modeling Pharmacokinetic/Pharmacodynamic Variability

Lewis B. Sheiner

Department of Laboratory Medicine and Division of Clinical Pharmacology, Departments of Medicine and Pharmacy, Schools of Medicine and Pharmacy, University of California, San Francisco, California 94143

Variability in a dependent variable (y) can be of two types: that which correlates with other observables (x) and that which does not. To deal with the first kind, structural models are proposed that link x to an expected value [$E(y)$] or prediction of y via a functional form $f(x, \phi)$, quantified by parameters ϕ. To deal with residual variability, one is usually content simply to model its typical magnitude as a function of the observables x. The typical magnitude of residual variability can be measured by its variance, the expected squared deviation of y from its expectation. A variance model links x to the variance of y via a functional form $\sigma^2 v(x,\phi,\zeta)$, quantified by parameters σ^2 and ζ.

The two models, structural and variance, together will here be called the regression model of y on x, and each model will be called a submodel of the regression model.

REGRESSION MODELS

Univariate Responses and Models for Individuals

A simple type of regression model that has only one type of dependent variable will illustrate interesting structural and variance submodels and will be the basis for a subsequent extension to the multivariate case.

Consider a series of observations of the dependent variable y_i, $i = 1, n$. Associated with each y_i is a vector of independent variable values, x_i [for example, $x_i = $ (dose, time)]; y_i can be written

$$y_i = f(x_i, \phi) + \epsilon_i \qquad (1)$$

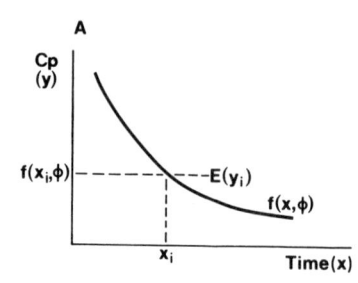

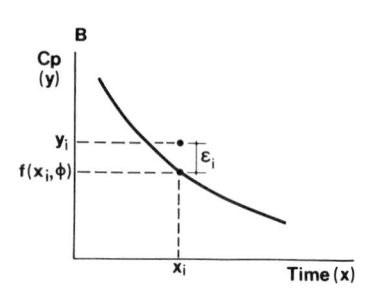

FIG. 1. **A:** The relationship of a plasma drug level (C_p) to time after a bolus dose is used to illustrate the structural submodel of a regression model. The expected value of y_i is given by the structural model evaluated at x_i and the true parameter values ϕ. **B.** The observed value of y at time x_i, y_i (filled circle), differs from its expected value by an error ϵ_i. A model for the variance of ϵ_i is required to fully specify the regression model. (From Sheiner, ref. 6, with permission.)

where the structural model $E(y_i)$ (for example, the monoexponential model) is written $f(x_i, \phi)$, so that its dependence on x_i and ϕ is made explicit.[1] It is further assumed that ϵ_i and ϵ_k are independent for $i \neq k$. One or more arguments will sometimes be omitted when writing $f(x_i, \phi)$; for example, the symbols f_i or $f_i(\phi)$ will sometimes be used instead. Figure 1 further illustrates the concept of a structural model.

Variance models are generally less familiar to kineticists than structural models. Consider Fig. 2A, in which multiple measurements of y_i (r of them) are indicated. Then

$$y_{ik} = f(x_i, \phi) + \epsilon_{ik}; \quad k = 1, r \qquad (2)$$

where the variances of all the ϵ_{ik}, $k = 1, r$, are equal because x_i is constant. Let this variance be $\text{Var}(\epsilon_i)$. Now consider Fig. 2B, where i is allowed to vary; clearly, $\text{Var}(\epsilon_i)$ does not equal $\text{Var}(\epsilon_k)$. The variance appears to decrease with increasing time. It seems possible that this dependence could be modeled by

---

[1] It should be noted that x and ϕ, for example, are lists of items, called vectors—not to be confused with the directional vectors of physics. To deal with these, vector and matrix notation will frequently appear in this chapter. A vector, for our purposes, is a column of scalars (numbers), and a matrix is a table of them. These columns and tables can be combined (e.g., added or multiplied) by the rules of linear algebra. The notation for such operations is similar to that used for scalar arithmetic. The reader unfamiliar with linear algebra should read vector and matrix notation as though it referred to scalars: The sense of the indicated operations and expressions will be clear, even if the multivariate details are not. For example, if X is a vector and A is a matrix, $X^t A^{-1} X$ (read "X-transpose times A-inverse times X," but ignore the superscript t, indicating the transpose operation, as this operation, which switches rows and columns of a matrix, does not affect scalars) accomplishes, in a multivariate sense, much the same thing as $XA^{-1}X$, i.e., X^2/A, does in a univariate one.

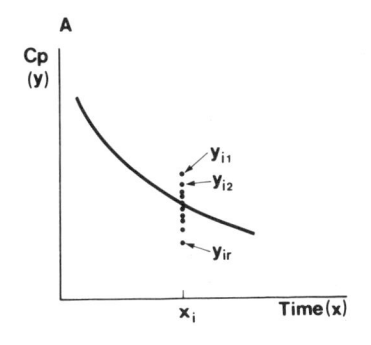

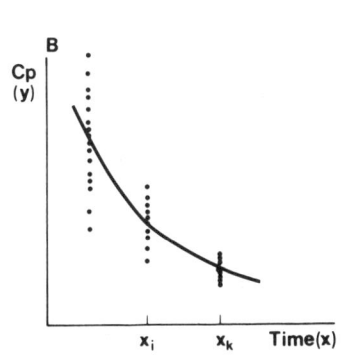

FIG. 2. The model of Fig. 1 is used to illustrate the following: **A:** The distribution of r_i measurements all taken at x_i. The sample variance of such measurements could be used to estimate the variance of ϵ_i. **B:** The fact that $\mathrm{Var}(\epsilon_i)$ need not equal $\mathrm{Var}(\epsilon_k)$. Here the variance of observations of y about its expected value appears to decrease as time (x) increases, or $E(y_i)$ itself decreases. A model linking $\mathrm{Var}(\epsilon_i)$ to $E(y_i) = f_i$ is commonly used when the data look like this. (From Scheiner, ref. 6, with permission.)

expressing the variance of ϵ at any given x as a function of x, or, perhaps, as a function of $f(x_i, \phi)$. To do the latter will usually require the definition of several new parameters; these can be collected in a new parameter vector, ζ. The important point is that $\mathrm{Var}(\epsilon_i)$ need not equal $\mathrm{Var}(\epsilon_k)$; each is an expectation, just as $E(y_i)$ is, and can be modeled. That model, like $f(\cdot)$, will be a function of independent variables and parameters. Formally, the dependence of $\mathrm{Var}(\epsilon_i)$ on x_i and ϕ can be expressed in terms of the variance (submodel) of the regression model. This can be written

$$\mathrm{Var}(\epsilon_i) = \delta^2 v(x_i, \phi, \zeta) \tag{3}$$

where the parameter δ^2 is introduced to make the variance model per se $[v(x_i, \phi, \zeta)]$ scale-invariant. The variance model has parameters ϕ and ζ. The latter vector, as previously indicated, contains parameters that appear in the variance model, but not in the structural model.

The entire (univariate) regression model can now be written:

$$y_i = f(x_i, \phi) + \epsilon; \quad i = 1, n$$
$$E(\epsilon_i) = 0 \tag{4}$$
$$\mathrm{Var}(\epsilon_i) = \delta^2 v(x_i, \phi, \zeta)$$
$$\epsilon_i, \epsilon_k \text{ independent for } i \neq k$$

If ϕ is of length p and ζ of length q, then the number of parameters of the regression model (4) is $p + q + 1$. The parameters are

$$\phi_1, \phi_2, \ldots, \phi_p, \zeta_1, \zeta_2, \ldots, \zeta_q, \delta^2$$

What is missing from the foregoing is the detail as to the functional forms of $f(\cdot)$ and $v(\cdot)$. These "details" obviously express the understanding of the underlying relationships between $E(y_i)$ and $\text{Var}(y_i)$ and x_i. The parameters of those models are what the kineticist wants to know.

Multivariate Responses and Population Models

Kineticists often measure more than one kind of response in a single experiment; for example, they may measure both plasma and urine drug concentrations. If plasma and urine levels both are measured, then the "response" at any time could be a plasma level or a urine level or both. Thus, the response is a vector and can be modeled as before using model (4), but where now a second subscript is introduced to index the type of observation. That is, y_i consists of the two elements y_{i1}, y_{i2}; $f_i(\phi)$ is vector-valued (i.e., predicts both plasma and urine concentrations), and ϵ_i also consists of ϵ_{i1}, ϵ_{i2}. For purposes of illustration, assume $v_i = 1$ for all i. Despite this radical simplification, the variance model is still potentially more complicated than previously in that δ^2 is now a (covariance) matrix. That is, not only is the variance of the plasma-level observations a parameter, but so are both the variance of the urine-level observations and the covariance of plasma- and urine-level observations.

The covariance will, for example, be positive and greater than zero if, for some reason, observed plasma levels higher than their expected values tend to be associated with simultaneous urine-level observations also above their expectations. The covariance matrix will be square (have the same number of rows as columns; in this case, two of each) and symmetric (a square matrix, A, is symmetric if the element in row i and column j, a_{ij}, equals a_{ji} for all i, j). The variances of the two types of observations will be the diagonal elements (elements a_{ii} of square matrix A are the diagonal elements), and the covariance of the observations will appear in both off-diagonal positions.

An even more complex situation exists when one is interested in mean parameters in a population, and a multivariate approach is needed. A population model is a model that describes not only the relationship of observations in an individual to his parameters but also the population relationships of individuals' parameters to other observable patient features.

To begin to define a population model, model (4) is recognized as applying to the observations on a single individual among many in a total population. If similar data are available from each of N individuals, and the individual from whom each datum originated can be explicitly noted, then a model treating the set of individual observations as a single unit of response can be stated. Assuming the ith response in the jth individual is univariate (e.g., only plasma, not urine, levels are measured), the model for the set of responses from a single individual is similar to model (4):

$$y_j = f(x_j, \phi_j) + \epsilon_j; \quad j = 1, N$$
$$E(\epsilon_j) = 0$$
$$\text{Cov}(\epsilon_j) = \delta_j^2 \, \text{Diag}[v(x_j, \phi_j, \zeta_j)]$$
$$\epsilon_j, \epsilon_k \text{ independent for } j \neq k$$
(5)

Now, however, y_j and ϵ_j are vectors with elements y_{ji} and ϵ_{ji}, $i = 1, n_j$, respectively; x_j is a matrix with columns x_{ji}; $f(\cdot)$ and $v(\cdot)$ are vector-valued functions; and $\text{Diag}[v(x_j, \phi_j, \zeta_j)]$, where $v(x_j, \phi_j, \zeta_j)$ is a vector of length n_j, is a square $n_j \times n_j$ matrix with diagonal elements equal to the elements of $v(x_j, \phi_j, \zeta_j)$ and all off-diagonal elements equal to zero. Note that model (5) is multivariate not because of different types of observations but because the unit of observation has shifted to the individual, and consequently the single "observation" on each individual has become the complete vector of all observations taken on him. These, as will be seen, are correlated from a population viewpoint.

Each individual contributes an entire parameter vector, $(\phi_j, \zeta_j, \delta_j^2)'$, to the total list of parameters of model (5). Indeed, the major step in writing a population model is to provide a model for the individual parameter vector. Consider the following model:

$$\phi_j = g(x_j, \theta) + \eta_j$$
$$\zeta_j = \zeta; \quad \delta_j^2 = \delta^2$$
$$E(\eta_j) = 0; \quad \text{Cov}(\eta_j) = \Omega$$
$$\eta_j, \eta_k \text{ independent for } j \neq k$$
(6)

In this model, θ is a vector of population parameters; the η_j are independent vectors (each of length p) of differences of individual structural-model parameters from their mean, each with identical symmetric $p \times p$ covariance matrix Ω; and $g(x_j, \theta)$ is a vector-valued function equal to $E(\phi_j)$. Some simple examples of such models will be given shortly. Note that model (6) assumes that all ζ_j and δ_j^2 are equal to common values, ζ and δ^2, without individual variation. This assumption is not required, but it simplifies the exposition for the present. One final assumption completes model (5,6); viz., η_j and ϵ_j are independent.

STRUCTURAL-MODEL FORMS

Functional forms for structural models (and, in the next section, for variance models) are first discussed, for simplicity, in the context of modeling separate univariate responses within a single individual. Some multivariate (and population) extensions are considered afterward.

Empirical Models

Mechanistic models (often expressed as differential equations) are often used when detailed descriptions of pharmacokinetics or pharmacodynamics are desired. These are beyond the scope of this chapter. A few generally useful simple empirical models particularly relevant to pharmacokinetic modeling will be mentioned.

The most important independent variable relevant to individual pharmacokinetic data is a continuous-valued variable, time. Occasionally, concentration itself acts as an independent variable (when, for example, the model concerns pharmacodynamic responses).

Linear and Log-Linear Models

These are the most popular empirical models in many fields. The basic linear model states

$$f(x, \phi) = \phi_0 + \phi_1 x \qquad (7)$$

whereas the basic log-linear model has

$$\ln f(x, \phi) = \phi_0 + \phi_1 \ln x \qquad (8)$$

Note that (a) if $E[\ln(y)]$ is modeled by model (8), then $y = \exp(\phi_0 + \phi_1 x) = \exp(\phi_0) x^{\phi_1}$, a power model, and (b) model (7), with $\ln(x)$ substituted for x, is sometimes called the log-linear model, but it will not be so called here.

Sums of Exponentials

The most commonly used empirical model in pharmacokinetics is undoubtedly the sum-of-exponentials model, which for univariate x and m exponentials is

$$f(x, \phi) = \sum \phi_{2k-1} \exp(-\phi_{2k} x); \quad k = 1, m \qquad (9)$$

Note that there are twice as many parameters as exponentials. Model (9) provides a flexible family of functions for approximating monotone-decreasing, monotone-increasing, and unimodal functions. The appeal of model (9) is not only its flexibility but also that it is the form of the integrated solution to the most common type of mechanistic model used in pharmacokinetics (a set of linear differential equations).

The Hill Model

A useful form for a monotone function of a single continuous variable arises from the Michaelis-Menten model:

$$f(x, \phi) = \frac{V_m x}{K_m + x}$$

for x, a concentration. More generally, of course, the model is

$$f(x, \phi) = \frac{\phi_1 x}{\phi_2 + x}$$

where $\phi = (\phi_1, \phi_2)$ is simply a parameter list and ϕ_1 need not be V_m, nor ϕ_2 K_m. The model assumes its final (Hill) form with the introduction of a third parameter:

$$f(x, \phi) = \frac{\phi_1 x^{\phi_3}}{\phi_2 + x^{\phi_3}} \tag{10}$$

If $x' = \log(x)$ and $\phi'_2 = \log(\phi_2)$, model (10) can be written

$$f(x, \phi) = \frac{\phi_1}{1 + \exp(\phi'_2 - \phi_3 x)} \tag{11}$$

and is a symmetric sigmoid-shaped function eual to 0 at $x' = -\infty$, and ϕ_1 at $x' = \infty$.

Indicator Variables

A simple means to express the relationship between a dependent variable and a categorical independent variable is by use of an indicator variable. Suppose the clearance of a drug (per kilogram of body weight) is studied in a group of men and a group of women, and the possibility of a difference in clearances due to gender is to be investigated. A structural model such as the following might be used:

$$CL_j = \theta_0 + \theta_1 x_j$$

where

$$x_j = \begin{cases} 1, & \text{if individual is female} \\ 0, & \text{otherwise} \end{cases}$$

This model states that the mean clearance for males is θ_0, whereas that for females is $\theta_0 + \theta_1$. The indicator-variable idea can easily be extended to more than two classes. In general, $l - 1$ indicator variables are needed for l groups.

One or more indicator variables can also be used in place of a continuous-valued variable when detailed knowledge of a structural model is lacking. For example, if the relationship of clearance to age was under investigation, but the form of the relationship was in doubt, one could use

$$CL_j = \theta_0 + \sum \theta_k x_{jk}; \quad k = 1, l - 1 \tag{12}$$

where

$$x_{jk} = \begin{cases} 1, & \text{if } A_k \le \text{age} < A_{k+1} \\ 0, & \text{otherwise} \end{cases}$$

and, perhaps, where $l = 4$ and $A_1 = 0.25$ years, $A_2 = 15$ years, and $A_3 = 60$ years. Figure 4 illustrates this model. The mean clearance for individuals 0 to 0.25 year of age is given by θ_0; that of individuals older than 0.25 year but not older than 15 years is given by $\theta_0 + \theta_1$, etc. The model allows (as illustrated in Fig. 4) clearances to be different for various age groups (as a function, perhaps, of neonatal immaturity, sexual maturation, and senescence), while avoiding the need for specification of an arbitrarily exact functional form.

As a final example of the versatility of indicator variables, reconsider the previously discussed case in which both urine and plasma levels are being measured. But now, assume that at any particular time only one concentration, not both, can be measured. This is no longer, strictly speaking, a multivariate situation, because no covariance between C_p and C_u is possible, as they are never measured simultaneously. An indicator variable can profitably be used to deal with this simpler model as follows. Let x_{ik}, the kth element of the vector x_i, be defined as

$$x_{ik} = \begin{cases} 1, & \text{if level } i \text{ is a plasma level} \\ 0, & \text{otherwise} \end{cases}$$

The model can now be written as

$$f(x_i, \phi) = f_1(x_i, \phi)x_{ik} + f_2(x_i, \phi)(1 - x_{ik}) \tag{13}$$
$$v(x_i, \phi, \zeta) = x_{ik} + (1 - x_{ik})\zeta$$

where $f_1(\cdot)$ is the pharmacokinetic model for the plasma levels, $f_2(\cdot)$ is the model for the urine levels, δ^2 is the variance of the plasma levels, and ζ is the ratio of the variance of urine levels to that of plasma levels. Note (a) that $f_1(\cdot)$ and $f_2(\cdot)$ will share many of the same parameters, (b) that by using a term involving 1

FIG. 3. The theoretical relationship between clearance of a hypothetical drug and age is depicted by the curve. Lacking a functional form to describe this, and, indeed, lacking knowledge of the relationship, an investigator might nonetheless wish to entertain a model allowing distinct mean clearances for various age groups. Model (12) allows this. This model is depicted by horizontal lines whose heights are related to the four model parameters θ_0 through θ_3, as shown. The model is poor for age greater than 60, but a minor modification to the model could compensate for this: The term $\sum \theta_k x_{jk} + x_3[\theta_2 - \theta_3(\text{age}_j - 60)]$, with $k = 1, 2$, could be substituted for $\sum \theta_k x_{jk}$, with $k = 1$, 3, in model (12). This would cause the model above age 60 to follow a line with (negative) slope θ_3 beginning at height $\theta_0 + \theta_2$ and age 60. (From Sheiner, ref. 6, with permission.)

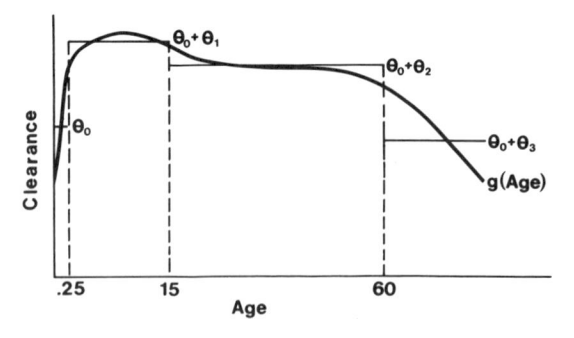

minus the indicator variable, the model can be caused to switch between the two submodels depending on the value of the indicator variable, rather than [as in model (12)] choosing the sum of the submodels for the case that the indicator variable = 1, and (c) how neatly the indicator variable allows the variance model to select the appropriate variance term for each observation.

Structural Models for Populations

Reconsider now model (6), and to simplify matters, consider only a single element of ϕ_j, ϕ_{jk}. Let $g_k(x_j, \theta)$ denote the expectation of this kth "element" of ϕ. An example of a population structural model for $g_k(x_j, \theta)$ was given earlier as model (12). This model is typical of such models: They are usually simple and empirical. Indeed, the most common such models choose $g_k(x_j, \theta) = \theta_k$, a constant, or $g_k(x_j, \theta)$ to be a model such as (12) (i.e., different patient groups, as indicated by the value of some indicator-variable element of x, have different mean parameters). Occasionally, a linear relationship between a parameter and some x is used. For example, the renal clearance of drug for the jth patient. CL_{Rj}, might be modeled as

$$CL_{Rj} = \phi_{j1} \cdot CL_{Crj}$$

where CL_{Crj} is creatinine clearance for the jth patient. Also, it is not unusual to model the logarithm of an element of ϕ, or, equivalently, to model the element as the exponential of $g_k(x_j, \theta)$. The usefulness of such a transformation will be apparent soon, when the population variance model is discussed.

Simple structural population models are usual. The lack of more complex population models is probably due more to the difficulty of studying large members of individuals for subtle relationships between pharmacokinetic parameters and independent variables than to a lack of interest in more detailed and powerful models.

VARIANCE MODELS

Several (semiempirical) variance models are in common use and will be discussed. The importance of the variance model is that it determines the appropriate means of fitting the structural model to the data so as to estimate ϕ. Most such fitting procedures choose their estimate, $\hat{\phi}$, of ϕ as that value minimizing some measure of distance between the model and the data. The distance measure is often the (weighted) sum of squared deviations (residuals) of observations from predictions. To properly combine the separate squared residuals, each should be normalized to its expected size, so that large residuals from imprecise measurements are not counted more than moderate residuals from more precise ones. The expected size of a squared residual is, of course, its variance, and this is given by the variance model. Consequently, the appropriate weighting of squared residuals depends on the variance model. When this model has unknown parameters, the weights are unknown, and certain adaptations of standard least-squares methods are needed. The least-squares type of fitting procedure appropriate for each type of variance model to be discussed will be mentioned later. The models will be discussed first as they pertain to observations taken from a single individual and then as they pertain to parameters of individuals within a population (i.e., population models).

Variance Models for Data from a Single Individual

Homoscedastic Case

The simplest possible variance model has

$$v(x_i, \phi, \zeta) = 1 \quad \text{for all } i \tag{14}$$

In this case the variance of y_i is simply δ^2 and is independent of x_i and ϕ; ζ is empty. Clearly, $\text{Var}(y_i) = \text{Var}(\epsilon_i) = \delta^2$. The appropriate least-squares method for estimating ϕ when model (14) holds is ordinary (unweighted) least squares (OLS).

Heteroscedastic Case with Known Weights

In this model, prior knowledge of the inhomogeneities in the variances of the various y_i (up to a proportionality constant) is claimed. Accordingly, the model is

$$v(x_i, \phi, \zeta) = v(x_i) = w_i^{-1} \tag{15}$$

where the weights, w_i, are assumed known and are therefore regarded as part of x_i. The model is again independent of ϕ, and ζ is again empty. The reason for writing the weights as reciprocally related to v_i is that the appropriate least-squares method of estimating ϕ when model (15) holds is weighted least squares (WLS), with weight w_i. Note that according to model (2), w_i^{-1} need not be the variance of y_i; the (unknown) parameter, δ^2, will scale all weights appropriately. All that is required of the w_i is that $\text{Var}(y_i) / \text{Var}(y_k) = w_k / w_i$ for all i, k. Note that model (15) reduces to model (14) when all $w_i = 1$.

Limited Heteroscedastic Case

Here, the general model has

$$v(x_i, \phi, \zeta) = v(x_i, \phi) \tag{16}$$

Again, ζ is empty. The most common example of this model is the constant-coefficient-of-variation (constant-CV) model that states

$$v(x_i, \phi, \zeta) = f_i^2 \tag{17}$$

This model corresponds to the example given at the beginning of the earlier section, Regression Models. Note that v_i is a function of ϕ because f_i is.

Model (17) is called the constant-CV model because it states that the coefficient of variation of y_i is a constant, δ. This is seen from

$$CV(y_i) = \frac{SD(y_i)}{E(y_i)} = \frac{\delta f_i}{f_i} = \delta$$

When model (16) holds, an appropriate least-squares procedure for estimating ϕ is iteratively reweighted least squares (IRLS). In this procedure, the WLS method is used repetitively until no further change in the estimate of ϕ occurs. Before each iteration the weights are recomputed as $v(x_i, \phi)^{-1}$ using ϕ equal to the estimates from the just-completed iteration. IRLS works for the general case of model (16). When model (17) in particular holds, approximate procedures can be used. One can (a) use OLS to regress $\ln y$ on $\ln f(x_i, \phi)$, or (b) use WLS with $w_i = y_i^{-2}$. The latter, although popular in pharmacokinetics, is particularly treacherous and is not to be relied on.

General Heteroscedastic Case

This is the general case in which $v(x_i, \phi, \zeta)$ is chosen as some preferred functional form. Until the form is chosen, little more can be said. A particular functional form that generalizes the homoscedastic and constant-CV models is

$$v(x_i, \phi, \zeta) = f_i^\zeta \tag{18}$$

The model is illustrated in Fig. 4. It states that the variance of y_i is proportional to some power, ζ, of f_i. When $\zeta = 2$, model (18) is identical with model (17), and when $\zeta = 0$, it is identical with model (14). When $0 < \zeta < 2$, the model compromises between the homoscedastic and constant-CV models and thus offers greater flexibility than either. Model (18) was first suggested for use with nonlinear regression models by Box and Hill (2) and has been advocated and used for radioimmunoassay calibration (4,5) and analysis of chemical kinetic experiments (3). When the general heteroscedastic model holds, a maximum-likelihood-based least-squares procedure, extended least squares (ELS), can be

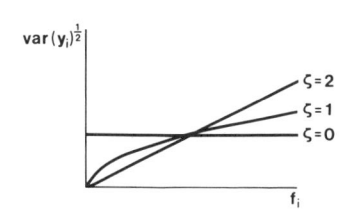

FIG. 4. A graph of the variance model, model (18), $Var(y_i) = \delta^2 f_i^\zeta$. The graph is of $Var(y)^{0.5}$ (the standard deviation of y) versus f, so that the units of both axes are the units of the independent variable, y, itself. Three functions are shown: $\zeta = 0$, $\zeta = 1$, and $\zeta = 2$. Note that when $\zeta = 0$, the model is identical with model (14), and when $\zeta = 2$, it is identical with model (17). (From Sheiner, ref. 6, with permission.)

applied (1). Other methods are also possible, but they do not have the generality of ELS.

Variance Model for an Individual's Parameters

Model (6) is essentially the simple homoscedastic case [model (14)] applied to the vector ϕ_j. The only difference is that here the homoscedastic model is multivariate, as ϕ is a vector, not a scalar, and covariances between elements of ϕ may be nonzero. For example, let the individual parameters for some drug's structural model be volume of distribution (V) and clearance (CL). If the drug is highly protein-bound and is cleared solely by renal filtration, then individuals with lesser protein binding than others will tend to have larger volumes of distribution and also larger clearances (all other things being equal). Hence, V_j and CL_j will correlate positively. If protein binding is unmeasured, unknown, and not modeled, this correlation will "show up" as correlation between the random aspects of CL and V, expressed as a positive off-diagonal term in Ω, the covariance matrix of ϕ_j. More generally, the matrix Ω expresses the covariance of ϕ_j, i.e., the variability of ϕ_j about its expected value, $g(x_j, \theta)$. Although the latter accounts for those interindividual differences due to known causes, residual interindividual variability in the kinetic parameters from unknown sources (protein binding in the foregoing example) is expected, and the diagonal elements of Ω express this.

Consider, as before, a single element of ϕ_j, ϕ_{jk}. If model (6), limited to this element, is taken as a model not of ϕ_{jk} but of $\ln \phi_{jk}$, then ϕ_{jk} is given by the exponential of the right-hand side of the expression. This model has several attractive features. First (if it applies separately to each element of ϕ_j), the elements of Ω become (nearly) dimensionless, expressing expected (squared) fractional deviations (i.e., squared CVs) rather than absolute ones. This can be seen by noting that for random variable δ, a (first-term) Taylor-series approximation to $\ln \delta$ is

$$\ln \delta \approx \ln E(\delta) + \frac{1}{E(\delta)} [\delta - E(\delta)]$$

from which

$$\mathrm{Var}(\ln \delta) \approx \left(\frac{1}{E(\delta)}\right)^2 \mathrm{Var}(\delta) = \mathrm{CV}(\delta)^2$$

Second, if a reasonably symmetrical distribution for η is assumed, then the distribution of η_j [the exponential of model (6)] is skewed to the right, and larger (absolute) deviations from the mean are expected for larger means. Both of these are commonly observed features of distributions of pharmacokinetic parameters. Lastly, most pharmacokinetic parameters must be strictly positive (e.g., clearance, volume of distribution), and the log-transform model accomplishes this: No matter what the (finite) value of expression (6), its exponential is strictly greater than zero.

CONCLUSIONS

Variability can be explained or simply measured. Explanation allows better predictions, within the limits quantified by the measurement of inexplicable variation. Predictions are useful in drug develpment, regulation, and therapy. It is important to know, for example, mean bioavailability, and when beginning therapy, it is useful to know that doses should be reduced if renal impairment is present.

Unexplained variability has received less attention; yet it is of equal interest. Large, unpredictable interindividual variation in drug clearance in some particular patient group, for example, might prompt a search for its cause. It would also be important to know about it for therapeutic reasons: If the variability is large relative to the therapeutic range, then the drug may be particularly unsafe to use in the particular population.

The relative magnitude of residual variations of observed drug levels about their expectations can give clues as to how a pharmacokinetic model may be in error, can be used to assess the relative merits of contending drug assays, and can fix a meaningful upper bound on requirements for tablet-to-tablet content uniformity, to cite some examples. Finally, all sources of random variability must be quantified in order to use observed drug levels for feedback dosage adjustment in an optimal fashion (7).

ACKNOWLEDGMENTS

This work was supported in part by NIH grants GM-26676 and GM-26691.

REFERENCES

1. Beal, S.L., and Sheiner, L.B. (1982): Estimating population kinetics. *CRC Crit. Rev. Bioeng.*, 8:195–222.
2. Box, G.E.P., and Hill, W.J. (1974): Correcting inhomogeneity of variance with power transformation weighting. *Technometrics*, 16:385–389.
3. Endrenyi, L. (1981): *Kinetic Data Analysis.* Plenum Press, New York.
4. Finney, D.J., and Phillips, P. (1977): The form and estimation of a variance function with particular reference to radioimmuno-assays. *Appl. Statist.*, 26:312–320.
5. Raab, G.M. (1981): Estimation of a variance function, with application to immunoassay. *Appl. Statist.*, 30:32–40.
6. Sheiner, L.B. (1984): Analysis of pharmacokinetic data using parametric models. 1. Regression models. *J. Pharmacokinet. Biopharm.*, 12:93–117.
7. Sheiner, L.B., and Beal, S.L. (1982): Bayesian individualization of pharmacokinetics: Simple implementation and comparison with non-Bayesian methods. *J. Pharm. Sci.*, 71:1344–1348.

DISCUSSION[2]

Discussant 1 (D1): I agree with you completely on the necessity of weighting the residuals and not naively using unweighted least squares. I think a point to be borne in mind, however, is that, especially when you have very great range in the weights you are using, you are inevitably estimating almost entirely from the precise observations. With little loss, you could throw away observations that had weight less than one-thousandth of the general run; you may then be putting undue faith in the mathematical formulation that you have adopted, because you will be omitting observations that relate to extreme conditions.

Speaker (S): In pharmacokinetics the squared residual associated with the imprecise observation is also 1,000 times bigger than the more precise one. For example, drug levels may vary, in an experiment, by three orders of magnitude. Because the weights associated with these are approximately proportional to the squared observations in the constant-coefficient-of-variation model, what this weighting accomplishes is to prevent loss of the information in the low-concentration data.

D1: I think there is still a problem if you have misspecified your expectation model, quite apart from the variance model.

S: I agree that weighting will not save you from the problems caused by an incorrect structural model.

---

[2] The points about population models raised in this chapter on the modeling of pharmacokinetic variability are discussed together with the following chapter on estimation of pharmacokinetic variability, and that discussion appears after the following chapter (J.-L. Steimer et al., *this volume*).

*Variability in Drug Therapy:
Description, Estimation, and Control,*
edited by M. Rowland et al.
Raven Press, New York © 1985.

Estimating Interindividual Pharmacokinetic Variability

[1] Jean-Louis Steimer, Alain Mallet, and France Mentré

INSERM U194, Department of Biomathematics, F-75634 Paris Cedex 13, France

Interindividual differences exist at all steps of interaction between the body and the drug. Investigating the overall ("mean") pharmacokinetic behavior of a given drug is the objective of most studies, but close attention should also be paid to between-subject variations in measured responses. Estimating interindividual pharmacokinetic variability involves extracting quantitative information about the pharmacokinetic similarities and differences between individuals from measurements of drug levels in biological fluids (often blood) of subjects or patients arising from some population of interest.

In general, the variability of a given parameter in a group of subjects can be described by statistical quantities such as mean, standard deviation, median, percentiles, etc. The calculation of these population characteristics as a summary of the data is the basic goal of applied statistics. Computer software, including up-to-date statistical data-analysis techniques, is available (35). However, despite the early work of Sheiner et al. (43) in 1972, statistical methods for estimating variability in kinetic processes from indirect and "noisy" observations (e.g., variability in pharmacokinetic parameters from plasma-level data) are not yet commonly available and applied; for a survey, see Beal and Sheiner (9).

This chapter will focus on estimation of interindividual variability, in the context of regression models relating pharmacokinetic parameters to a measured output (e.g., serum levels). The independent variables will generally reduce to the time-variate. Identification of variability sources through the detection of relationships between kinetic parameters and easily measurable subject characteristics like age, sex, weight, renal function, etc., is also of primary concern for drug therapy. The statistical aspects of that problem have been addressed in a systematic way in several articles (6,36); for an example, see chapter by D. J. Finney (*this volume*). Herein we shall present methods for

---

[1] On sabbatical leave: Biopharmaceutical Department, Sandoz Ltd., CH-4002 Basel, Switzerland.

estimating unexplained or, more precisely, not-yet-explained interindividual pharmacokinetic variability. The topic will be covered with the following objectives in mind:

1. To show the specificity of the estimation problem from the point of view of data analysis. In the first section a traditional statistical approach is presented and rebutted. In the second section a more appropriate approach relying on a pharmacostatistical model is recalled; for more details, see Sheiner (36) and the chapter entitled Modeling Pharmacokinetic/Pharmacodynamic Variability (L. B. Sheiner; *this volume*). In the third section we distinguish between experimental and routine pharmacokinetic data as requiring different approaches for data analysis.
2. To present various methods available for estimating pharmacokinetic variability. The methods described in the fourth section can be applied only when reasonably high numbers of data points are available for each individual, i.e., in experimental drug studies. Methods applicable to any type of kinetic data, experimental as well as routine, are presented in the fifth section. A novel maximum-likelihood approach for analysis of fragmentary kinetic data is described in the sixth section.
3. To discuss each estimation procedure in the course of its presentation and contrast the various approaches.
4. To illustrate the relevance of knowledge of pharmacokinetic variability for drug development and drug therapy.

IDEAL (UNREALISTIC) CASE: PRECISE KNOWLEDGE OF THE PARAMETERS IN A LARGE SAMPLE OF INDIVIDUALS

As a starting point, we are interested in the distribution[1] of one single parameter ϕ in a population. A sample[2] of N individuals has been drawn at random from the population. The parameter value for each individual is assumed to be known without error. The individual values $\phi_j, j = 1, \ldots, N$, build a sample of independent, identically distributed random variables. Or, otherwise stated, $\phi_1, \ldots, \phi_N$ is a random sample of size N from an unknown probability distribution F. For a large N, the histogram of individual values gives a picture of the parameter's underlying distribution (Fig. 1). Trying to summarize the variability in such data is a standard statistical problem. At a first step, graphic methods can be used to investigate whether or not the distribution can be considered as Gaussian. A probit plot (Fig. 1) should produce a straight line if the

---

[1] The term *distribution* is mainly used in the statistical sense (the distribution of a parameter in a population) throughout this chapter; incidentally it will have pharmacokinetic meaning (e.g., in "volume of distribution").

[2] The term *sample* will be used with two different meanings: a sample of individuals from a population; a blood sample in a drug study. The significance is generally clear from the context.

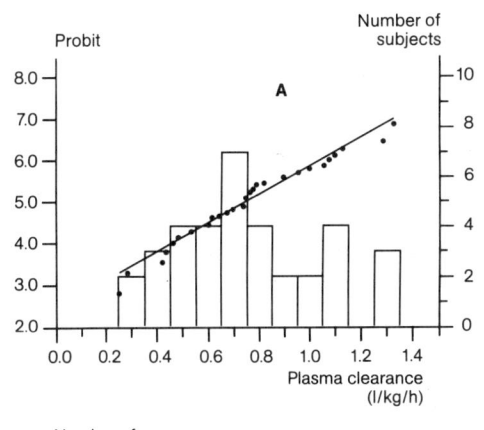

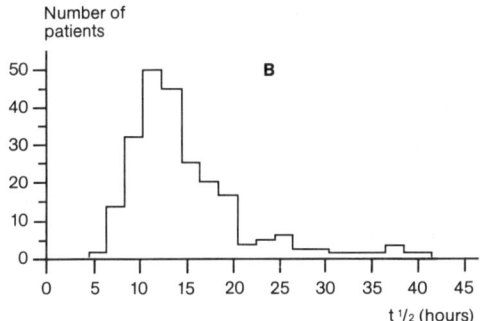

FIG. 1. Two examples of histograms showing the distribution of a pharmacokinetic parameter in a sample of individuals. The relative frequency, which is analogous to a probability, is the ratio of the number of individuals in a given class to the total number N of individuals in the sample. **A:** Plasma clearance of nortriptyline in 35 subjects. (From Alvan, ref. 1, with permission.) **B:** Apparent half-life of lithium, derived from data between 12 and 20 hr after last drug intake in 226 patients. (From Amdisen, ref. 2, with permission.) Part A includes a probit plot, a graphic technique for exploring whether or not the probability distribution of the parameter is reasonably Gaussian. In general, histograms of pharmacokinetic parameters incorporate variability from many other sources, because the parameters are not precisely measured but are estimated from concentration data. The picture they give of pharmacokinetic variability is distorted to an unknown extent.

data arise from a normal distribution. Graphic methods can be completed by statistical tests for skewness and/or kurtosis of the data that are available in most recent statistical software packages, e.g., SAS (35). Sometimes the attractive Gaussian distribution can be obtained after a transformation (e.g., logarithmic) of the original data. Once an assumption about the distribution has been postulated, appropriate "summary statistics" can be calculated from the sample as estimates of population characteristics, e.g., the expected value and the variance of the parameter in the population.

The classic maximum-likelihood estimates of mean ($\hat{\mu}$) and variance ($\hat{\Omega}$) for Gaussian data are the following:

$$\hat{\mu} = \frac{1}{N} \sum_{j=1}^{N} \phi_j \qquad (1a)$$

$$\hat{\Omega} = \frac{1}{N} \sum_{j=1}^{N} (\phi_j - \hat{\mu})^2 \qquad (1b)$$

The estimate of the standard deviation ($\hat{s}$) is easily derived as

$$\hat{s} = (\hat{\Omega})^{1/2} \qquad (1c)$$

It is well known that $N - 1$ should replace N in the denominator of the variance formula to render the estimate of that characteristic unbiased. If significant skewness is apparent in the data, equations (1a) and (1b) can be used after preliminary logarithmic transformation of the data. Accordingly,

$$\hat{\mu}_{\ln} = \frac{1}{N} \sum_{j=1}^{N} \ln \phi_j \qquad (2a)$$

$$\hat{\Omega}_{\ln} = \frac{1}{N} \sum_{j=1}^{N} (\ln \phi_j - \hat{\mu}_{\ln})^2 \qquad (2b)$$

In this case the most meaningful population characteristics are $\hat{\mu} = \exp(\hat{\mu}_{\ln})$, which is an estimate of the median value, and $(\hat{\Omega}_{\ln})^{1/2}$, which is an (approximate) coefficient of variation (9); see chapter entitled Modeling Pharmacokinetics/Pharmacodynamic Variability (L. B. Sheiner, *this volume*). From equation (2a) it can be seen that $\hat{\mu}$ is just the geometric mean of the parameters:

$$\hat{\mu} = \left(\prod_{j=1}^{N} \phi_j \right)^{1/N} \qquad (3)$$

This set of standard calculations of the first two moments of the distribution of a parameter from a sample of individual values is referred to in the literature on pharmacokinetic data analysis as the standard two-stage (STS) method (40,45). We shall comment on application of the STS method to real-world pharmacokinetic data later.

Investigation of a parameter's distribution through simple standard methods should be considered as valid only when individual values of the parameter of interest are known without error or, at least, with a high degree of precision. When the parameters are derived from kinetic-process investigations, especially from pharmacokinetic studies, these strong assumptions are generally unrealistic. Individual pharmacokinetic parameters are unknowns. They are not easily and precisely measurable quantities. The existence of significant deviations between the sample values and the true values will generally extend the range of the histogram and might frequently distort its shape. It therefore reflects pharmacokinetic variability, but also variability from many other sources. The presence of this additional "nuisance" variability renders the validity of the sample mean, the variance, and the percentiles derived from the histogram questionable. The straightforward statistical data-analysis scheme must be reconsidered, and new approaches must be developed, first for modeling variability in pharmacokinetic data, second for estimating it.

PHARMACOSTATISTICAL MODEL

In practice, pharmacokinetic parameters cannot be directly measured in an individual. The "measurement device" provides indirect data, namely levels of drug and/or metabolites in some easily accessible biological fluids, typically plasma or blood and/or urine, often as serial measures at different times after drug intake. Accordingly, some mathematical transformation of the original data (the drug levels) to the attributes we are interested in (the parameters) is necessary. The connection between the original data and the parameters is made through the pharmacokinetic model.

The usefulness of pharmacokinetic models assessed after ad hoc studies in animals and humans is widely recognized. A model not only is useful for a simplified though global description of drug pharmacokinetics but also is essential for forecasting purposes. Knowledge of the values of the pharmacokinetic parameters that enter the mathematical model is a prerequisite to study the sensitivity of drug therapy (or at least of drug concentrations) to input modifications (e.g., changes in dosage and/or route of administration in a given patient) and/or to alterations in pharmacokinetics (e.g., a disease-state-induced modification of a pharmacokinetic parameter).

Let y_{ij} be the ith measurement in subject j; let y_j be the n_j-vector of the total n_j measurements obtained for this subject. Let ϕ_j be the p-vector of the parameters.[3]

We assume the existence of a mathematical model relating the data to the parameters in the following way:

$$y_j = f_j(\phi_j) + \epsilon_j \qquad (4)$$

where f_j is the structural model, a vector-valued functional relationship allowing computation of data-analogue-predicted values for any given set of parameters (ϕ_j); in pharmacokinetic data analysis, f_j is generally a nonlinear function of the parameters; ϵ_j is the random residual-error n_j-vector (herein supposed additive) that accounts for the deviations between the model predictions and the actual observations. It is generally admitted that ϵ_j has mean zero and that its components ϵ_{ij} ($i = 1, \ldots, n_j$) are all independent. The variance of the error term may be known, postulated, or just incorporated in the full model through

---

[3] About linear algebra notations (vectors, matrices, transposition, inversion) that will be used throughout this chapter, readers are referred to the chapter entitled Modeling Pharmacokinetic/Pharmacodynamic Variability (L. B. Sheiner, *this* volume). Superscript t will be used to denote matrix transposition.

a variance model including additional unknown parameters [see the chapter entitled Modeling Pharmacokinetic/Pharmacodynamic Variability (L. B. Sheiner, *this volume*)].

As an example, consider a drug whose pharmacokinetics are described by a one-compartment open model. Successive serum levels of unchanged drug at times t_{ij} ($i = 1, \ldots, n_j$) after the start of drug administration are predicted according to the following equations. For subject j' (where an intravenous bolus dose D_j' was given),

$$y_{ij}' = \frac{D_j'}{V_j'} \exp(-\frac{\text{CL}_j'}{V_j'} t_{ij}') + \epsilon_{ij}' \quad \text{for } i = 1, \ldots, n_j' \tag{5}$$

For subject j'' (where an intravenous infusion at rate R_j'' was started and maintained),

$$y_{ij}'' = \frac{R_j''}{\text{CL}_j''} [1 - \exp(-\frac{\text{CL}_j''}{V_j''} t_{ij}'')] + \epsilon_{ij}'' \quad \text{for } i = 1, \ldots, n_j'' \tag{6}$$

Each equation is associated with an experimental design and is therefore specific to each individual. On the other hand, the underlying pharmacokinetic model, as a fundamental characteristic of the drug, is the same for both subjects. For a given drug, the pharmacokinetic parameters [in this case clearance (CL) and volume of distribution (V)] build a basic set of descriptive attributes. These parameters are independent of input (dosage regimen) and measurement (sampling design); they can be used to summarize any type of individual pharmacokinetic data.

The existence of interindividual variability can be taken into account as follows. The individual parameters ϕ_j, for $j = 1, \ldots, N$, are independent realizations from a p-valued random variable with unknown probability distribution F on some domain D of the real space IR^p. F is the p-dimensional joint distribution that characterizes the interindividual variations of pharmacokinetic parameters in the population by means of probabilities. For a given parameter value ϕ_0 and for a small vector-valued increment Δ [with $\Delta = (\Delta_1, \ldots, \Delta_p)'$], $F(\phi_0)|\Delta_1| \ldots |\Delta_p|$ is the probability that ϕ will lie in a domain centered at ϕ_0, with volume $|\Delta_1| \ldots |\Delta_p|$. As exemplified by Fig. 2 in a bivariate case (two parameters), a histogram of individual parameter values is basically a staircase approximation to the probability distribution of the random-variable "parameter" (in the example, a normal probability distribution).

To emphasize this statistical aspect, the pharmacokinetic model for an individual, equation (4), is expanded to a global pharmacostatistical model for the sample of subjects:

$$y_j = f_j(\phi_j) + \epsilon_j \quad \text{for } j = 1, \ldots, N \tag{7}$$

with ϕ_j random with probability distribution F.

The single equation (7) accounts for a very general model formulation. A detailed description of pharmacostatistical models involving various types of independent variables is available (6). For present purposes we shall consider

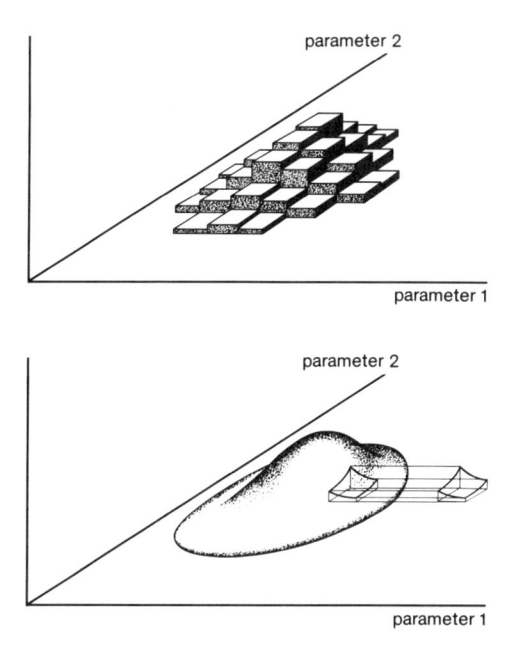

FIG. 2. The analogy between a (staircase) histogram of relative frequencies **(top)** and a probability density function **(bottom)** describing the continuous distribution of a two-dimensional random-parameter vector is shown by means of a theoretical example: a bivariate normal distribution. The relative frequency distribution is constant in each square. For comparison, the actual shape of the probability density in a square is shown in the lower panel. Note that for graphic purposes the distribution and the histogram have been truncated; only the domain within two standard deviations from the mean is displayed.

models with one unique independent variable. Because the processes we deal with are kinetic, the independent variable will be time, except in one particular example later in the chapter in which steady-state pharmacokinetic data (with concentration as the independent variable) will be used for illustrative purposes.

PHARMACOKINETIC DATA

The problem of describing and estimating interindividual pharmacokinetic variability can be more precisely stated with regard to the commonly available data from drug studies. In a broad sense, "population pharmacokinetic data" will be any data in which evident interindividual variability in drug kinetics is observable.[4]

---

[4] It is obvious that one cannot expect very accurate inferences from samples of 6, or even 12 or 24, individuals. We think, however, especially for drug development, that precise assessment of between-subject variability even in small "populations" can be useful.

At present, pharmacokinetic information comes from two major sources: experimental studies in animals and human subjects, on one hand, and routine monitoring of patients, on the other hand. A detailed contrasting argumentation about these two types of pharmacokinetic data-collection procedures has been given by Sheiner and Beal (39). The salient features that have direct relationships with data analysis are herein recalled. The usefulness of a third type of data, fictive pharmacokinetic data obtained through computer simulation, is also pointed out.

Pharmacokinetic Data from Experimental Studies

Experimental pharmacokinetic studies (EP studies) are mainly performed during drug development, often on normal volunteers, sometimes on patients with diseases likely to cause therapeutic problems (e.g., renal failure). Measurements in each individual include numerous blood samples and/or urine collections that are assayed for unchanged drug and/or metabolite(s). Short-term (often single) administration is the rule. The number of individuals in a study is generally small for practical, economic, and ethical reasons. Typical examples are given in Figs. 3 and 4 for a given drug (lithium) in two different studies.

Figure 3 shows the pharmacokinetics of the lithium ion in 3 volunteers after two oral ingestions of a lithium chloride solution. Data were obtained through frequent and extensive plasma sampling and urine collection over several days. These data were part of a study of 24 normal volunteers to whom other dosage forms were also administered (19). Figure 4 shows data obtained after oral administration of two types of tablets to 12 individuals (3). The well-known high degree of variability in drug absorption is well reflected in these data. Both sets of data document the typical (significant) between-subject variability that is observed in the serum levels of healthy volunteers in controlled experimental conditions.

EP studies provide valuable basic information about drug disposition (Fig. 3) and absorption (Fig. 4) kinetics. Elaboration and testing of pharmacokinetic assumptions about the behavior of the drug in the body and estimation of associated parameters are possible through fitting of a given model to the data for each individual. This procedure has become standard practice in pharmacokinetic data analysis; see Balant and Garrett (4) for a recent survey.

At a first glance, the information content of EP data regarding pharmacokinetic variability appears very limited. At least two major impediments to any variability assessment should be mentioned: (a) Clinical cases that will later be treated with the drug are generally not included. A sample composed of healthy volunteers is far from being representative of a patient target population. (b) The typical sample size for a given study is, from a statistical point of

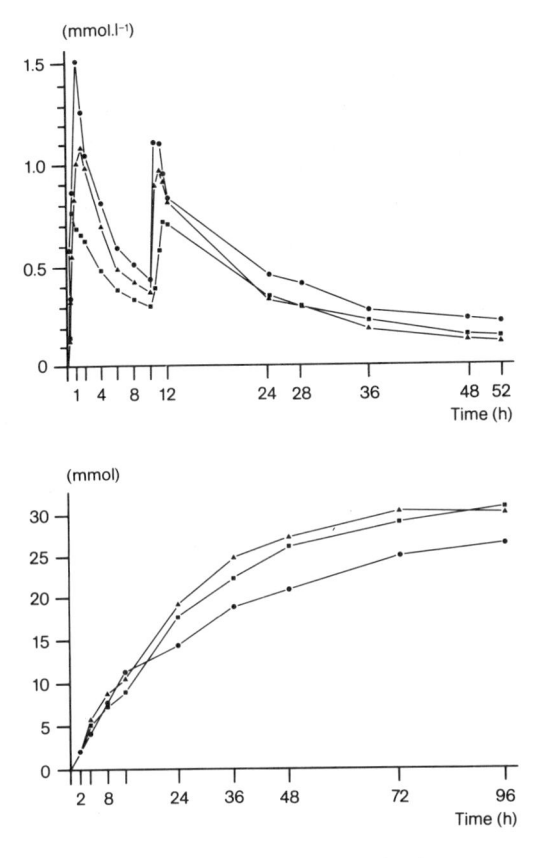

FIG. 3. Serum lithium levels **(top)** and accumulated urinary amounts **(bottom)** in 3 subjects after oral administration of a lithium chloride drinkable solution (24 mmol at time zero and 12 mmol 10 hr later). The resemblance in the shapes of the curves reflects the standardized design but also suggests that a unique pharmacokinetic model is valid for the 3 subjects. The differences between individuals in the achieved levels and in the rates of increase and decrease can be accounted for by differences in the parameter values of the common pharmacokinetic model.

view, small (always less than 30, often less than 15). However, the following should be kept in mind: (a) Kinetic differences may be striking even in normal healthy volunteers (Figs. 3 and 4), because individual variations in pharmacokinetics may result as well from biological or environmental differences as from clearly defined pathophysiological alterations. Even in a subpopulation of normal healthy volunteers, accurate description and estimation of variability may be of interest. (b) Whereas the number of subjects in a given study is small, the numbers of studies performed during the development and subsequent marketing of a compound are often tremendous. The total number of people who took the drug is actually large. The studies are, however, sequentially per-

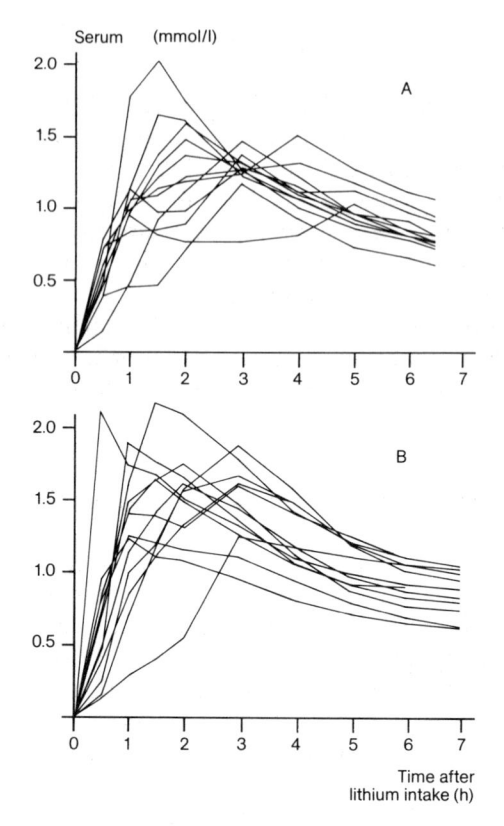

FIG. 4. Serum lithium curves over the first 6–7 hr after intake of ordinary tablets. **A:** Eleven volunteers given lithium at about 0.7 mmol/kg body weight as ordinary lithium carbonate tablets. **B:** Twelve volunteers given about 0.85 mmol/kg body weight as ordinary lithium citrate tablets. These concentration profiles document the typical (rather wide) interindividual pharmacokinetic variability observable even in healthy volunteers, especially in absorption. (From Amdisen, ref. 3, with permission.)

formed over years. In addition, some strategy is needed for combining results from several small-sample studies in a meaningful way. Suggestions for proper compilation of pharmacokinetic parameter estimates have been given (42).

Although sampling bias is likely, precise assessment of variability in pharmacokinetic data from normal volunteers might be useful in several ways: (a) Information about variability could be profitably taken into account in order to plan properly or avoid future experiments. (b) The variability in normal subjects is likely to be smaller than in patients with respect to a given parameter; the variance estimate derived from a study in normals can be reasonably expected to give some lower bound for the actual variance in the target patient population. (c) With growing experience, information about the likely sign, and possibly the amplitude, of the bias in the mean values between normals and patients may be available, allowing realistic extrapolations from one compound to another (e.g., that the average plasma clearance in patients is 50% less than in normals).

Furthermore, when a drug-related therapeutic problem is anticipated or detected, EP studies are the means of choice for a clear-cut answer to be obtained. Crossover designs can be used for bioavailability comparisons, for drug interaction studies, and, in general, for studying the influence of a factor under the investigator's control. Case–control protocols are necessary for most other studies, e.g., to compare young normals with elderly "normals" or to investigate a genetic influence on drug disposition.

All these data from EP studies contribute to document interindividual variations. Accordingly, methods for evaluation of pharmacokinetic variability from classic experimental data are of interest. They will be presented in a later section.

Pharmacokinetic Data from Population Studies

Although the concept of population pharmacokinetic studies (PP studies) has not yet gained wide influence, we shall use it in this chapter to describe, essentially, pharmacokinetic investigations in which the numbers of data per individual are limited (in general, much less than in EP studies; at the extreme, one observation). A PP study generally involves patients treated with the drug and relies on occasional drawing of blood, which is then assayed for active compound. Routine monitoring of patients on chronic dosing is one example of PP studies. Such pharmacokinetic data collection is generally performed after release of the drug on the market when the control of plasma levels through such follow-up appears to be (a) realistic as an intermediate therapeutic target because of knowledge of an optimal concentration range for the drug and (b) necessary because the small therapeutic index of the drug implies individual dosage adjustment.

The observational data gathered during PP studies exhibit specific drawbacks:

1. The time of blood sampling may occur randomly (for necessity or temporary convenience) with respect to the time of dosing. Also, the number of individual observations may be highly variable between subjects. Accordingly, interpretation of data from PP studies requires a kinetic model, just as do data from EP studies. "Simple" statistical techniques are not adapted.
2. Unbalanced data from PP studies contain less "pure" kinetic information than data from carefully designed EP studies. When the number of measurements in a given patient is less than the number of parameters, the model is actually unidentifiable. If a unique level has been measured in a patient, an infinite number of combinations of pharmacokinetic parameters will exactly predict this level; because many values are equally likely,

the parameters of the individual cannot be estimated from only that fragmentary information.
3. Because the data are routinely collected, the level of "noise" is likely to be higher than in carefully controlled studies, incorporating (a) all inaccuracy related to routine collection, manipulation, and assay of the samples at the hospital and the laboratory and that due to mistakes in the recording of the data and (b) patient noncompliance, leading to errors in the amount(s) of drug taken in previous administrations or errors in the timing of the blood sample relative to the previous dose(s).

For a statistical analysis of data from PP studies to be valid, it must cope with the previously mentioned specificities of these data. Despite the difficulties involved, these observational pharmacokinetic data are worth the effort, because they arise from patients receiving the drug for therapeutic purposes. It seems reasonable to admit that such a sample is representative, at least at the level of a hospital or some geographic region. If relevant *a priori* selection criteria are applied, and if the data are collected with reasonable accuracy, such a sample of patients may provide a fairly good picture of pharmacokinetic variability in the target population of people intended to receive the drug.

Bias problems related to the unbalanced design may exist (e.g., an excessively large proportion of blood samples arises from critically ill or noncompliant patients). In our opinion, this point is of minor concern.

In summary, for the question of pharmacokinetic-variability assessment to be adequately addressed, the following items are required: (a) a model for the pharmacokinetics of the drug; this information should be available from the controlled studies in volunteers in an early phase of drug development, (b) a statistical model for description of individual variations in pharmacokinetic parameters, and (c) an ad hoc method for estimation of the distribution of the parameters in the population.

The distinction betwen EP data and PP data is important, because the methods presently available differ depending on the nature of the data. Some methods are restricted to analysis of kinetic data from EP studies; on the other hand, methods dedicated to data analysis from PP studies have general applicability, as will be described later.

Pharmacokinetic Data from Computer Simulations

Because examples based on simulated pharmacokinetic data will be referenced throughout this chapter, the creation and manipulation of fictive data deserve a comment. With the increasing development and widespread diffusion of powerful machines, computer simulation has become one method of choice for investigation of issues in which "randomness" (variability) plays a dominant role. A so-called Monte Carlo simulation relies, in the case of pharmacokinetic data, on choices of (a) a pharmacokinetic model, (b) a population distribution of pharmacokinetic parameters, (c) an experimental design, and (d) a distribution of measurement errors. Appropriate choice of these items allows *in numero* creation of fictive data that can nicely mimic those collected in real *in vivo* studies. Computer-generated individuals are easily obtained as independent realizations from the theoretical population distribution, using computer random generators. For large numbers of fictive individuals, the histogram of the parameters will conform to the (assumed) population distribution. Exact pharmacokinetic data, e.g., plasma levels, are then calculated according to a predefined design. Eventually, random noise is added if the issue is to mimic actual data. A typical example of artificially created concentration data is shown in Fig. 5. The drug and the administration route are different from the experimental data shown previously (Figs. 3 and 4). However, the resemblance in the "variability patterns" of responses between simulated data and real data is remarkable. Figures 13 and 14 allow further comparison.

Computer simulations can be used to make pharmacokinetic predictions including variability. An example using clearance models is given in the chapter by M. Rowland (*this volume*). We shall comment later on these applications. Of primary importance for the estimation topic is the use of raw computing power for investigating the properties of statistical methods. The almost unlimited ability to create data allows us to perform and repeat quasi-costless pharmaco-

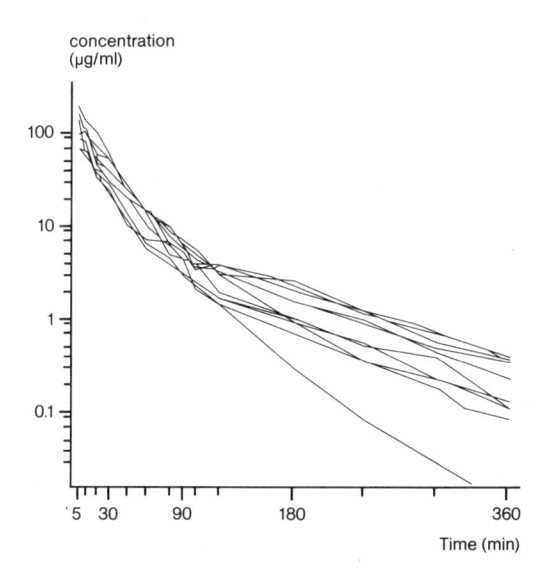

FIG. 5. A typical set of simulated data for chlorothiazide. Each line represents the data for a fictive "individual." The simulated noisy drug-level values are connected by straight lines. There is no peculiarity in the plot that would allow us to ascertain whether these are actual data after a 1-g bolus injection of the drug in 10 volunteers or fictive data calculated according to a two-exponential equation with pharmacokinetic parameters from 10 computer-generated individuals, with added measurement noise. (Adapted from Sheiner and Beal, ref. 38, with permission.)

kinetic pseudostudies. Furthermore, the parameters underlying the simulated data (among others, the characteristics that define the population distribution) are known. This allows evaluation of data-analysis techniques by means of statistical criteria (absence of bias, accuracy). A meaningful comparison of the performances of rival methods in (almost) real situations can thereby be warranted. Of course, for a very general result to be obtained, numerous and diverse simulation studies are required.

SPECIFIC METHODS FOR ANALYZING EXPERIMENTAL PHARMACOKINETIC DATA

Several methods are available for estimating population characteristics of pharmacokinetic parameters from EP data. A brief presentation of the classic and recent methods will help to illustrate the basic differences between the various approaches. Fitting a pharmacokinetic model to the data is generally the basic step. The methods and the statistical aspects of nonlinear parameter estimation are well documented, although the field of kinetic data analysis is still moving (15). The number of available computer packages is steadily increasing (4). The fitting criterion can be least squares, weighted least squares, extended least squares (30), or any other. Good computer programs provide as standard output the p-vector $\hat{\phi}$ of optimal parameter values and the (approximate) $p \times p$ variance-covariance matrix of the estimate M. This matrix depends both on the level of error in the data and on all aspects of the experimental design (input and measurement strategy). The standard error on each parameter can be computed as the square root of the corresponding diagonal element of matrix M. The precision of the estimate may vary widely across individuals even in a given study. For details, see the chapter by E. M. Landaw (*this volume*).

Naive-Averaging-of-Data Approach

It is common practice in pharmacokinetics to perform experiments in which the study design, with respect to drug input as well as to measurement schedule, is identical for all individuals. At each measurement time, as many data (e.g., serum levels) as there are individuals in the sample are available.

For analyzing such data, a widely used procedure, which we shall call here NAD for naive averaging of data, consists in the following:

1. Calculating the average value of the data for each observation time

$$\bar{y}_i = \frac{1}{N} \sum_{j=1}^{N} y_{ij} \tag{8}$$

for $i = 1, \ldots, n$, where n is the standard number of individual data. Averaging the data across individuals apparently makes sense, because all y_{ij} for $j = 1, \ldots, N$ have been measured under identical conditions.
2. Fitting a model $y^m = f(\phi)$ to the mean-data n-vector $\bar{y} = (\bar{y}_1, \ldots, \bar{y}_n)^t$ and estimating the best-fit parameter values ϕ^*. The notation ϕ^* is used to distinguish from individual estimates, denoted $\hat{\phi}$.

The NAD method is attractive and commonly used by kineticists. The main reason may be its simplicity: One unique fitting is sufficient to get estimates of parameters describing a mean response. The components of ϕ^* are then, quite often, interpreted as "mean" parameter values. Accordingly, $\hat{\mu}_{NAD}$ will be used for ϕ^* in the latter. Because standardized designs are commonplace in EP studies, as well for dose dependence, bioavailability, and bioequivalence assessment, the method is widely applicable in that context. Furthermore, mean data "look nicer" than individual data because of the smoothing effect of the averaging, and better fitting than with individual data often results.

The method, apparently, provides an estimate $\hat{\mu}_{NAD}$ of the sample mean. In this respect, several fundamental limitations of the NAD approach must be stressed:

1. With respect to modeling, the use of NAD to establish a kinetic model may be misleading. Averaging of the data can, quite often, produce a distorted picture of the response. The creation of false information, especially in small samples, was early suggested by Levy and Hollister with a simple example: Averaging of monoexponential data from 2 subjects with very different half-lives will produce a mean curve that exhibits an apparent biexponential decay (24). Most frequent is the opposite situation, in which the smoothing effect of the averaging will tend to obscure peculiarities that can be seen in individual data. A similar argument has recently been developed by Boxenbaum (11) for evaluation of sustained-release dosage forms. A phenomenon like the existence of secondary peaks in the plasma-level time course for all individuals may be undetectable in the average curve if the rebounds occur at different time points. A striking but not extreme example based on fictive data from 6 "individuals" is shown in Fig. 6. Note the relative smoothness of the mean profile (Fig. 6, lower panel) and the absence of any resemblance to the individual curves (Fig. 6, upper panel). The basic features of the individuals' profiles (time lags and secondary peaks) have been wiped out through the averaging. A simple one-compartment model fits the mean data reasonably as well with zero-order absorption as with delayed first-order absorption. None of the predicted curves bears any relationship to the individual data. Both models clearly result from "averaging artifact."
2. With respect to parameter estimation, NAD also performs poorly. After averaging, the reference to individual data has disappeared. All sources of

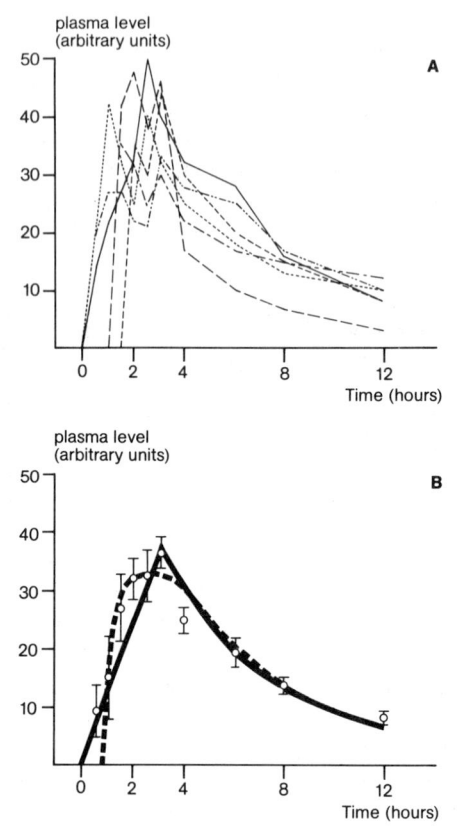

FIG. 6. NAD applied to fictive time–concentration data intended to mimic a set of data from a conventional pharmacokinetic study (oral intake, 6 individuals, 10 observations) with typical interindividual variability. **A:** Plasma-level data after single oral dose in the 6 "individuals." Note the systematic presence of a secondary peak in individual data 2.5–3.0 hr after drug intake. With respect to onset of absorption, two groups of 3 "individuals" each can be distinguished with respect to the presence/absence of a significant time delay (at least 1 hr). **B:** Fitting of mean data (represented as means ± SEM without connecting line) with a one-compartment model: (a) with first-order absorption (*broken line*) and (b) with zero-order absorption (*continuous line*). The mean profile obtained through averaging the data across subjects exhibits none of the striking analogies (secondary peaks) and differences (delayed absorption in three data sets) that exist in individual data. Both models fit the mean data "reasonably well." Neither model accounts for individual data.

random variation are confounded. The NAD estimate $\hat{\mu}_{NAD}$ should not, in general, be regarded as a valuable estimate of the expected value of kinetic parameters. This holds even if the true model, i.e., the one adequately describing individual data, has been used for the fitting. This lack of performance is mainly related to the essential parametric nonlinearity of pharmacokinetic models. Exceptions occur when the signal-to-noise ratio is small, i.e., when interindividual variability contributes less to the spread in the observations than other sources of random fluctuation (measurement error and random intraindividual variation). This unusual situation might be seen when concentrations are measured in standardized laboratory animals (small interindividual variation) or when drug effects are measured in humans (high level of additional variability). Then preliminary averaging of the data across individuals contributes to "remove" the noise. Averaging methods other than the straightforward arithmetic mean may improve the quality of the estimates to some extent (12). However, these ad hoc solutions do not fundamentally solve the problem. In addition, because NAD tends to mask variability rather than to shed light on it, no estimate of pure interindividual variability is obtained.

In conclusion, NAD cannot be recommended as a reliable method for kinetic data analysis, either for modeling or for parameter estimation.

Two-Stage Methods

The basic philosophy of the previous method is, first, to combine the data through averaging and, second, to perform one estimation step to get the parameter values. In the so-called two-stage methods, individual parameters estimated in the first stage are combined in the second. Individual estimates are obtained through separate fitting of each subject's data. The data are summarized in the set $[(\hat{\phi}_j, M_j), j = 1, \ldots, N]$; $\hat{\phi}_j$ is the p-vector of parameter estimates and M_j is the $p \times p$ symmetric variance-covariance matrix of the corresponding individual estimate. In a second stage the individual estimates are combined to derive values for population characteristics according to a given strategy. In this chapter we shall present only the salient features of the methods. More detailed presentations and comparisons are available (36,45).

Standard Two-Stage Method

The esoteric name standard two-stage (STS) method actually refers to a well-known and widely used procedure. Estimates of the population characteristics for each parameter are computed as the empirical mean (either arithmetic or geometric) and variance of the individual estimates $\hat{\phi}_j$ according to equation (1) or (2), or, more generally, to their multivariate analogues. Estimates for the mean vector μ and the $p \times p$ symmetric variance-covariance matrix describing the population distribution are computed as

$$\hat{\mu}_{STS} = \frac{1}{N} \sum_{j=1}^{N} \hat{\phi}_j \tag{9a}$$

$$\hat{\Omega}_{STS} = \frac{1}{N} \sum_{j=1}^{N} (\hat{\phi}_j - \hat{\mu}_{STS})(\hat{\phi}_j - \hat{\mu}_{STS})^t \tag{9b}$$

Algebraically, the analogy of equation (9) with equation (1) is straightforward. As in the monovariate case, $N - p$ can be used instead of N in the denominator of the variance estimate $\hat{\Omega}_{STS}$. However, there is a major difference between equations (9) and (1) that ought to be stressed. Equation (1) assumed the true values ϕ_j to be available. In equation (9) the (computed) estimated value $\hat{\phi}_j$ for each individual is used instead of the (unknown) true value. The consequences of this difference will be discussed later.

Global Two-Stage Method

In fact, the $\hat{\phi}_j$ can be viewed as observations of the individual parameters. The estimate for a subject may deviate widely from the true value, especially in case of poor experimental design or a high level of measurement error. The matrices $\{M_j, j = 1, \ldots, N\}$, which reflect these deviations, are used extensively in the global two-stage (GTS) method, together with the estimates $\{\hat{\phi}_j, j = 1, \ldots, N\}$. Under general assumptions, the expectation $E(\cdot)$ and the variance-covariance $\text{Var}(\cdot)$ of each (random) $\hat{\phi}_j$ can be computed as

$$E(\hat{\phi}_j) = \mu \quad \text{for } j = 1, \ldots, N \tag{10a}$$

$$\text{Var}(\hat{\phi}_j) = M_j + \Omega \quad \text{for } j = 1, \ldots, N \tag{10b}$$

where μ is the true population expectation and Ω the true population variance-covariance.

The previous equations show in which way the expected value and the variance of each $\hat{\phi}_j$ (i.e., the first two moments of the observations) depend on the population characteristics μ and Ω. In such a case, the extended least-squares method (5,6) can be used to estimate the unknowns μ and Ω. The population parameters θ are the p components of the vector μ and the $p(p + 1)/2$ independent components of the symmetric matrix Ω. The objective function to be minimized is the following:

$$O_{GTS}(\mu, \Omega) = \sum_{j=1}^{N} [(\hat{\phi}_j - \mu)^t (M_j + \Omega)^{-1} (\hat{\phi}_j - \mu) + \ln \det(M_j + \Omega)] \tag{11}$$

Extended least squares is equivalent to maximum likelihood in a "Gaussian world." The first term in O_{GTS} is the summation (over individuals) of weighted squared deviations of individual estimates from the expected value μ. The weighting matrix depends on the "quality" of the estimate through the factor $(M_j + \Omega)^{-1}$. The latter term is the logarithm of the determinant of the $(M_j + \Omega)$ matrix. It prevents the variance-covariance matrix (through its determinant) from going to infinity.

Minimization of O_{GTS} can be performed through an ad hoc simple recursive algorithm suggested by Prevost (31) and described elsewhere (45). A computationally "heavier" two-stage method that relies on repeated fittings of individual data [the iterated two-stage method (ITS)] has also been described (31,45).

Comments Regarding the Two-Stage Methods

Two-stage methods derive estimates of the first two moments of the population distribution from parameter values of individual subjects. The STS approach combines estimates of individual parameters as if the set of estimates were a true N-sample from a multivariate distribution. Rodda recommends it as a very simple and valuable approach for pooling individual estimates of pharmacokinetic parameters derived from EP studies (33). The simplicity of the calculation involved in STS should be stressed. On the other hand, the general validity of STS results should not be overemphasized.

Evidence for the behavior of STS in real practice has been provided by numerous computer simulation studies reported in the pharmacokinetics literature (37,38,40,45). In most cases the STS estimate of the expected value is acceptable, i.e., not significantly inferior to the estimate provided by other more complex methods. No systematic deviation of the estimate from the true mean value was detected. On the other hand, with respect to the estimate of dispersion (the variance-covariance matrix), simulation investigations confirmed the predictions from statistical theory. STS provides upward biased estimates of the variances (38,45). The bias is generally relevant, except when individual values are precisely estimated. Lack of bias in variance estimates can be achieved only through very well designed and performed EP studies. The typical performance of STS is shown graphically in Fig. 7, where results from repeated analyses of simulated data are summarized. The existence of the bias in the variance estimate should at least be kept in mind when STS estimates of population characteristics are used for comparative or predictive inference purposes.

The refinement of the GTS approach over STS is that the individual covariances M_j are taken into account at the second stage. It is well known from nonlinear estimation theory that these (asymptotic) covariance matrices are approximate. Various aspects of the problem for pharmacokinetic data analysis have been recently documented by Metzler (29) by means of Monte Carlo simulations. GTS will probably fail in situations in which the picture that the matrices M_j give of the imprecisions of the estimates is misleading. The Michaelis-Menten model furnishes a well-documented example (47). The experience with GTS is presently limited, though promising (45). In addition, Prevost's problem-tailored algorithm relies on simple algebraic calculations. It is therefore easy to program and to implement even on microcomputers.

Analysis of simulated data from a one-compartment model after bolus intravenous injection, with individual parameters arising from a Gaussian distribution, showed the GTS estimate of the population variance-covariance matrix to

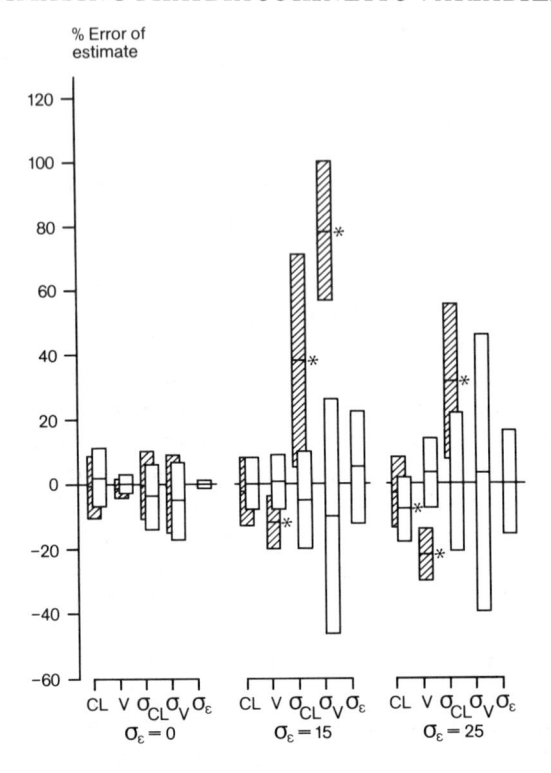

FIG. 7. Bias and precision of population-parameter estimates by the standard two-stage (STS) method (*shaded bars*) and the nonlinear mixed-effect model (NONMEM) (*open bars*). Routine pharmacokinetic data were simulated according to a simple monoexponential model with repetitive bolus dosing. One sample is composed of 50 individuals, with two serum levels measured in each. A Monte Carlo simulation involving 30 replications of each data set was performed. The ordinate is in units of percentage error (%E) defined as (estimate/true value − 1) × 100. The average %E over the 30 replications measures the bias in the estimator. It is indicated by the horizontal line in the middle of the bar corresponding to the parameter and the method. Significant ($p > 0.05$) biases are indicated by *asterisks* in the bars. The full height of each bar is two standard deviations of the %E. This measures the precision of the estimator. Each panel shows the results for each population parameter for both methods. The distribution is assumed log-normal. The parameters are as follows: CL, clearance; V, volume of distribution; σ_{CL}, interindividual (approximate) coefficient of variation of CL; σ_V, interindividual (approximate) coefficient of variation of V; σ_ϵ, approximate coefficient of variation of residual error. The three panels represent simulations with increasing residual-error magnitudes $\sigma_\epsilon = 0\%$, 15%, and 25%. (From Sheiner and Beal, ref. 40, with permission.)

be significantly better than its STS analogue (45). On the other hand, no improvement over the GTS estimates was achieved by the computationally more demanding ITS method. This may be due to the excellent performance of GTS on this particular data set.

To definitely assess the superiority of GTS over STS and to reach a conclusion regarding the usefulness of the complex ITS approach with respect to the two simpler two-stage methods, additional work will be required, especially further simulation studies on data with other types of kinetic models, drug inputs, and experimental designs.

GENERAL METHODS FOR ESTIMATION OF PHARMACOKINETIC POPULATION CHARACTERISTICS

For pharmacokinetic data gathered in situations other than experimental drug studies, the number p of parameters in the kinetic model might be larger than the number of data n_j from a given individual. This might even be the rule for routinely collected patient data. The model is unidentifiable. No meaningful estimates of individual parameters can be obtained using conventional fitting procedures. Note in passing that one usefulness of population-characteristics estimates is that once interindividual pharmacokinetic variability has been quantified, the situation is different. Taking this knowledge into account, empirical Bayes estimates of individual parameters can be computed from as few as one serum level for a subject. This technique is known as "Bayesian feedback" in the pharmacokinetics literature (41,46); see the chapters by D. Katz, and S. Vožeh et al. (*this volume*).

Two-stage methods cannot deal adequately with fragmentary individual data. The methods to be presented next rely on a population approach to the problem. The population characteristics are estimated directly using the original data from all subjects, without an attempt to calculate individual parameter values. These methods directly address the population-kinetics issue.

Naive-Pooled-Data Method

Naive pooled data (NPD) is a term proposed by Sheiner and Beal (37) for the procedure in which all data from all individuals are considered as arising from one unique experimental unit. This reference individual is characterized by a set of parameters $\tilde{\phi}$. For example, in the case of a least-squares fitting, $\tilde{\phi}$ will be the parameter vector minimizing the global objective function

$$O_{\text{NPD}}(\phi) = \sum_{j=1}^{N} \left\{ \sum_{i=1}^{n_j} [y_{ij} - f_{ij}(\phi)]^2 \right\} \quad (12)$$

where $\{f_{ij}, i = 1, \ldots, n_j\}$ is the set of components of f_j; the summation is over all individuals and all measurements for a given individual.

The NPD approach is far more general than NAD. It can deal easily with nonstandard data and as well with experimental as with routine pharmacokinetic data. Estimates are available after a unique fitting (of all data at once). NPD may perform well when variations between subjects are small. This might occasionally be the case in a group of very homogeneous laboratory animals from a given strain, but it is rarely true for humans. However, NPD's basic faults are the same as those of NDA, as has been repeatedly pointed out (37,38,40). In a different way, but with similar (negative) consequences as NAD, the NPD method tends to "forget" the individual differences in the data and to confound diverse sources of randomness. Although the consequences of that omission can be minor (16), the NPD estimate for the reference individual $\tilde{\phi}$ should be considered as a rough approximation ($\hat{\mu}_{NPD}$) of the population expectation μ. Furthermore, no estimate for the dispersion of the parameters in the population is provided. Therefore, caution is necessary when one extrapolates mean outcomes on the basis of the set of estimates $\hat{\mu}_{NPD}$. An example showing the significant bias between the NPD predicted mean curve (solid line) and the true underlying mean curve (dotted line) is shown in Fig. 8.

Nonlinear Mixed-Effect Model

The nonlinear mixed-effect model (NLME) was the first attempt to estimate interindividual pharmacokinetic variability without neglecting any of the difficulties associated with data from patients undergoing therapy (43): fragmentary individual measurements, absence of a schedule for drawing of blood samples, subject-specific dosing history, and so forth. The vector θ of popula-

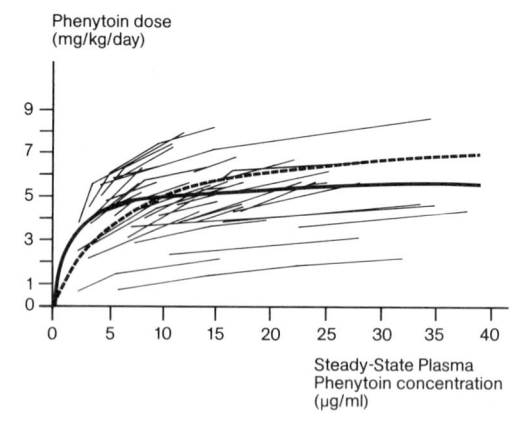

FIG. 8. An example of the respective estimates of a mean relationship by the NPD approach (*solid curve*) and by NONMEM (*broken curve*). The data are phenytoin daily doses R_{ij} and steady-state concentrations C_{ij}. Line segments connect data points ($n_j = 2$ to 4) for individual patients ($N = 49$). Using the dose per day R as the dependent variable leads to the classic Michaelis-Menten formulation for the model $R_{ij} = (V_m C_{ij})/(K_m + C_{ij})$ with pharmacokinetic parameters $\phi = (V_m, K_m)^t$. Note that the population-estimation problem is typical, although the independent variable is not time. Major discrepancies between the NPD-predicted and the NONMEM-predicted curves are apparent. This results from the differences in the estimates of the population means for NPD and NONMEM: 5.55 vs. 7.22 for V_m (mg/kg/day) and 1.57 vs. 4.44 for K_m (μg/ml), respectively. Computer simulations with the Michaelis-Menten model confirmed that the NONMEM-predicted mean relationship did not significantly differ from the true population mean curve. (Adapted from Sheiner and Beal, ref. 37, with permission.)

tion characteristics is composed of all quantities defining the first two moments of the distribution of the parameters: the mean values, or fixed effects, and the elements of the variance-covariance matrix that characterize random effects. The NLME approach has been described in numerous sources (6,36–38,40,41, 43). A brief presentation follows.

Extended Least Squares

As previously mentioned, the information content of individual data may not be sufficient to allow derivation of parameter estimates $\hat{\phi}_j$. Adopting the population point of view, one might attempt the following:

1. Calculate the first two moments of the raw observations, $E(y_j)$ and $\text{Var}(y_j)$, as functions of the population characteristics μ and Ω, in a way similar to the procedure used for the GTS approach for the individual parameters.
2. Optimize the following extended least-squares (ELS) criterion built from the observations, with respect to the parameters μ and Ω:

$$O_{\text{ELS}}(\mu, \Omega) = \sum_{j=1}^{N} [(y_j - \psi_j)' v_j^{-1}(y_j - \psi_j) + \ln \det v_j] \quad (13)$$

where $\psi_j = E(y_j)$ and $v_j = \text{Var}(y_j)$. The objective function depends on μ and Ω through the n_j-vector ψ_j and the $n_j \times n_j$ matrix v_j, which are (complex) functions of the population characteristics, as will soon become clear. The parameters to be estimated through minimization of O_{ELS} are the population characteristics μ and Ω, just as with the objective function of the GTS method [equation (11)]. In ELS, however, the data themselves (the y_j) are used. This is in contrast to GTS, in which ELS is applied to pseudoobservations, the individual estimates of pharmacokinetic parameters $\hat{\phi}_j$ that result from a previous calculation step.

Knowledge of (or, more precisely, "the ability to calculate") the first two moments ψ_j and v_j of each individual data set y_j as a function of the population characteristics is a necessary condition for the ELS approach to be applicable. According to the model, equation (7), the expected value of the jth observation vector is

$$\psi_j = E[f_j(\phi) + \epsilon_j] \quad (14)$$

where the expected value has to be taken with respect to both random variables ϕ and ϵ_j. Because of the nonlinear dependence of the observations on the parameters through the vector-valued function f_j, a closed-form solution for ψ_j and v_j involving μ and Ω can be obtained only for specific kinetic models. An example is provided by exponential models (6).

A general (approximate) solution is provided by first-order method. Note that the presentation that follows differs slightly from that given by the promoters of the method in several sources (37,41,43).

Consider the model for a given observation in a given individual y_{ij}:

$$y_{ij} = f_{ij}(\mu + \eta_j) + \epsilon_{ij} \quad \text{for } i = 1, \ldots, n_j, j = 1, \ldots, N \tag{15}$$

where $\mu + \eta_j = \phi_j$. The population mean (μ) is the fixed effect; η_j is the (random) individual shift (from the mean) for individual j. By definition, the random effects η_j have a zero mean and variance-covariance Ω. ϵ_{ij} is the additive error. To derive the moments of y_{ij}, Sheiner et al. (43) suggested linearizing the model using a first-order Taylor-series expansion in the random effect η_j, evaluated at the expected value (i.e., zero). Accordingly,

$$y_{ij} = f_{ij}(\mu) + \frac{\partial f'_{ij}(\mu)}{\partial \eta_j}(\eta_j = 0) \cdot \eta_j + \xi_{ij} + \epsilon_{ij} \tag{16}$$

$[\partial f'_{ij}(\mu)/\partial \eta_j](\eta_j = 0)$, which is subsequently denoted G_{ij}, is the p-vector of partial derivatives of the model equation for the ith measurement in the jth subject with respect to the elements of η_j, evaluated for $\eta_j = 0$. Clearly, each G_{ij} is a function of the fixed effect μ.

ξ_{ij} accounts for the approximation error between the true value and the forecast of the linearized version of the model.

In vector notation, for subject j, equation (16) translates into

$$y_j = f_j(\mu) + G_j(\mu) \cdot \eta_j + \xi_j + \epsilon_j \tag{17}$$

where $G_j(\mu)$ is the $n_j \times p$ Jacobian matrix whose ith line contains the same elements as the p-vector G_{ij}, and ξ_j is the n_j-vector of the approximation errors.

Computation of the expected value ψ_j for the profile of the jth subject is straightforward:

$$\psi_j = E(y_j) = f_j(\mu) + G_j(\mu) \cdot E(\eta_j) + E(\xi_j) + E(\epsilon_j) \tag{18}$$

Because $E(\eta_j) = 0$ by definition, and $E(\epsilon_j) = 0$ as a reasonable assumption, one obtains

$$\psi_j = f_j(\mu) + E(\xi_j) \tag{19}$$

According to the previous equation, provided the approximation error has a zero mean [$E(\xi_j) = 0$], the expected value for the profile of subject j is the profile calculated according to the same design equation f_j for the population mean μ. The approximation $\psi_j \simeq f_j(\mu)$ corresponds to the assumption that

$$E[f_j(\phi_j) + \epsilon_j] \simeq f_j[E(\phi_j)] \tag{20}$$

The variance-covariance matrix of y_j can be derived in a similar way. Just remember that the variance of a linear combination of random variables [so is the term $G_j(\mu) \cdot \eta_j$] is a linear combination of the variances and covariances of its constituent variables. For any j, $\text{Var}(\eta_j) = \Omega$ (the population $p \times p$ variance-covariance matrix), and η_j and ϵ_j are assumed independent. If all terms including the approximation error ξ_j vanish in the variance calculations, the variance-covariance matrix v_j of y_j is given by

$$v_j = \text{Var}(y_j) = G_j(\mu) \cdot \Omega \cdot G_j(\mu)^t + \text{Var}(\epsilon_j) \tag{21}$$

Any assumption about the variance of the residual error ϵ_j can be simply incorporated. The constant error variance model would be written as $\text{Var}(\epsilon_j) = \sigma_\epsilon^2 \cdot I(n_j)$, where $I(n_j)$ is the $n_j \times n_j$ identity matrix.

One should recognize in equation (21) that the covariances of the serial observations in an individual (the off-diagonal elements of the matrix v_j) are nonzero. As well as the variances at a given time point, the covariances of the observations are a function of interindividual variability (as summarized in Ω) and of subject-specific design [as approximately expressed in $G_j(\mu)$]. This is the way in which the NLME method combined with the first-order approximation keeps track of the individual information in its attempt to estimate population characteristics. The crucial improvement in this method over NPD resides in these covariances, because with respect to the average response, the model is the same for both methods (the expected value of the response across individuals is approximated by the response calculated for the "average" individual). The moments μ and Ω of the distribution are estimated through extended least squares [equation (13)] after replacement of ψ_j and v_j by their expressions (19) and (21).

Comments

The nonlinear mixed-effect model with first-order approximation (henceforth called NONMEM) is presently the best-documented method for population-kinetics data analysis. It is available from its authors as computer software (7,8). The initial IBM-specific program has recently been supplemented by a portable FORTRAN 77 version (10). NONMEM relies on the assumption that the contribution of second- and higher-order terms in the expectation and variance calculations is negligible. From a theoretical point of view, this assumption could appear as too strong at a first glance. To assess how NONMEM performs in practice, the results from computer simulation studies, especially those aiming to investigate the influence of the approximation, are helpful. Lindstrom and Birkes (26) analyzed extensive computer-generated data that had been simulated according to a destructive sampling design (one unique data point per individual) for a one-compartment model. Those authors concluded that an approximation higher than the first order to the mean response function seemed to be "asking too much." The algebraic manipulations for writing the second-order approximate model are cumbersome. The computing time for data analysis is significantly increased. A similar exponential example was studied by Beal, who also concluded that no significant improvement over the first-order method was obtained with higher-order approximations (6). Numerous simulation studies have confirmed that NONMEM provides reasonable estimates for the first two moments of the population distribution of pharmacokinetic parameters. The investigated examples have included different pharmacokinetic models [one-compartment (40), two-compartment (38), Michaelis-Menten (37)], various types of drug input [single-intake (38) and chronic dosing (37,40)], and several experimental designs, with respect to number of patients and sampling schedule, in one study (40). A graphic illustration of NONMEM's accuracy and precision in estimating pharmacokinetic population characteristics is given in Fig. 7. The picture is typical of the good estimation properties reported to date. Figure 8 shows the mean relationship between dosage and steady-state phenytoin concentrations derived by NONMEM from routinely collected serum levels in patients. Simulation studies performed after real data analysis showed that the NONMEM-predicted curve was superimposed with the true mean curve (37). In another simulation study, a high population correlation was assumed between the two parameters clearance and volume of distribution in a one-compartment model (45). The study design was of the EP type, with single intravenous bolus input and 10 blood samples in each of 10 individuals. In this example, a significant bias was observed in the NONMEM estimates of random effects. Whether this problem was specific to the example or might be general has not yet been determined.

To be applicable for data analysis, the extended least-squares method requires only the first two moments of the distribution of each observation. This requirement is not so easy to fulfill. In practice, no model for the mean and the covariance of the data can be stated *a priori* as a function of the population characteristics. The associated formulations need to be derived in several steps [equations (16)–(21)] from the initial "full" pharmacostatistical model [equation (15)]. In fact, the calculation not only involves a linearization procedure (which we discussed earlier) but also requires assumptions about the distributions of the parameters in the population (or, equivalently, the distribution of the random effects, the η_j's) and of the residual errors, the ϵ_j's. If the distribution of the pharmacokinetic parameters is assumed log-normal instead of symmetric, the model for interindividual variability of a given parameter, or, equivalently, the structural model for the population [see the chapter entitled Modeling Pharmacokinetic/Pharmacodynamic Variability (L. B. Sheiner, *this volume*)], might rather be

$$\ln(\phi_j^l) = \ln(\mu^l) + \eta_j^l \quad \text{for } j = 1, \ldots, N \text{ and } l = 1, \ldots, p \quad (22)$$

where ϕ_j^l, μ_j^l, and η_j^l are the *l*th components of ϕ_j, μ_j, and η_j, respectively.

In case of multiplicative noise, the dependence of a given observation on the parameters is modeled as

$$\ln(y_{ij}) = \ln[f_{ij}(\phi_j)] + \varepsilon_{ij} \quad (23)$$

The choice between additivity and log-additivity influences all subsequent calculations. Therefore, although the approach of estimating just the first two moments of the distribution may appear very general, NONMEM estimates should not be regarded as distribution-independent. Precise assumptions about the underlying distributions are required. As a matter of fact, all reported NONMEM analyses on simulated data as well as on real data have relied on classic assumptions of normality or log-normality for the population distribution of pharmacokinetic parameters.

Because of the analogy between the extended least-squares objective functions used in NONMEM and GTS, the possibility for NONMEM users to take advantage of this package to obtain two-stage estimates with the GTS approach may exist (L. B. Sheiner, *personal communication*). For a GTS analysis, the input data would be the parameter vectors $\hat{\phi}_j$ and the covariance matrices M_j. The model would be the identity model, because we use the estimates $\hat{\phi}_j$ as observations of the true parameters ϕ_j. The model is the simplest one possible, but the structure of the data is multivariate and very different from the standard situation. It is therefore likely that this "deviant" application of NONMEM may require expertise or at least a high level of skill in use of the software. The possibility to perform constrained optimization (with lower and/or upper bounds on the population characteristics) might also be useful. Prevost's simple algorithm for GTS estimation does not allow incorporation of constraints in its present form.

Despite the good performance of NONMEM in simulation studies, the software is, apparently, not yet widely used for kinetic data analysis. The (past) IBM specificity, the lack of "user-friendliness," and the computational burden with respect to time and therefore cost are software-specific reasons (16). Other general reasons may be the lack of appropriate population-kinetics data because of data-collection problems and the high level of combined "statistical-kinetic-computing" expertise required of the user. Good data and user expertise will still be required in the future for estimation of pharmacokinetic variability, regardless of the method or the software.

NEW APPROACH TO POPULATION-KINETICS ESTIMATION: NONPARAMETRIC MAXIMUM LIKELIHOOD

The nonparametric maximum-likelihood (NPML) approach for estimation of the distribution of kinetic parameters in a population has been proposed recently (27). The method will be briefly described, together with preliminary results from a simulated example. Details about the statistical background of NPML can be found elsewhere (27,28).

Maximum-Likelihood Estimation of the Parameter Distribution

The basic conceptual framework, the pharmacostatistical model, remains the same as before [equation (7)]. However, the estimation step will be completely different.

Let us first restate the population-kinetics estimation problem in general terms. Individual parameters ϕ_j, $j = 1, \ldots, N$, are assumed to be independent realizations of a given random variable Φ, whose probability distribution $F(\phi)$ is defined on a domain D of the real space IR^p. Let y be the n_{tot}-vector grouping all observations y_j from all individuals ($j = 1, \ldots, N$), with $n_{tot} = \sum_{j=1}^{N} n_j$. The likelihood of the whole set of observations, y, can be written in concise form as the joint distribution of the data. With the usual assumption of independence, the likelihood of the data $L(y)$ is just the product of individual contributions, according to

$$L(y) = \prod_{j=1}^{N} F_{Y_j}(y_j) \qquad (24)$$

where F_{Y_j} is the probability distribution of the n_j-vector of observations for subject j.

The observations depend on two random variables: the parameters, which are random to express kinetic variability, and the noise, which incorporates all the other sources of random fluctuations in the data. The likelihood can be expressed using the population distribution F and the distribution of the observations conditional to Φ, $F_{Y_j/\Phi}$, in the following way:

$$L(y) = \prod_{j=1}^{N} \int_D F_{Y_j/\Phi}(y_j; \phi) \cdot F(\phi) \, d\phi \qquad (25)$$

where D is the domain of definition of the parameter Φ (*vide supra*), and $F_{Y_j/\Phi}(y_j; \phi)$ recalls that this probability should be computed for the actual observation (y_j) and for any ϕ.

In equation (25), $F_{Y_j/\Phi}$ is "known" or, at least, can be calculated after appropriate assumptions have been stated. Denoting the probability density function of the noise ϵ_j by F_{ϵ_j}, and assuming a pharmacostatistical model, as in equation (7) (with additive error), $F_{Y_j/\Phi}(y_j; \phi)$ simply appears as $F_{\epsilon_j}[y_j - f_j(\phi)]$. This is the way in which the pharmacokinetic model (f_j) and the measurement noise (via F_{ϵ_j}) "enter" the likelihood. Furthermore, equation (25) expresses the dependence of the sample data on the unknown distribution F. Note that the dependence of the likelihood on the population distribution is complex, because L appears as a product of integrals involving F.

In his approach to population-kinetics estimation through maximum likelihood, Mallet (27,28) stated two assumptions:

1. A restrictive assumption about the noise statistics; namely, that the distribution of the error terms ϵ_j, $j = 1, \ldots, N$, is known.
2. Soft assumptions about the population distribution F; namely, that F takes only positive values and that its integral over the D domain is equal to unity. These are the weakest possible assumptions in order to warrant that F is a probability distribution. This level of generality justifies calling the approach nonparametric.

Mallet proved that the maximum-likelihood solution is a discrete distribution (27). Otherwise stated, the function F is zero almost everywhere. F is nonzero in N' parameter values, with N' less than or equal to N, the number of individuals in the sample. According to this specification of the solution, the NPML distribution estimate is searched in the class of discrete measures in the space IR^p. In the NPML approach, the primary "parameters" of the distribution, i.e., the population characteristics θ, are the number N', a set of p-vectors $(q_l; l = 1, \ldots, N)$ defining the locations, and a set of corresponding scalar "masses" $[\alpha_l; l = 1, \ldots, N]$. Some masses will be zero if $N' < N$, and the number of locations will accordingly be reduced. Subscript l is used instead of j because there is no direct connection between a given location and a given individual, although the numbers of locations and individuals might be identical. The likelihood is a function $L(y; q, \alpha)$ of the pN-vector q (grouping all locations) and of the N-vector α (the masses). After substitution of q and α in equation (25), the following log-likelihood is obtained:

$$\ln L(y; q, \alpha) = \sum_{j=1}^{N} \sum_{l=1}^{N} F_{Y_j/\Phi}(y_j; q_l) \cdot \alpha_l \qquad (26)$$

This expression has to be maximized with respect to α and q, with the constraints

$$\sum_{l=1}^{N} \alpha_l = 1 \quad \text{and} \quad \alpha_l \geq 0 \quad \text{for all } l = 1, \ldots, N$$

The algorithm specifically developed for the constrained optimization of the log-likelihood [equation (26)] is described elsewhere (28). The maximum-likelihood nonparametric estimate of the population distribution of kinetic parameters is finally written as

$$\hat{F} = \sum_{l=1}^{\hat{N}' \leq N} \hat{\alpha}_l \cdot \delta(\hat{q}_l) \qquad (27)$$

where $\delta(x)$ denotes the Dirac probability distribution, which takes the value 1 at x and 0 elsewhere.

The solution is described by $\hat{N}'$, the number of masses, $\{\hat{q}_l, l = 1, \ldots, \hat{N}'\}$, the set of locations ($p\hat{N}'$ parameters), and $\{\hat{\alpha}_l \neq 0, l = 1, \ldots, \hat{N}'\}$, the associated nonzero weights ($\hat{N}' - 1$ linearly independent parameters).

In order to give a feeling for the NPML solution, a representation of the discrete distribution provided by this method is shown in Fig. 9 in the case of a fictive two-dimensional example. The univariate distributions of each single parameter (the p marginal distributions) are also discrete. A simple procedure analogous to a projection (exemplified by the dotted lines in Fig. 9) is used to derive each marginal distribution. When the joint probability distribution is

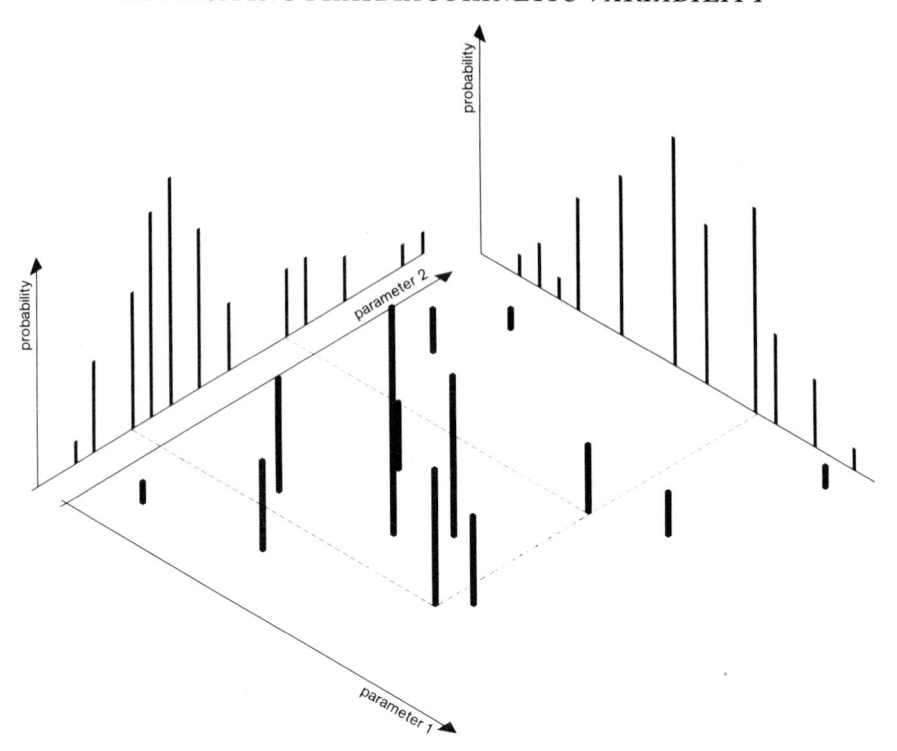

FIG. 9. Graphic representation of the NPML estimate of the population probability distribution (two-dimensional example). The joint distribution in the plane is composed of a set of locations (the vertical pillars) with associated unequal masses (the heights of the pillars). The usual (here also discrete) univariate distributions of each single parameter (the marginal distributions), which are derived from the joint (bivariate) distribution (as exemplified by the broken line segments), are shown in the upper right (parameter 1) and upper left (parameter 2) of the figure.

continuous (the usual case), the latter is obtained for a given parameter through integration over all other components of the parameter vector.

To give further insight into the NPML solution, the following comparison might be useful. Consider N independent realizations of the random variable Φ that constitute a pure sample $(\phi_1, \ldots, \phi_N)$. This situation arises when the pharmacokinetic parameters are known very precisely for all N subjects in the sample (*vide supra*). The data can be described exhaustively by the empirical probability distribution $\tilde{F}$, obtained by putting a standard mass $1/N$ on each observed value. With the terminology introduced for the NPML approach, the empirical probability distribution is a discrete distribution composed of a set of locations $[\tilde{q}_l = \phi_l, l = 1, \ldots, N]$ with associated equal weights $[\tilde{\alpha}_l = 1/N, l = 1, \ldots, N]$.

The empirical probability distribution for a sample from a fictive bivariate distribution is represented in the same way as the NPML estimate in Fig. 10.

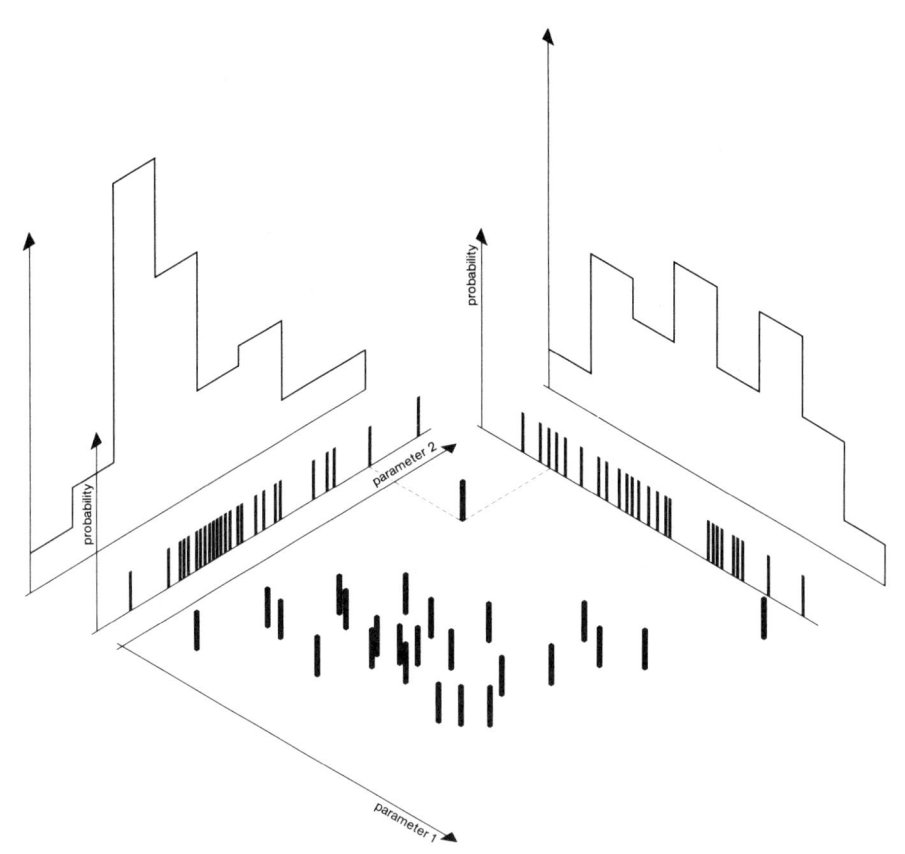

FIG. 10. A pure sample of a bivariate distribution displayed as the joint and marginal empirical distributions and the frequency distribution. The empirical distribution is a multidimensional representation of the data. Each pillar reflects one individual from the sample with a given combination of exactly known parameter values (see the broken line segments for an example). Histograms in the format of Fig. 1 show the univariate frequency distributions for each parameter, derived by calculating the proportion of individuals in equally spaced intervals.

The pictures that the NPML estimate and the empirical distribution give of the joint distribution of the parameters in the population are, in essence, of the same nature (compare Fig. 10 with Fig. 9).

In the case of a sample of independent realizations of a parameter vector from a population, the statistical analysis then actually starts. The empirical distribution stays so close to the observations that it is not generally an appropriate statistical endpoint. More useful summary statistics are obtained by studying the shape of the marginal distributions (of each component of the parameter vector), by investigating the joint distribution (e.g., for detection of correlations), by calculating estimates of the mean vector and the covariance matrix, by evaluating the median and other percentiles, by constructing univariate frequency histograms, etc. Figure 10 shows the link between the marginals of the empirical distribution and the derived univariate histograms. For further inference in practical applications, a continuous solution is often useful. In general, a distributional assumption (e.g., of normality) is postulated. Another possibility is multidimensional smoothing of the empirical distribution with kernel-based methods (18).

In the case of population-kinetics data, only indirect evidence on the distribution of the parameters, through a nonlinear (with respect to the parameters) mathematical model, is provided by the observations at hand. A first, rather complex estimation step is required to derive the discrete NPML estimate of the population distribution from the raw data. As we have shown, the NPML solution is not as unrealistic and irrelevant as it might appear initially. Most conventional statistical techniques can subsequently be applied to the NPML distribution to get derived statistical descriptors: calculation of conventional population characteristics like the two first moments (as in the GTS and the NONMEM methods), analysis of the discrete marginal distributions (Fig. 9) to detect skewness or other peculiarities, smoothing of the NPML distribution to get a continuous solution, etc.

Simulated Example

To illustrate application of the NPML method to pharmacokinetic data, the following simulated example is investigated.

Data

The computer-generated data arise from a model accounting for monocompartmental drug pharmacokinetics after intravenous bolus injection of a 1,000-unit dose. The two parameters are clearance (CL) and volume of distribution (V). Accordingly, the model is

$$f(\phi) = \frac{1{,}000}{V} \exp\left(-\frac{\text{CL}}{V} t\right) \tag{28}$$

with $\phi = (V, \text{CL})^t$.

The assumptions about the distribution of the parameters in the population are the following:

1. V is Gaussian, with expected value $\mu_V = 5$, and with standard deviation $\sigma_V = 2$, hence with a coefficient of variation CV_V of 40%.
2. The distribution of CL is an equal mixture of two Gaussian distributions with respective expectations 0.5 and 1.3 and standard deviation 0.2. Accordingly, the distribution of CL is bimodal, with two maxima close to 0.5 and 1.3 and a minimum at 0.9. This minimum is in fact the expected value

μ_{CL} of the parameter. The coefficient of variation CV_{CL} in the population is 50%.

3. V and CL are independent.

All random samplings were performed using the pseudo-random-number generator of a VAX-780 digital computer. The prototype FORTRAN program for NPML estimation runs on the same computer. A sample of fictive individuals of size $N = 50$ was considered. Individual parameters $\phi_j = (V_j, CL_j)^t$ were drawn in accord with the population distribution. For each individual, a unique serum level was computed with the model of equation (28), then corrupted with a sample ϵ_j of measurement noise from a Gaussian zero-mean distribution. The standard deviation of the noise was assumed proportional to the true level, with a 5% coefficient of variation. The pharmacostatistical model is the following:

$$y_j = \frac{1{,}000}{V_j} \exp(-\frac{CL_j}{V_j} t_j) + \epsilon_j \quad for\ j = 1, \ldots, 50 \qquad (29)$$

with (V, CL) distributed as stated earlier.

Note that in this particular example y_j is scalar. Subscript i has been dropped in equation (29) because one single observation (a unique measurement at time t_j) is taken on each individual. The simulated example reproduces an extreme situation in population kinetics: where the model is not identifiable for any individual at all. Measurement times are different across individuals; each t_j is taken as a realization from a uniform distribution over the range (0, 20). The fictive data set is displayed in Fig. 11. Note that the strong bimodality of the clearance distribution (almost a clustering into two groups) is not easily detectable in the scattering of the data.

Results

The NPML method was used to analyze the simulated data. The distribution of the measurement noise assumed at the data-analysis step was the one used to generate the data (Gaussian, zero mean, with a 5% coefficient of variation). This reflects the (ideal) situation in which the statistics of the noise are known exactly.

The discrete NPML estimate of the population distribution is displayed in Fig. 12 (lower right panel). The NPML estimate can be compared with the postulated theoretical distribution and with the empirical distribution. The true individual parameter values on which the latter relies are known in the simulation. The three marginal densities (theoretical, empirical, and NPML estimate) are shown in the upper panel (clearance) and the left panel (volume). The empirical probability distribution and the NPML solution have been smoothed with Gaussian kernel functions. Note that for both parameters the overall agreement among the smoothed NPML estimate, the (identically smoothed)

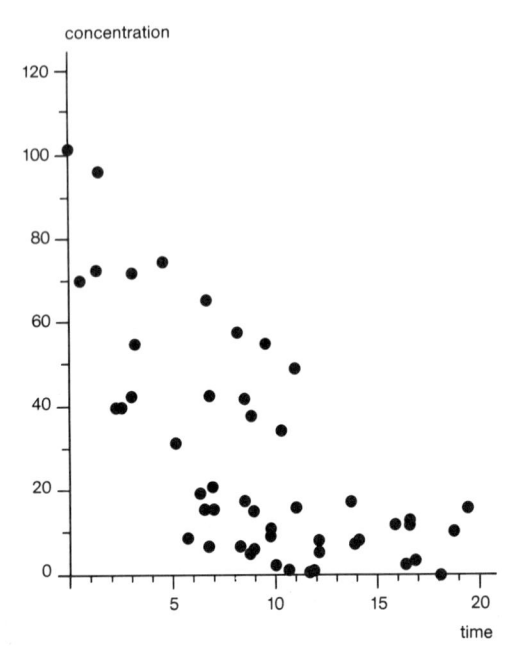

FIG. 11. Fictive data generated according to a monocompartmental model with standard bolus input. The population distribution of pharmacokinetic parameters is (a) Gaussian for volume of distribution and (b) bimodal for clearance. The dots represent 50 time–concentration measurements. A "population approach" is necessary because each data point arises from a different computer-generated individual.

empirical distribution, and the theoretical probability density function is satisfactory. The ability of the nonparametric approach to detect the bimodality in the clearance distribution is remarkable even if the estimated heights of the peaks are slightly different. Estimates of the two first moments are also in good agreement with the true values (Table 1).

Comments

The NPML method is a new approach for estimating interindividual pharmacokinetic variability and, more generally, for population-kinetics data analysis. We shall first discuss some inherent limitations of this approach, then focus later on its positive aspects.

In its present version, NPML assumes that the statistics of the measurement noise are known. This may not necessarily be realistic in practice, especially for analysis of routine data. The sensitivity of the approach to misspecification of the error-variance model should be studied in the future. A certain level of robustness of the method with respect to this assumption is required, at least

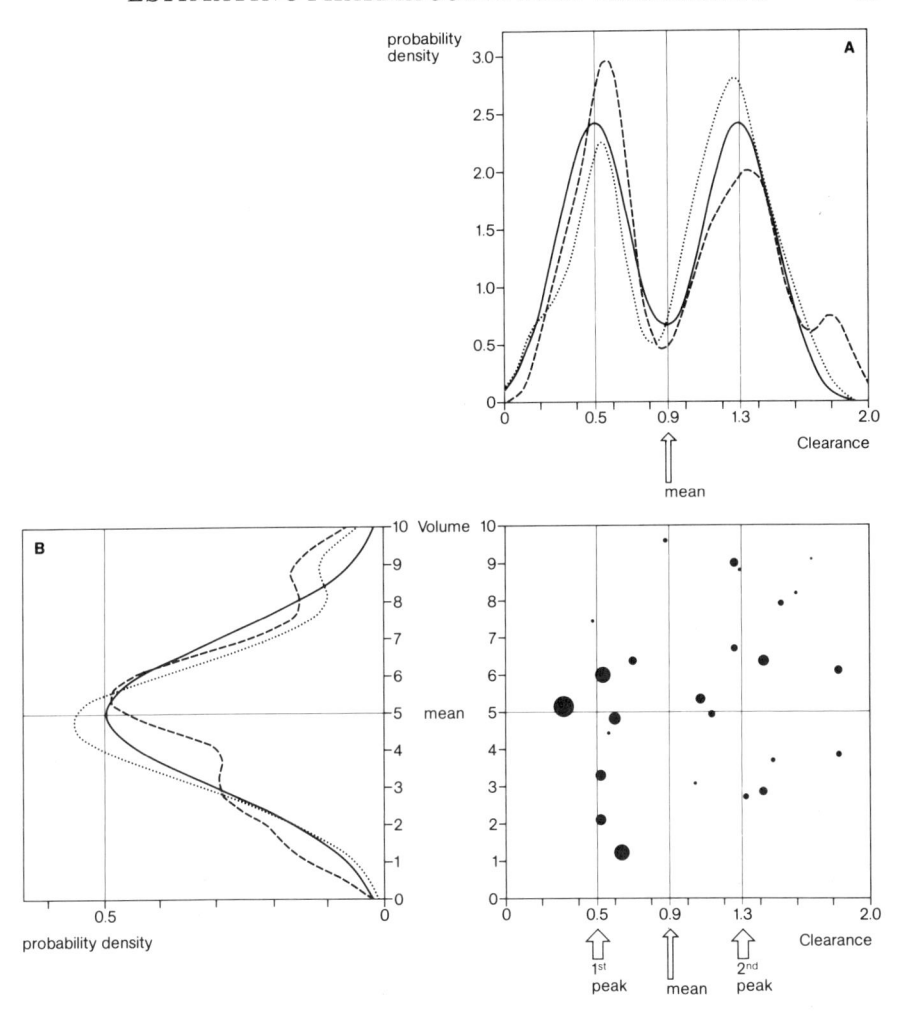

FIG. 12. NPML estimate of the distribution of pharmacokinetic parameters (clearance and volume of distribution) from the time–concentration data of Fig. 11 is shown in the lower right panel. The (discrete) solution is displayed as full circles. For graphic purposes, the circles are centered on estimated locations, with radius proportional to the corresponding estimated mass. Note that the number of locations ($N' = 25$) is less than the number of individuals in the sample ($N = 50$). Panels A and B display the theoretical (*solid line*), empirical (*dotted line*), and estimated (*broken line*) univariate distributions for clearance and volume of distribution, respectively, after smoothing of the latter two probability distributions. Note for both parameters the good agreement in location and shape of the estimated marginal density with the theoretical one.

TABLE 1. *Estimates of means and variances of volume and clearance (in arbitrary units) by NPML from computer-simulated concentration data*[a]

Pharmacokinetic parameters	Population characteristic	True	Sample	NPML estimate
Volume	Mean	5.0	4.8	4.6
	Variance	4.0	4.2	4.6
	(Standard deviation)	(2.0)	(2.05)	(2.14)
Clearance	Mean	0.90	0.88	0.88
	Variance	0.20	0.19	0.23
	(Standard deviation)	(0.45)	(0.44)	(0.48)

[a] Pharmacokinetic model, one compartment open; drug administration, intravenous bolus; observation, one serum level for each individual; measurement noise, coefficient of variation of 5%; population distribution, Gaussian for volume, bimodal for clearance; sample size, 50 individuals.

when applied to standard pharmacokinetic models and experimental designs, in order to make this approach applicable and useful.

The optimization of the likelihood criterion [equation (26)] raises complex numerical problems. How well the suggested ad hoc algorithm (28) will behave (with respect to numerical convergence and to the rate at which it occurs) when the size of the sample (N) and/or the dimension of the estimation problem (p) are increased is presently unknown. The method is costly with respect to computing time, probably as much as or even more than NONMEM. Because a NONMEM run already requires one to two orders of magnitude more time than the simple NPD approach (16), computing could be presently limiting for NPML.

The NPML estimate is a discrete distribution. If a continuous solution is necessary, the initial solution must be smoothed. This procedure is heuristic by nature; in general, a "tuning factor" allows us to smooth the discrete distribution, more or less. Visual inspection of the marginal densities and comparison with the initial discrete solution may help in choosing a realistic tuning factor. On the other hand, smoothing is not required to derive estimates of mean, variance, or percentiles. Furthermore, a discrete distribution can even be preferable to its continuous counterpart for stochastic prediction purposes [see the chapter by D. Katz (*this volume*)]. An application of that type based on the (also discrete) empirical distribution of pharmacokinetic parameters (more precisely a distribution of estimates of the parameters) has been reported for evaluation of theophylline dosage regimens (32).

The simplified extrapolation of the distribution of some variable of interest is one possible straightforward application of the discrete NPML solution. However, application of the approach to a given population estimation problem should rather be regarded as a preliminary step toward detection of the type of parametric distribution that should be assumed for further data analysis. The simulation relied on a peculiar but not unlikely distribution for the clearance (which might reflect genetically controlled drug metabolism). The results have shown the ability of NPML to suggest the shape of a parameter's distribution from indirect and fragmentary data. It is expected that NPML may help answer questions like the following: Is the probability distribution of a parameter unimodal or multimodal? Is it symmetric or skewed? Is it "long-tailed"? Are there some "outlying" individuals or subgroups? Answering these questions will help suggest a possible transformation of the parameter space in order for methods that require normality to be applicable. Once justified after the nonparametric step, parametric analysis may be more efficient than its nonparametric counterpart.

In this exploratory context, the fact that confidence limits on the solution and on other derived population characteristics cannot yet be assessed is of secondary concern.

COMPARISON OF METHODS AND ISSUES IN KINETIC-VARIABILITY ESTIMATION

Available Methods

Methods for estimating interindividual pharmacokinetic variability can be distinguished with respect to the information they actually provide, regardless of its quality. Basically, three types of methods are available:

1. Methods that provide only an estimate of central tendency (e.g., the mean): (a) averaging of the data across subjects and subsequent fitting of mean data (naive averaging of data, NAD); (b) fitting of all data in one step as if all observations arose from a single "reference individual" (naive pooling of data, NPD).
2. Methods that provide estimates of central tendency and dispersion (e.g., the first two moments of the parameter distribution): (a) two-stage methods, in which individual data are fitted in a first stage, and individual estimates are combined to derive population characteristics in a second stage; the latter can be performed through simple averaging (standard two-stage, STS), through optimization of an extended least-squares objective function (global two-stage, GTS), or may imply repeated fittings of individual data (iterated two-stage, ITS); (b) the nonlinear mixed-effect model with first-order approximation (NONMEM), in which the population characteristics are estimated in a unique stage through global analysis of all data.
3. Methods that provide information about the whole probability distribution of the parameters in the population: (a) the two-stage graphic method, in which the sample of individual parameter estimates obtained after the first-stage fitting is displayed as a histogram; (b) the nonparametric maximum-likelihood approach (NPML), in which the shape of the univariate

marginal distributions of each parameter can be detected after smoothing of the (discrete) estimate of the joint distribution.

From a practical point of view, all previously mentioned methods for population-kinetics analysis have advantages and limitations. "Better" information in the statistical sense is definitely related to increasing implementation and computing costs. As a general method for estimating mean values of pharmacokinetic parameters, NDA should be discarded. The performances of NPD, STS, and NONMEM have been compared in several studies on simulated data (37,38,40). A detailed comparison between the two-stage methods (STS, GTS, ITS) and NONMEM with respect to statistical and computational aspects is available (45). In all cases, the shape of the population distribution postulated for the parametric analysis was identical with that of the data-generating distribution. Conclusively, evidence exists that GTS (when applicable) and NONMEM perform reasonably well when the data satisfy the assumptions on which the methods rely. Up to now, no attempt has been reported to study the robustness of these estimation methods in cases of misspecification of the population distribution and/or of the kinetic model. The simple NPD and STS approaches, despite their drawbacks, are valuable alternatives to more ambitious methods when "rough" estimates will serve the purpose. The NPML approach should serve as an exploratory technique, intended to suggest the shape of the distribution for subsequent parametric analysis of the data.

Statistical Issues in Population-Kinetics Data Analysis

Kinetic data analysis based on a population approach actually started in pharmacokinetics (43). However, the underlying estimation problem is far more general. It arises not only in the investigation of biological processess in individuals but also every time serial measurements are performed in different experimental units. In the statistical literature, the problem is known as "stochastic parameter regression"; see Johnson (21,22) for a comprehensive bibliography on the topic. Econometrics is the application field in which most "current" statistical methods for between-unit variability estimation from serial observations were developed; see Dielman (14) for a review. The advocated models are generally linear with respect to the parameters. Furthermore, restrictions on the structure of the data are common. Observations should arise from designs standardized across the experimental units or from time-series, equally spaced measurements. Because these properties are unusual for pharmacokinetic and more generally for biokinetic data and models, transposition of the methods to biomedical data analysis is not straightforward. One exception is the analysis of growth curves. Linear mixed-effect models were early proposed (20) and are still being investigated (23).

Moreover, current methods usually deal with distributions belonging to given classes of parametric functions, generally Gaussian or derived ones. Such strong assumptions about the population distribution often cannot be reliably stated for pharmacokinetic parameters.

The lack of well-accepted statistical methods for population-kinetics estimation prompted the development of ad hoc techniques by data analysts in applied pharmacokinetics. However, most of the methods presented in this chapter do not pretend to statistical originality. For example, the basic ideas of the GTS approach were early suggested in the context of Bayesian linear estimation (25). The algorithm suggested by Prevost is an instance of a general statistical procedure, the EM algorithm proposed for maximum-likelihood estimation from incomplete data (13). In the case of population-kinetics data analysis, the missing data are the individual (unknown) parameter values. However, less attention has been paid in the statistical literature to the real problem with respect to biomedical applications, that of estimating a population distribution of parameters in a nonlinear model from indirect, noisy, and fragmentary observations. New ideas have recently appeared in maximum-likelihood estimation (27,28) and in Bayesian approaches (34).

It should be recognized that in the existing (and probably future) "sophisticated" methods, the price to be paid for generality, versatility, and statistical validity is a huge computational burden for the estimation step. For the development of the method, numerical difficulties will have to be solved, and complex programming will be required. For any application, extensive computing time, even on powerful machines, will be necessary. Therefore, there is no general answer to the question whether the improvement of costly methods over "rough and dirty" techniques like the simplest among the two-stage methods (the standard two-stage) is significant. A hierarchy based strictly on statistical criteria is not necessarily helping the practitioner.

IMPACT OF KNOWLEDGE OF KINETIC VARIABILITY ON DRUG DEVELOPMENT AND THERAPY

Estimating interindividual pharmacokinetic variability is not a goal per se, but has to serve a purpose. The connection between population-variability estimation and individual therapy (the ultimate goal) is clearly explained in several sources (41,43). In fact, the type of inference the kineticist has in mind when performing a pharmacokinetic study might dictate which level of accuracy in variability estimates is required and might influence the choice of the method for data analysis. Actually, one future prospect in population kinetics could be to incorporate in the estimation step, in some way, knowledge of what the population characteristics should serve for.

To a certain extent, the choice of the data analysis method for pharmacokinetic-variability assessment can depend on the nature of the drug. For a drug with a large therapeutic index, a crude estimate of the population mean clearance value may be sufficient for the choice of a standard intravenous infusion rate that will prove adequate therapy for all patients. Unfortunately, for many drugs, the picture is fairly different. Figure 13 displays steady-state plasma concentration data for the drug quinidine in a group of patients undergoing a standardized dosage regimen (17). The wide between-subject variability in the achieved drug levels reflects interpatient pharmacokinetic variation. The validity of the dosing scheme is questionable, because the standard dosage resulted in overdosage (in 1 patient) as well as in underdosage (in several). For drugs difficult to manage because of a poor balance between the therapeutic concentration range and the range of individual variations in the handling of the drug, quantitative knowledge of pharmacokinetic variability should lead to more rational patient care. This improvement in therapy will be significant if (and most likely only if) information about the basic population characteristics (fixed and random effects) and/or the population probability distribution is sufficiently accurate. For such drugs, estimation methods that are simple but biased must be used with caution.

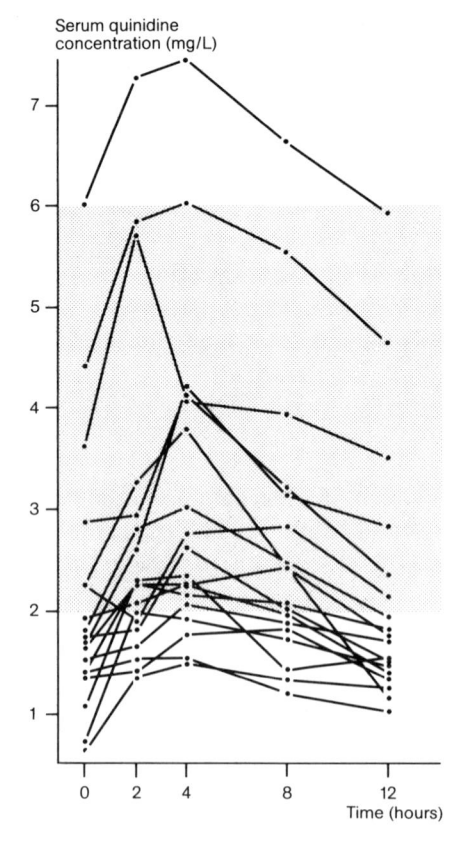

FIG. 13. Steady-state plasma-concentration profiles (experimental data) for quinidine in patients receiving a standard maintenance dosage of slow-release quinidine preparation. Dark area is the therapeutic range. (From Follath et al., ref. 17, with permission.)

Knowledge of the statistical distribution of pharmacokinetic parameters can be useful for rational decision making during drug development and later during clinical use of the drug for individual patient care.

During Drug Development

Knowledge of population characteristics can be incorporated in Monte Carlo simulations to predict the variability in some outcome of interest that depends on the pharmacokinetic parameters. *In numero* evaluation of dosage-regimen strategies can be useful for better design or even avoidance of experiments on patients. Different dosage forms and dosage regimens can be compared, and a hierarchy can be assessed not only by means of an average behavior but also by taking pharmacokinetic variability into account. The lithium dosage regimen was investigated in this way (19). Population characteristics of pharmacokinetic parameters for a two-compartment model were estimated from 24 normal volunteers. Surprisingly good agreement was observed between the computer extrapolations based on this limited group of subjects and the results from clinical serum-level monitoring in patients. A Monte Carlo simulation of steady-state drug levels is shown in Fig. 14 for a widely used standard dosage regimen of 350 mg lithium carbonate b.i.d. Note

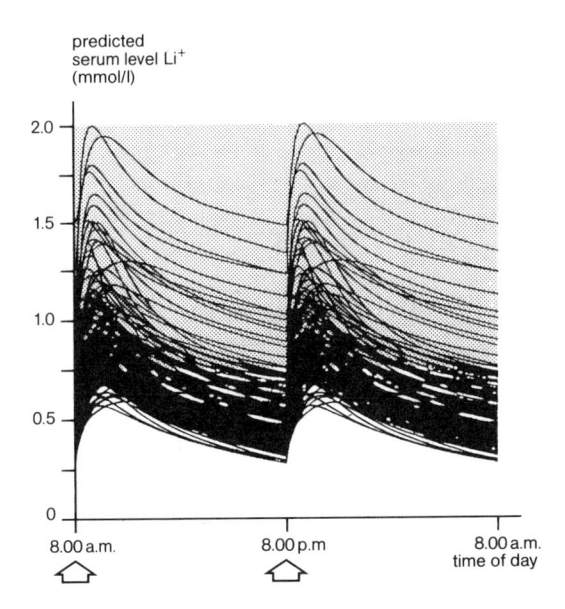

FIG. 14. Calculated steady-state plasma-level profiles (Monte Carlo computer simulation) of lithium in 100 fictive patients. The dosage regimen is 350 mg lithium carbonate b.i.d. The underlying population distribution of the pharmacokinetic parameters (two-compartment open model with first-order absorption) is multivariate normal (19). The dashed area is the therapeutic range (from 0.75 to 2.0 mmol/liter).

in passing the resemblance in the global patterns of serum levels over 12 hr between Fig. 13 (quinidine) and Fig. 14 (lithium). The ability of the simulation to reproduce the (skewed) distribution (across individuals) of the steady-state profiles is striking. Unlikely overdosage and very frequent underdosage probably reflect the widespread safety-first principle that led to the choice of the corresponding standard dosage regimens for both drugs. Lithium is well known as a problematic drug. Computer simulation, of course, did not prove that. However, based on reasonable estimates of population characteristics, computer simulation of pharmacokinetic models may help derive appropriate counterstrategies against variability in drug therapy. Precise suggestions for dosage-regimen adjustment procedures could have been made in the previously mentioned study (19) before the actual experiment in the clinical setting was undertaken.

During Drug Treatment for a Given Patient

The "open-loop" dosage regimen for starting therapy in a given patient is often standard. The choice is made according to the dosing guidelines accepted as "the best" after the drug-development step. Provided a relevant endpoint (a level of plasma concentration or effect) can be defined, knowledge about population characteristics of pharmacokinetic parameters can be incorporated in the decision process for the optimal dosage (19,32). If, in addition, covariates (e.g., sex, age, weight, genetic factors, concomitant therapy, smoking) are introduced in the analysis (which is possible with some of the estimation methods, e.g., NONMEM) and found significant, variability is not only estimated but also (at least partly) explained. Then, knowledge of the covariate data for a given individual allows patient-specific dosage-regimen adjustment.

During long-term therapy, knowledge of pharmacokinetic variability can be used to further adjust the individual dosage regimen with a target-concentration strategy (44). In the absence of a clear-cut clinical endpoint (e.g., in prophylactic therapy, or when a given therapeutic or toxic effect can be seen only after considerable delay), serum levels measured during routine monitoring provide meaningful feedback information for adjusting the dosage. Optimal individual forecasting combines general knowledge of population characteristics and patient-specific data. Both types of information are weighted according to their respective (estimated or assumed) variances. The more data are gathered on an individual, the less influential is the population distribution (the *a priori* knowledge). Various examples of Bayesian dosage-regimen adjustments have been reported in the literature (41,46); see chapter by S. Vožeh et al (*this volume*).

CONCLUSION

Pharmacokinetic variability is one major component of overall variability in response to drug therapy. In this chapter, widely used and recent data-analysis techniques for estimating average behavior and interindividual variability in pharmacokinetics from experimental and routine data have been presented, discussed, and contrasted. Simple methods (naive averaging of data, naive pooled data) often fail to provide unbiased estimates of the mean value of the pharmacokinetic parameters. Among the two-stage methods, which combine parameter estimates obtained through separate fitting of individual data, the global two-stage approach appears promising. The widely used standard two-stage procedure produces overestimates of the variance-covariance of the parameter distribution. All these simple techniques can be used for analyzing experimental data from pharmacokinetic studies in volunteers, which bring information about variability in the early phases of drug development. Observational data from population-pharmacokinetic studies in patients, which up to now have been gathered in late phases, require appropriate methods. The best-documented and -validated method to date is the nonlinear mixed-effect model with first-order approximation, which provides good estimates of the first two moments, mean and covariance, as population characteristics. A more recent procedure, the nonparametric maximum-likelihood approach, attempts to give also the shape of the distribution. Data and statistical methods for individual and population pharmacokinetics are complementary for the purpose of estimating pharmacokinetic variability. Taking knowledge of population characteristics into account will improve the relevance of pharmacokinetics for drug development and drug therapy.

ACKNOWLEDGMENTS

The authors are indebted to numerous persons who contributed in different ways to this chapter. We acknowledge the help of Martine Fréchelin, Margaret Nagel, and especially Anne Maurer for their efficient and clever typing, the input of Markfried Veit for design and drawing of the figures, and the criticisms and suggestions of several Sandoz colleagues regarding earlier drafts of the chapter.

Free access to the VAX computer of the Service d'Informatique Médicale (CHU Pitié-Salpêtrière, Assistance Publique des Hôpitaux de Paris) for the computing of the nonparametric example is gratefully acknowledged. This work was partly supported by a grant from the Caisse Mutuelle Provinciale des Professions Libérales.

REFERENCES

1. Alvan, G. (1978): Individual differences in the disposition of drugs metabolised in the body. *Clin. Pharmacokinet.*, 3:155–175.
2. Amdisen, A. (1973): Serum lithium estimations. *Br. Med. J.*, 2:240.
3. Amdisen, A. (1975): Monitoring of lithium treatment through determination of lithium concentration. *Dan. Med. Bull.*, 22:277–291.
4. Balant, L.P., and Garrett, E.R. (1983): Computer use in pharmacokinetics. In: *Drug Fate*

and Metabolism: Methods and Techniques, Vol. 4, edited by E.R. Garrett and J.L. Hirtz, pp. 1–150. Marcel Dekker, New York.
5. Beal, S.L. (1974): Adaptative M-estimation with independent not identically distributed data. Ph.D. dissertation, University of California, Los Angeles.
6. Beal, S.L. (1984): Population pharmacokinetic data and parameter estimation based on their first two statistical moments. *Drug Metab. Rev.*, 15:173–193.
7. Beal, S.L., and Sheiner, L.B. (1979): *NONMEM Users Guide. I. Users Basic Guide*. Division of Clinical Pharmacology, University of California, San Francisco.
8. Beal, S.L., and Sheiner, L.B. (1981): *NONMEM Users Guide. II. Users Supplemental Guide*. Division of Clinical Pharmacology, University of California, San Francisco.
9. Beal, S.L., and Sheiner, L.B. (1982): Estimating population kinetics. *CRC Crit. Rev. Biomed. Eng.*, 8:195–222.
10. Beal, S.L., and Sheiner, L.B. (1984): *NONMEM Users Guide. V. Users NONMEM 77 Guide*. Division of Clinical Pharmacology, University of California, San Francisco.
11. Boxenbaum, H. (1984): Pharmacokinetic determinants in the design and evaluation of sustained-release dosage forms. *Pharmaceutical Research*, 1:82–88.
12. Cocchetto, D.M., Wargin, W.A., and Crow, J.W. (1980): Pitfalls and valid approaches to pharmacokinetic analysis of mean concentration data following intravenous administration. *J. Pharmacokinet. Biopharm.*, 8:539–552.
13. Dempster, A.P., Laird, N.M., and Rubin, D.B. (1977): Maximum likelihood from incomplete data via the EM algorithm. *J. Roy. Statist. Soc. B*, 39:1–38.
14. Dielman, T.E. (1983): Pooled cross-sectional and time series data: A survey of current statistical methodology. *Amer. Statist.*, 37:111–122.
15. Endrenyi, L. (editor) (1981): *Kinetic Data Analysis*. Plenum Press, New York.
16. Fluehler, H., Huber, H., Widmer, E., and Brechbuehler, S. (1984): Experiences in the application of NONMEM to pharmacokinetic data analysis. *Drug Metab. Rev.*, 15:317–339.
17. Follath, F., Ganzinger, U., and Schuetz, E. (1983): Reliability of antiarrhythmic drug plasma concentration monitoring. *Clin. Pharmacokinet.*, 8:63–82.
18. Fukunaga, K. (1972): *Introduction to Statistical Pattern Recognition*. Academic Press, New York.
19. Gaillot, J., Steimer, J.L., Mallet, A., Thebault, J.J., and Bieder, A. (1979): A priori lithium dosage regimen using population characteristics of pharmacokinetic parameters. *J. Pharmacokinet. Biopharm.*, 7:579–628.
20. Grizzle, J.E., and Allen, D.M. (1969): Analysis of growth and dose response curves. *Biometrics*, 25:357–381.
21. Johnson, L.W. (1977): Stochastic parameter regression. *Int. Stat. Rev.*, 45:257–272.
22. Johnson, L.W. (1980): Stochastic parameter regression: An additional annotated bibliography. *Int. Stat. Rev.*, 48:95–102.
23. Laird, N.M., and Ware, J.H. (1982): Random-effects models for longitudinal data. *Biometrics*, 38:963–974.
24. Levy, G., and Hollister, L.E. (1964): Inter- and intrasubject variations in drug absorption kinetics. *J. Pharm. Sci.*, 53:1446–1452.
25. Lindley, D.V., and Smith, A.F.M. (1972): Bayes estimates for the linear model. *J. Roy. Statist. Soc. B*, 34:1–18.
26. Lindstrom, F.T., and Birkes, D.S. (1984): Estimation of population pharmacokinetic parameters using destructively obtained experimental data: A simulation study of the one-compartment open model. *Drug Metab. Rev.*, 15:195–264.
27. Mallet, A. (1983): Méthodes d'estimation de lois à partir d'observations indirectes d'un échantillon: application aux caractéristiques de population de modèles biologiques. Thèse pour le doctorat d'état es-sciences. Université Paris 6.
28. Mallet, A. (1984): A maximum likelihood estimation method for random coefficient regression models. (*in press*).
29. Metzler, C.M. (1981): Statistical properties of kinetic estimates. In: *Kinetic Data Analysis*, edited by L. Endrenyi, pp. 25–37. Plenum Press, New York.
30. Peck, C.C., Sheiner, L.B., and Nichols, A.I. (1984): The problem of choosing weights in nonlinear regression analysis of pharmacokinetic data. *Drug Metab. Rev.*, 15:133–148.
31. Prevost, G. (1977): Estimation of a normal probability density function from samples measured with non-negligible and non-constant dispersion. Internal report 6-77, Adersa-Gerbios, 2 avenue de 1er Mai, F-91120 Palaiseau.

32. Richter, O., and Reinhardt, D. (1982): Methods for evaluating optimal dosage regimens and their application to theophylline. *Int. J. Clin. Pharmacol.,* 20:564–575.
33. Rodda, B.E. (1981): Analysis of sets of estimates from pharmacokinetic studies. In: *Kinetic Data Analysis,* edited by L. Endrenyi, pp. 285–297. Plenum Press, New York.
34. Rodman, J.H., D'Argenio, D.Z., Katz, D., Cerra, F., and Jelliffe, R.W. (1984): Population analysis of tobramycin kinetics. *Clin. Pharmacol. Ther.,* 35:270 (*abstract*).
35. SAS Institute Inc. (1982): *SAS User's Guide.* SAS, Box 8000, Cary, NC 27511.
36. Sheiner, L.B. (1984): The population approach to pharmacokinetic data analysis: Rationale and standard data analysis methods. *Drug Metab. Rev.,* 15:153–171.
37. Sheiner, L.B., and Beal, S.L. (1980): Evaluation of methods for estimating population pharmacokinetic parameters. I. Michaelis-Menten model: Routine clinical data. *J. Pharmacokinet. Biopharm.,* 8:553–571.
38. Sheiner, L.B., and Beal, S.L. (1981): Evaluation of methods for estimating population pharmacokinetic parameters. II. Biexponential model and experimental pharmacokinetic data. *J. Pharmacokinet. Biopharm.,* 9:635–651.
39. Sheiner, L.B., and Beal, S.L. (1981): Estimation of pooled pharmacokinetic parameters describing populations. In: *Kinetic Data Analysis,* edited by L. Endrenyi, pp. 271–284. Plenum Press, New York.
40. Sheiner, L.B., and Beal, S.L. (1983): Evaluation of methods for estimating population pharmacokinetic parameters. III. Monoexponential model: Routine pharmacokinetic data. *J. Pharmacokinet. Biopharm.,* 11:303–319.
41. Sheiner, L.B., Beal, S.L., Rosenberg, G., and Marathe, V.V. (1979): Forecasting individual pharmacokinetics. *Clin. Pharmacol. Ther.,* 26:294–305.
42. Sheiner, L.B., Benet, L.Z., and Pagliaro, L.A. (1981): A standard approach to compiling clinical pharmacokinetic data. *J. Pharmacokinet. Biopharm.,* 9:59–127.
43. Sheiner, L.B., Rosenberg, B., and Melmon, K.L. (1972): Modelling of individual pharmacokinetics for computer-aided drug dosage. *Comp. Biomed. Res.,* 5:441–459.
44. Sheiner, L.B., and Tozer, T.N. (1978): Clinical pharmacokinetics: The use of plasma concentrations of drugs. In: *Clinical Pharmacology: Basic Principles in Therapeutics,* 2, edited by K.L. Melmon and H.F. Morelli, 71–109. Macmillan, New York.
45. Steimer, J.L., Mallet, A., Golmard, J.L., and Boisvieux, J.F. (1984): Alternative approaches to estimation of population pharmacokinetic parameters; comparison with the nonlinear mixed effect model. *Drug Metab. Rev.,* 15:265–292.
46. Vozeh, S., Muir, K.T., Sheiner, L.B., and Follath, F. (1981): Predicting individual phenytoin dosage. *J. Pharmacokinet. Biopharm.,* 9:131–146.
47. Watts, D.G. (1981): An introduction to nonlinear least squares. In: *Kinetic Data Analysis,* edited by L. Endrenyi, pp. 1–24. Plenum Press, New York.

DISCUSSION[5]

Discussant 1 (D1): One always recommends that raw data be plotted in various ways before applying models to fit it. In the two-stage methods, after the first stage, one can plot out the parameter values even though they don't have a high degree of certainty, and look at their distribution. It may not be symmetric, or may be otherwise unusual. In contrast, in the NONMEM method such distributions cannot be observed. Also, do you not assume they are normal?

Speaker (S): The first-order extended least-squares method doesn't assume any distribution. It does, however, focus exclusively on the first two moments of the parameter distribution. By so doing, one doesn't get any information about such things as skewness or other aspects of the distribution. Thus, your first point is correct; one doesn't get a look at the parameter distribution. However, let me ask whether it is worth look-

---

[5] This discussion concerns the points about population models raised in the previous chapter on the modeling of pharmacokinetic variability (L.B. Sheiner, *this volume*) as well as this chapter. The actual speaker was L.B. Sheiner; J.-L. Steimer agrees with all responses and opinions of the speaker.

ing at the distribution of parameter estimates when they are as poor as they are when they are derived from very little data from each individual? Won't that histogram have nothing to do with reality? In contrast, of course, if there are many data points per person from a well-designed pharmacokinetic experiment, then the individual parameter estimates are good, but the chances are that there are fewer than 15 individuals. In that case the mean is fairly well estimated, the variance is poorly to moderately well estimated, but higher moments are not. Consequently, the histogram will not be very much more informative than the first two moments. It's a dilemma. If one studies each individual well enough to trust individual parameter estimates, one can't study enough individuals to get a histogram that is informative; while if one studies many individuals poorly, I am very concerned (although I don't know for sure) that the histogram, though informative, will bear no relationship to biological reality.

D2: You mentioned that the intraindividual variability is about 10%. Do you quote these data from the work of Upton et al. (3,4), or do you have other sources for your estimate? Another question is related to the upward bias that distinguished the two-stage approach. From the point of view of a regulatory agency, this is a conservative bias and will not harm the patient. If this is the only disadvantage of the two-stage method, it doesn't seem very important. The advantage of the method is that it is very easy to use. Also, because there are many programs for multivariate analysis, it is a convenient approach.

S: Regarding intraindividual variability of 10 to 20%, what I am referring to is the residual variability of drug levels about the fitted function. When levels are measured over the course of several days, as is often the case for routine clinical data, I believe this variability is the intraindividual biological variability in kinetics. My information comes from several population analyses (1,2,6), but I don't know how general it is. Certainly some drugs, for example those whose kinetics vary day to day with changes in diet and so forth, will clearly show greater variability than others. Regarding your second point, I'm not sure that overestimation of interindividual variability is of little consequence. For example, it can lead us to try to investigate variability that doesn't exist. Using a greater number of subjects, by the way, does not decrease bias; one needs better design in each subject. Finally, however, I currently believe that modified two-stage methods (GTS, ITS) may obviate the problem. Moreover, the nonparametric approach may provide what a previous questioner wants: a "reasonable histogram" for the probability distribution of the parameter.

D3: I completely agree with you in the main principle that you must allow for intercorrelation of observations from the same individual. I want to raise a question, however, about your assumption of independence of errors for different individuals. I am worried that you may not really be taking random samples from the population on which you want to make inference, so that you may have interindividual correlations, possibly through close family relationships, close genetic relationships between individuals in your samples, and possibly because of other environmental factors.

S: That is a good point. One might hope to be able to identify, for example, environmental factors and put them in the regression. Then the correlation would go away, but the point is worrisome, as you note, especially when one is dealing with observational data. All I can say is that it is important to study the type of person who is going to receive the drug. One can't do very elaborate experiments on such people, because one must care for them. All I can think of is to use the data that are available and do the best one can with it, understanding that certain data-analysis assumptions may be violated.

D4: From a practical point of view in drug development, how applicable would a population approach (e.g., with NONMEM) be to a two-compartment or a three-compartment model? In other words, how much data must we generate in order to be able to use it for relatively complicated pharmacokinetic models?

S: First, it is rare in clinical practice that one has to deal with complicated kinetic models, especially for orally administered drugs. However, when the data suggest the need for a more complicated model, such can certainly be used. For example, Vozeh et al. (5) estimated population characteristics for two-compartment models from routine data.

REFERENCES

1. Grasela, T.H., Sheiner, L.B., Rambeck, R., Boenigk, H.E., Dunlop, A., Mullen, P.W., Wadsworth, J., Richens, A., Ishizaki, T., Chiba, K., Miura, H., Minagawa, K., Blain, P.G., Mucklow, J.C., Bacon, C.T., and Rawlins, M. (1983): Steady-state pharmacokinetics of phenytoin from routinely-collected patient data. *Clin. Pharmacokinet.*, 8:355-364.
2. Sheiner, L.B., Rosenberg, B., and Marathe, V.V. (1977): Estimation of population characteristics of pharmacokinetic parameters from routine clinical data. *J. Pharmacokinet. Biopharm.*, 5:445-479.
3. Upton, R.A., Thiercelin, J.F., Guentert, T.W., Wallace, S.M., Powell, J.R., Sansom, L., and Riegelman, S. (1982): Intraindividual variability in theophylline pharmacokinetics: Statistical verification in 39 of 60 healthy young adults. *J. Pharmacokinet. Biopharm.*, 10:123-134.
4. Upton, R.A., Thiercelin, J.F., Moore, J.K., and Riegelman, S. (1982): A method for estimating within-individual variability in clearance and in volume of distribution from standard bioavailability studies. *J. Pharmacokinet. Biopharm.*, 10:135-146.
5. Vozeh, S., Berger, M., Wenk, M., Ritz, R., and Follath, F. (1984): Rapid prediction of individual dosage requirements for lignocaine. *Clin. Pharmacokinet.*, 9:354-363.
6. Vozeh, S., Katz, G., Steiner, V., and Follath, F. (1982): Population pharmacokinetic parameters in patients treated with oral mexiletine. *Eur. J. Clin. Pharmacol.*, 23:429-433.

Variability in Drug Therapy:
Description, Estimation, and Control,
edited by M. Rowland et al.
Raven Press, New York © 1985.

Models, Formulations, and Statistics

David J. Finney

Department of Statistics and AFRC Unit of Statistics, University of Edinburgh, Edinburgh EH9 3JZ, United Kingdom

APOLOGIA

Although I have had some association with pharmacological matters for the past 40 years, this has been restricted to bioassay and drug toxicity. I have never worked on pharmacokinetic problems, and I have avoided involvement with the theory of time-series and stochastic processes. This volume is concerned with questions that are pharmacologically and physiologically complex, but that also have substantial mathematico-statistical difficulties. My impression is that few of those who work in this field are professionally trained in statistics, although many have developed a masterly skill in handling the complicated equations that arise. Some methods adopted may not always be consistent with general statistical practice, but with reasonably good data they work and help to carry understanding forward. In such circumstances, will introduction of a participant from the mainstream of statistical science be valuable? Perhaps that participant will see interconnections of methods, and will judge when and how a procedure that is heuristic in origin but inexact in theory may give misleading results. The desirable end of clarification and improvement will follow, however, only if the statistician is well chosen. I could suggest many who would be more suitable than I am.

Having agreed to participate in this volume, I asked two of the organizers to send me a few articles that might give me ideas. I was appalled by the result. Not, I hasten to add, appalled by bad science or unsound statistics, but appalled by my own inability to comprehend the methods, the aims, even the terminology. I finally fixed attention on one article that, because it had 16 authors, gave me hope that a seventeenth approach might not be totally irrelevant. Because Dr. Sheiner, who bears responsibility for asking me to contribute to this volume, was one author, I thought I could fairly inflict on him some of my fault-finding. I recognize that a Michaelis-Menten situation is not typical of the problems that concern most people here. I chose it in part because I thought I could understand it, and in part because it exhibits in simple form statistical features that are certainly relevant to other more complicated formulations of pharmacokinetic phenomena. I now realize that my initial reactions to that article were based on misunderstanding of its text, but I hope that I may still have points worth making. But before turning to this topic, I want to comment on two general statistical issues.

INDICES

Several authors have discussed aspects of their topics in terms of indices formed as ratios between pairs of measurements or other derived quantities. I have no wish to condemn this, but I want to point out the danger that an entirely irrelevant correlation may be induced. Take the simplest case of two indices:

$$I_1 = x_1/y_1, \quad I_2 = x_2/y_2 \tag{1}$$

Suppose that x_1, x_2 are uncorrelated with one another and with y_1, y_2, but y_1 and y_2 are correlated. If the coefficient of variation of x_i is small relative to that of y_i ($i = 1, 2$), the correlation coefficient between I_1 and I_2 will be almost as great as that between y_1 and y_2. Of course, as an extreme, y_1 and y_2 may be identical; the danger then will be magnified if y_1 has large errors of measurement. If there are other correlations among x_1, x_2, y_1, and y_2, the consequences for the correlation coefficient between I_1 and I_2 are more complicated, but even the simple example serves to emphasize the need for care in interpretation.

COEFFICIENTS OF VARIATION

In the foregoing, I used coefficients of variation, because they aid concise statements of results relating to quotients and products of variables. In general, I deprecate use of this statistic because it confuses different aspects of data in an arbitrary manner. Some practitioners of statistical analysis appear to believe, and indeed some textbooks may seem to teach, that the coefficient of variation provides an uniquely correct way of comparing variabilities of different measurements. If σ_x is the standard deviation for the frequency distribution of x, the coefficient of variation is

$$100\sigma_x/\mu$$

where μ is the mean; in practice, μ and σ_x usually must be replaced by $\bar{x}$ and s_x, estimates from a sample. To use this as a standardized (and dimensionless) measure of variability is a legitimate convention, and no more than a convention, that can be adopted for positive reasons but not for any belief that it is ordained by statistical theory.

Consider three comparisons:

1. Is height more variable among men than among women? Mean heights are not very different, and if I had to respond to this question I would prefer to

answer in terms of the standard deviations; for all I know, the order may be reversed by coefficients of variation. Either way of answering, like others that could be suggested, is arbitrary, because variability is not uniquely defined as a property of quantitative measurements.

2. Is body weight more variable among elephants than among mice? Comparison of standard deviations is unlikely to be helpful, because the conclusion is so obvious. I am not clear that any numerical answer is useful unless a specific purpose is defined. There is nothing wrong with the convention that variability will be interpreted as standard deviation relative to mean, but there is no reason for this other than convention.

3. Is creatinine clearance rate more variable than systolic blood pressure? Now the two quantities have totally different units, and numerical comparisons of standard deviations are meaningless. Here, perhaps, lies the strongest attraction of the coefficient of variation: It permits a comparison of variabilities when quantities are not measured in the same units. My retort to this is that it is wiser not to attempt any comparison unless in accordance with a specific objective.

There is indeed danger in adopting the coefficient of variation if the user then assumes that he or she has a good indicator of which of several variables should receive most attention in respect of improving precision. A trivial example can illustrate the point. Suppose that quantities a and b are measured on members of a population (and are uncorrelated) and that the function interesting the investigator is

$$f = Ae^{-\lambda t} \tag{2}$$

where t is time. Write μ_A and μ_λ for the population means and σ_A and σ_λ for the standard deviations of A and λ. Write

$$\text{CV}_A = \frac{\sigma_A}{\mu_A}, \quad \text{CV}_\lambda = \frac{\sigma_\lambda}{\mu_\lambda} \tag{3}$$

Then, to the first-order approximation, which is all that can be stated in respect of a function such as equation (2), the standard deviation of f can be shown to be

$$\psi(\text{CV}_A^2 + \mu_\lambda^2 t^2 \cdot \text{CV}_\lambda^2)^{1/2} \tag{4}$$

where

$$\psi = \mu_A e^{-\mu_\lambda t} \tag{5}$$

Then the relative magnitudes of CV_A and CV_λ do not tell whether improved precision in determination of A will benefit the precision of f more or less than improvement in determination of λ; the simultaneous dependence on $\mu_\lambda t$ is inescapable. Of course, the position is no better if equation (4) is written in terms of σ_A and σ_λ, or in terms of any other measures of variability. The fault with forming coefficients of variation is not that they themselves are wrong, but that their users too readily assume that they suffice to indicate where improved precision is most needed.

DATA

Grasela et al. (2) incorporated into a single analysis data from three different populations; the data relate to daily dose of phenytoin and steady-state phenytoin concentration in plasma. Sex, age, weight, and height were recorded for 322 patients; each patient provided at least two dose–concentration data points, the total number of points being 780. Table 1 summarizes the situation

TABLE 1. *Summary of data from patients treated with phenytoin*

Characteristic	Data set A	Data set B	Data set C
Source	Germany	Japan	England
No. of patients	178	104	40
No. of observations	385	236	159
Proportion of data from males	0.53	0.50	0.54
Means and standard deviations			
Age (years)	29.5 ± 15.2	6.0 ± 3.9	1.3 ± 0.5
Weight (kg)	54.4 ± 16.7	22.9 ± 11.6	11.8 ± 2.1
Height (cm)	160 ± 16	115 ± 24	?
Daily dose, R (mg/day)[a]	238 ± 72	157 ± 70	101 ± 26
Steady-state concentration, c (mg/liter)[a]	13.8 ± 8.5	9.2 ± 9.0	8.9 ± 6.6

[a] I do not know whether standard deviations for R and c were calculated from patient means or from all observations; this affects the extent to which they represent a mixture of interpatient and intrapatient variability. Purely as a broad description of the character of the data, the values shown should be adequate.

From Grasela et al. (2), with permission.

MODELS AND FORMULATIONS

These authors stated that, for any patient, the relation between R, the dose of phenytoin (mg/day), and C, the steady-state concentration (mg/liter), will be given by the Michaelis-Menten equation. That is to say, for observation i on patient j,

$$R_{ij} = \frac{V_{mj} \cdot C_{ij}}{K_{mj} + C_{ij}} \qquad (6)$$

V_{mj} is the maximum elimination rate (mg/day), and K_{mj} is the Michaelis-Menten constant (mg phenytoin per liter) for patient j. I accept the authors' claim that this is a *model* of the relation between R and C, which I take to mean that it is an exact equation for true dose and true concentration. Because R is a dose chosen for administration and C is a measured consequence of R, I find it more natural to write the dependence as

$$C_{ij} = \frac{K_{mj} \cdot R_{ij}}{V_{mj} - R_{ij}} \qquad (7)$$

If equations (6) and (7) are exact, in the sense of being disturbed only by errors of measuring C and R, there is little to choose between them; even so, my guess is that measurement errors in R, an administered dose, are small relative to those in C. To be a complete description of how a system behaves, the error structure ought also to be specified; this is certainly important if there are other sources of uncontrolled statistical variation. As the simplest possibility, I write the observed concentration as c_{ij}, where

$$c_{ij} = C_{ij} + \epsilon_{ij} \qquad (8)$$

C_{ij} is as in equation (7), and ϵ_{ij} has an error distribution with mean zero. One might take the distribution of ϵ to be Normal (or Gaussian), with variance either constant or dependent on the expectation C; however, any such statement about ϵ is almost certainly more a tentative *formulation* (*vide infra*) than part of the model, for I doubt whether biological theory can say any more than statistical theory on the necessity for the error distribution to have a particular form. Moreover, the error distribution will be troublesome if any doses R_{ij} approach closely to V_{mj}, but this complication is not important for the discussion that follows. [If I am wrong in preferring equation (7) to (6), I can still develop essentially the following argument in terms of an observed r_{ij} with expectation R_{ij}.]

Grasela et al. (2) sought to predict values for individuals by "modeling" the influences of various factors on V_{mj} and K_{mj}. They did so by regarding V_{mj} (and similarly K_{mj}) as a product of a standard value V_{m0} (or K_{m0}), with numerical factors representing effects of sex, age, body size, and origin of data; in fact, they wrote

$$\ln V_{mj} = \ln V_{m0} + \sum_{p=1}^{4} \ln FV_{mp} \qquad (9)$$

$$\ln K_{mj} = \ln K_{m0} + \sum_{p=1}^{4} \ln FK_{mp} \qquad (10)$$

where FV_{mp} and FK_{mp} are functions of the four factors stated. I see one point to dislike and another as a potential danger.

The practice of calling every equation used in relations among biological quantities a "model" is widespread, but I deplore it as bad and possibly misleading terminology. I think no one believes that equation (9) has the same status as equation (6); it is not a statement of exactly how V_{mj} is determined by sex, age, etc., but is rather a conveniently flexible expression that may be capable of describing much (but not all) of the patient-to-patient variation in V_{mj}.

The true determinant of V_{mj} is unlikely to be a simple addition of factors [the effect of sex may change with age, the effect of body size may be far more complicated than a single term in equation (9) can allow], and other factors (concomitant medication, diet, etc.) may be relevant. Equation (9) may be an adequate *mathematical formulation* for approximating to V_{mj} for the purpose in hand, but it cannot be a *model* of a complex chain of biological interrelations.

I believe the distinction between a model and a formulation to be of far more than philosophical importance. Newton and Mendel produced models of how sectors of our universe behave, excellent approximations to reality despite the subsequent need to generalize, modify, and refine. Both the originals and the improvements were powerful aids to fundamental understanding and to extrapolation far outside the range of observations. Michaelis-Menten may, for all I know, have the same authority. Equations (9) and (10) do not; to say otherwise would take us toward regarding every fitted regression, every linear dose–response relation as a model. Those who adopt this terminology do not always realize that, for some purposes, simple formulations with no theoretical basis may have the advantage. In a field better known to me, that of radioimmunoassay, models for the ratio of bound to free counts have been devised with the aid of the law of mass action applied to multiple binding sites. These may be important to the full understanding of binding, but, for routine estimation of hormones in samples from patients, cruder formulations are more satisfactory, because they are more amenable to sound estimation procedures. Rodbard (4) has surveyed many different functions that have been used as alternative formulations: Whereas specification of a model must always aim at theoretical correctness, choice of a formulation can depend on what is adequate for interpolatory purposes in a particular context. Finney (1) and Raab (3) have compared the four-parameter logistic formulation with the complicated mass-action model, and have shown the former to have the advantage for routine assays. On this analogy, I suggest that, even if improved theory were to lead to a theoretical model for the influence of age or body size on V_{mj} and K_{mj}, a formulation such as Grasela et al. (2) adopt could prove more suitable for predicting dosage intended to obtain a desired plasma concentration in a new patient—not least because a model might involve too many parameters for satisfactory estimation.

ESTIMATION

My second concern about Grasela's analysis was that I thought it to have employed a two-stage estimation. I have been brought up to distrust the calculation of a regression of y on x followed by calculation of a regression of z on the fitted values of y; it is a procedure capable of producing serious biases. Separate estimations for V_{mj} and K_{mj}, followed by insertion of the equations so obtained into equation (6) or (7), are similarly dangerous as a definitive analysis. I prefer to attempt simultaneous estimation of all parameters. Even though

V_{mj} and K_{mj} are believed independent in the whole population, chance association among the 322 patients may have important consequences. Moreover, assessment of errors of estimation and study of expanded or reduced formulations of the whole problem become easier when estimation is seen as an integrated process. Dr. Sheiner has told me that the actual analysis was essentially as I would advocate, and indeed he has outlined the underlying statistical model in his chapter entitled Modeling Pharmacokinetic/Pharmacodynamic Variability (*this volume*). Nevertheless, I see that issue as so important that I believe myself justified in describing my own outlook on the problem.

Grasela et al. (2) made several simplifying assertions about the factors they studied, presumably on the basis of previous experience and preliminary examination of the data. These are

1. The effect of age is determined solely by whether the patient is younger or older than 15 years.
2. The effect of body size on V_{mj} can be expressed by the factor

    $$(\text{weight}/70)^{\theta_W}(\text{height}/175)^{\theta_H}$$

    this ensuring that the factor is 1.0 for a "standard individual" who weighs 80 kg and is 175 cm tall. The parameters θ_W and θ_H are unknown; $\theta_W = 1$ and $\theta_H = 0$ give proportionality to weight, and $\theta_W = 0.425$ and $\theta_H = 0.725$ give approximate proportionality to surface area.
3. Size has no effect on K_{mj}.
4. The only distinction in sources of data needing recognition is that between Japanese and northern Europeans.

I do not query these assumptions, but a comprehensive analysis should be able to examine each of them. The authors introduced parameters for sex, age, and source in a manner equivalent to

$$FV_{m1} = \begin{cases} 1 & \text{for males} \\ \theta_{v1} & \text{for females} \end{cases} \qquad (11)$$

$$FK_{m1} = \begin{cases} 1 & \text{for males} \\ \theta_{k1} & \text{for females} \end{cases} \qquad (12)$$

$$FV_{m2} = \begin{cases} 1 & \text{if age} \leq 15 \\ \theta_{v2} & \text{if age} > 15 \end{cases} \qquad (13)$$

$$FK_{m2} = \begin{cases} 1 & \text{if age} \leq 15 \\ \theta_{k2} & \text{if age} > 15 \end{cases} \qquad (14)$$

$$FV_{m3} = (\text{weight}/70)^{\theta_W}(\text{height}/175)^{\theta_H} \qquad (15)$$

$$FK_{m3} = 1 \quad \text{identically} \qquad (16)$$

$$FV_{m4} = \begin{cases} 1 & \text{for Europeans} \\ \theta_{v4} & \text{for Japanese} \end{cases} \qquad (17)$$

$$FK_{m4} = \begin{cases} 1 & \text{for Europeans} \\ \theta_{k4} & \text{for Japanese} \end{cases} \qquad (18)$$

The dummy variables in equations (11)–(14), (17), and (18) are a standard device for taking account of subclassifications of regression data. An obvious method of analysis would be first to obtain numerical values for V_{mj} and K_{mj} for each patient. Most of the 322 patients contributed only two pairs of R and C values, so that equation (6) would uniquely determine estimates of V_{mj} and K_{mj}. Next, equations (9) and (10) might be fitted by least squares, assuming constant variance for all log V_{mj} or log K_{mj} and disregarding any possible correlation of V_{mj} with K_{mj}. Equation (9) is linear in θ_W and θ_H and the logarithms of the other θ parameters, so that the calculations can easily be carried out as a multiple-regression analysis with the dummy variables for sex, age, and source. Subsequently, the values for V_{mj} and K_{mj} predicted by these two fitted equations for any specified patient could be regarded as appropriate for insertion in the Michaelis-Menten equation for that patient.

I dislike this procedure for several reasons. One is the use of expectations of V_{mj} and K_{mj} as input into equations (6) and (7). Equation (9) is at best a representation of an average V_{mj} predicted from other factors; if body size, for example, affects the parameters of the Michaelis-Menten equation, is it not likely to do so on an individual basis, rather than merely to be mediated through the average V_{mj} for a specified size? Second, I see little basis for an error structure in equations (9) and (10); moreover, if any statement is to be made about errors in C predicted from R, there is awkwardness in having population variances in V_{mj} and K_{mj} as contributors, and it is not easy to see how these combine with the error variance implied by equation (8). Third, no allowance is made for sample correlation of V_{mj} and K_{mj}, which could cause serious distortion in any final assessment of error variance. In so large a sample, trouble from this last source is unlikely unless there exists a true interperson correlation of V_{mj} and K_{mj}. Can even that possibility be rejected *a priori*?

My preference would be to express equations (9) and (10) as

$$V_{mj} = V_{m0}(FV_{m1})(FV_{m2})(FV_{m3})(FV_{m4}) \tag{19}$$

$$K_{mj} = K_{m0}(FK_{m1})(FK_{m2})(FK_{m3})(FK_{m4}) \tag{20}$$

with definitions as in equations (11)–(18), write these into equation (7), and then minimize

$$\sum_i \sum_j (c_{ij} - C_{ij})^2 \tag{21}$$

where c_{ij} is the observed concentration corresponding to the applied dosage R_{ij}. If I made a preliminary study of the data, I might infer that σ^2 increases markedly as C increases, and in consequence prefer to work with least squares on $\ln(c_{ij})$ and $\ln(C_{ij})$ or to use weighted least squares in equation (21). Grasela et al. (2) used a maximum-likelihood estimation technique, which may indeed be more appropriate to these data. This analysis may look unpleasant. It involves estimating nine parameters, which enter C_{ij} nonlinearly and therefore demand an iterative minimization. However, there ought to be no technical difficulty with any computer for which a good nonlinear optimization subroutine is available; the process may be relatively slow, because at each step summation over 780 observations is needed. The advantage is that the whole analysis is now well integrated, so that an (asymptotic) variance-covariance matrix for all parameters (V_{m0}, K_{m0}, and the other θ's) is obtained and can be used in assessing the precision of prediction for other patients.

Of course, it is easy to perform various modified analyses. For example, the effect of sex can be constrained to be zero by writing $\theta_{v1} = 1$ and $\theta_{k1} = 1$; differences in residual sums of squares permit approximate significance tests. Having a suspicious attitude toward assumptions, I would want to extend the analysis by defining FK_{m3} analogous to FV_{m3} or by introducing another parameter to differentiate between the English and German sources. I think it likely that Grasela et al. (2) explored their data in this way before deciding on the limitations implicit in equations (11) to (18). Further variations in parametric formulation are easily made in order to accommodate not only such possibilities as a more complicated age effect but also a dependence of size parameters on whether the patient is European or Japanese and other interactions. My chief concern is to urge the need to look at a single comprehensive analysis appropriate to a full formulation of the data in terms of parameters.

Finally, I want to draw attention to strengths and weaknesses of estimation procedures. Maximum likelihood has various optimal properties for large data sets. The estimates are consistent, in the sense that they tend to the true values as the number of observations increases; also, the error distribution tends to normality, with a variance matrix obtainable from the data. Iteratively weighted least squares does not in general have the consistency property, although commonly the numerical estimates are close to those from maximum likelihood. But consistency is meaningful only if the model or formulation is correctly specified. Moreover, large-sample optimal properties need not hold for small sets of data—and in general we do not know whether 100 or 100,000 observations is about the minimum that can be taken as "large"! In all but the simplest situations, no alternative is available, but both statisticians and users of statistics need to be aware of the logical weaknesses.

CONCLUSIONS

As compared with any two-stage analysis, I believe analysis along the lines of the preceding section to be conceptually easier, more easily adapted to changing needs, and above all nearer to using a correct formulation of the pattern of variability; the price is almost certainly an increase in computer time. It would be gratifying to be able to state conditions under which, for a new problem, the two methods will give results that for practical purposes are the same. I see little prospect of this without expenditure of human time and computer time greater than for what I regard as the better method.

SUMMARY

I have used an article on steady-state pharmacokinetics of phenytoin to illustrate two themes. I begin by confessing my near-total ignorance of pharmacokinetics, whence it follows that my themes are based on other experience.

First, I emphasize the need to distinguish between a (mathematical or statistical) *model* of a process that attempts to be a symbolic representation of exactly what is happening and a *formulation* in symbols that should prove adequate for particular interpolatory purposes and that is subject to tests of its adequacy. Second, I urge the desirability of putting together the various parts of a formulation (including some that may be model-like) into a comprehensive statement of how observations are represented by functions of parameters and random errors. Only then should standard estimation methods (such as least squares or maximum likelihood) be used to estimate all parameters and the variance–covariance structure of the estimates. This may be impracticable in some more complicated problems, but it should always be in mind as an ideal.

REFERENCES

1. Finney, D.J. (1983): Response curves for radioimmunoassay. *Clin. Chem.*, 29:1762–1766.
2. Grasela, T.H., Sheiner, L.B., Rambeck, B., Boenigk, H.E., Dunlop, A., Mullen, P.W., Wadsworth, J., Richens, A., Ishizaki, T., Chiba, K., Miura, H., Minagawa, K., Blain, P.G., Mucklow, J.C., Bacon, C.T., and Rawlins, M. (1983): Steady-state pharmacokinetics of phenytoin from routinely collected patient data. *Clin. Pharmacokinet.*, 8:355–364.
3. Raab, G.M. (1983): A comparison of logistic and mass-action curves for radioimmunoassay data. *Clin. Chem.*, 29:1757–1761.
4. Rodbard, D. (1978): Data processing for radioimmunoassays: An overview. In: *Clinical Immunochemistry*, edited by S. Natelson, A.J. Pesce, and A.A. Dietz, pp. 477–494. American Association for Clinical Chemistry, Washington, D.C.

DISCUSSION

Discussant 1 (D1): I wonder about single comprehensive analyses. I remember about 15 to 20 years ago I was marveling at the insight that "old-fashioned" biochemists obtained turning enzyme-kinetic data inside out: plotting, replotting, etc. The insight they gained during this process was quite remarkable, and I suspect their quantitative results were probably not off the mark very much. Nowadays, studies often generate large data sets, and analysts may immediately perform a huge analysis of variance, but not be able to interpret it. I wonder whether or not having access to computers, which offer the temptation of doing large, comprehensive but misguided analyses, may not actually cause us to be losing something.

Speaker (S): I certainly will not disagree with that. We have, I think, no good rules for how you look at data and gain insight. Except perhaps the first rule: "You begin by being rather clever." That is not a very easy rule to implement, for some of us. Nevertheless, I would suggest that, important as it is to have the bright ideas, most important of all, after you have had the bright ideas, is to go back to the data, or to extend the data set and undertake a more comprehensive analysis, so that estimates of whatever it is you want to estimate will be most efficient. The way this step is done may be entirely different from the "being clever" step; conceivably, on occasion, it will eventually tell you that your initial insight was wrong.

D2: I appreciate what you said about coefficients of variation, but in certain circumstances it is certainly a useful parameter, it is not?

S: Oh yes. What I argue against is the totally uncritical use of the coefficient of variation that may seem to be encouraged by some textbooks on statistics. The uncritical use can lean to such abuses as calculating a coefficient of variation, for example, for temperatures. Should this be in degrees Celsius or in degrees absolute? It makes a lot of difference. You will even find the abuse going still further. Consider an observation on the change of some quantity, where quite a number are negative, but rather more are positive. Consequently their mean is a small positive number, and the coefficient of variation may very well be 300%. That, I would maintain, is totally meaningless.

*Variability in Drug Therapy:
Description, Estimation, and Control,*
edited by M. Rowland et al.
Raven Press, New York © 1985.

Variability in Animal and Human Pharmacodynamic Studies

Gerhard Levy

Department of Pharmaceutics, School of Pharmacy, State University of New York at Buffalo, Amherst, New York 14260

Variability in the pharmacokinetic characteristics of drugs due to genetic, pathophysiologic, and environmental factors is well recognized and constitutes the basis for the monitoring and control of therapeutic plasma concentrations of a number of widely used medicinal agents (7,8). Much less attention has been given to assessment of the variability in the relationship between drug concentration and pharmacologic response. In fact, the prevailing dogma that the intensity of a pharmacologic effect is usually better correlated with drug concentration in plasma than with the drug's dose is often interpreted to mean that most of the variability in the pharmacologic response to a drug is due to pharmacokinetics. That reasoning is unwarranted, if only because so little is known about interindividual and intraindividual differences in the pharmacodynamics of drugs. It would seem that the proteins that constitute the drug receptors should be as sensitive to genetic or environmental factors as are the proteins that catalyze drug biotransformation reactions or serve as components of specialized transport systems for drugs.

Interestingly, none of the 10 most prescribed (based on acquisition cost) drugs in the United States during 1983 is among those for which plasma-concentration monitoring is customary or considered advisable (Table 1). There are different reasons for this, but an important one that applies at least to the three nonsteroidal, nonsalicylate antiinflammatory agents on the list is that the variability in their pharmacodynamic characteristics is greater than the variability in their pharmacokinetics. That may not be the case for all drugs in this class, nor is this always a good reason not to undertake pharmacokinetic monitoring, as experience with benoxaprofen has shown. The immediate problem presented by the relative lack of pharmacodynamic information (concentration–effect relationships as well as their variability) is that it greatly limits our ability to interpret and utilize pharmacokinetic data. For example, an awareness of the effect of renal failure on the elimination kinetics of a drug is not sufficient for optimizing the dosing regimen for an anephric patient unless the

TABLE 1. *Most prescribed drug products in the United States, 1983*[a]

Cimetidine, SK&F
Propranolol, Ayerst
Hydrochlorothiazide-triamterene, SK&F
Ibuprofen, Upjohn
Methyldopa, Merck
Diazepam, Roche
Piroxicam, Pfizer
Cephalexin, Dista
Naproxen, Syntex
Chlorpropamide, Pfizer

[a] Based on retail acquisition cost.
Source: APhA Weekly, March 30, 1984.

effect of renal failure on the drug's therapeutic plasma-concentration range is known. In the case of the barbiturates, we have found that renal failure is associated with increased sensitivity to the hypnotic effects of these drugs (2). The clinical implications of interindividual differences in pharmacokinetics and of altered bioavailability, and the potential advantages of controlled drug delivery, cannot be determined without knowing the nature and degree of variability of the relationship between drug concentration and pharmacologic effect.

Measurements of pharmacologic effects are usually more difficult than determinations of drug concentrations. This is one reason why so little information is available on pharmacodynamic variability. However, the typically wide range of 95% confidence limits of LD_{50} and ED_{50} values provides a clue that this variability is not trivial. We now know that receptor density is subject to rapid up- or down-regulation in response to environmental factors, another reason for expecting appreciable interindividual and intraindividual variations in pharmacodynamics. There have been examples of genetically based differences in responses to drugs, notably the hereditary transmission of pronounced resistance to the anticoagulant effect of the coumarin anticoagulants that is unrelated to and independent of any change in their pharmacokinetics (11).

A major problem in determining pharmacodynamic variability, in addition to the difficulty of measuring most pharmacologic effects in a graded manner, is that of distinguishing between pharmacodynamic and pharmacokinetic variabilities. If, for example, a certain pharmacologic effect arises, wholly or in part, from a minor metabolite of a drug, then a twofold or threefold increase in the formation of that metabolite could cause a substantial increase in pharmacologic effect without any apparent change in the drug's pharmacokinetics. The increased pharmacologic effect may be interpreted as an example of pharmacodynamic rather than pharmacokinetic variability if the role of the quantitatively minor metabolite has not been recognized. We have developed experimental strategy to avoid or minimize this kind of problem as well as other complexities arising from pharmacokinetic factors, such as variability in clearance, distribution, protein binding, and formation or elimination of interactive metabolites (3). This strategy involves intravenous infusion of the drug at various rates to the onset of a defined pharmacologic endpoint and, in the case of drugs that act on the central nervous system (CNS), sampling of blood, cerebrospinal fluid, and brain tissue for determination of drug concentrations at onset of action. The animals must obviously be killed to obtain brain tissue and can only be studied once. Consequently, there remains the problem of assessing intraindividual variability, which requires that sampling be limited to those tissues and fluids that can be obtained from animals without affecting their survival and from humans without causing them harm. Moreover, it is often difficult to distinguish pharmacodynamic variability from methodologic variability due to instrumentation or technique.

A striking example of pharmacodynamic variability in humans is the concentration of disoprofol in the blood necessary to produce general anesthesia (1). When 6 subjects were given a 1-mg/kg injection followed repeatedly by the same dose on awakening, the mean blood concentration on awakening varied fourfold between subjects, but very little within subjects (Table 2). In a larger group of subjects, the concentrations varied more than 10-fold between subjects (1). The fact that the disoprofol concentration in the blood at the time of awakening was apparently independent of the size of the dose (1–3 mg/kg) and the number of consecutive doses (up to 11) provides a strong indication that the interindividual differences in effective concentrations are not due to active or interactive metabolite(s).

What follows are examples of our own experiences with respect to interindividual and intraindividual variations in the pharmacodynamics of drugs. Most of the studies to be described were not originally designed or intended to explore variability per se, except that considerable care was taken to distinguish between pharmacokinetic and pharmacodynamic perturbations, and an effort was made, whenever possible, to assess intraindividual variability. We believe that studies of interindividual variability are of limited usefulness unless it can be shown that this variability is consistent and reproducible, i.e., that it is not an artifact of experimental technique.

TABLE 2. *Mean waking concentrations of disoprofol in patients given 1 mg/kg, followed by the same dose repeated at each awakening*

Subject	Concentration (μg/ml) Mean	SE	Number of doses
1	2.16	0.12	9
2	1.48	0.20	6
3	1.04	0.07	6
4	0.51	0.05	10
5	1.30	0.24	7
6	1.58	0.15	11

From Adam et al. (1), with permission.

HEPARIN

Clinical and experimental studies suggest that the therapeutic efficacy of heparin can be optimized by adjusting the rate of administration of this parenteral anticoagulant to maintain the activated partial thromboplastin time (APTT), an index of the blood clotting rate, within a defined range. This optimization may also decrease the incidence of hemorrhagic complications. Clinical studies have shown that heparin is subject to considerable variability in both its pharmacokinetic and pharmacodynamic characteristics (4). We carried out a study to assess the magnitude of interindividual and intraindividual variations in the relationships between heparin concentration and anticoagulant effect in normal adults and to determine if these variations are associated with, and therefore predictable from, certain physiologic characteristics of individual subjects (17). Citrated plasma was obtained from 12 men and 5 women, 21 to 35 years old. Heparin was added to the plasma to yield concentrations of 0.05 to 1.0 U/ml, and the APTT was determined. These studies were repeated once or twice over 65 days. Baseline APTT values (i.e., APTT without added heparin) ranged from 25.6 to 36.2 sec and showed little intrasubject variation

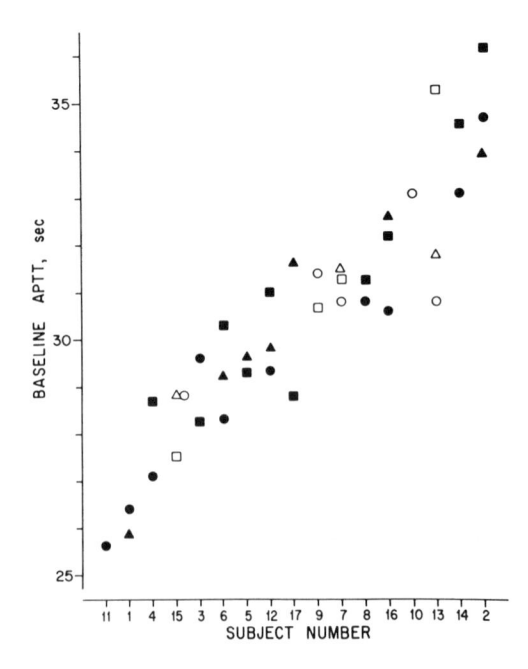

FIG. 1. Intersubject and intrasubject variability of baseline APTT in normal subjects: men (*filled symbols*); women (*open symbols*); day 1 (*circles*); day 38 (*squares*); day 65 (*triangles*). (From Whitfield and Levy, ref. 17, with permission.)

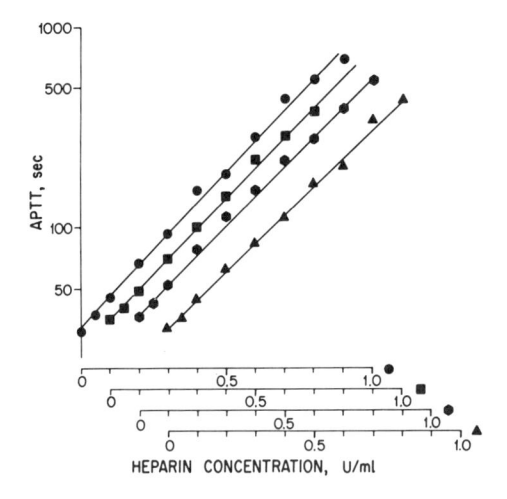

FIG. 2. Relationship between APTT and concentration of added heparin in the plasma of a normal female subject: first determination (*circles*); second determination (*squares*) (plasma obtained 38 days later); third determination (*triangles*) (plasma obtained 65 days after first determination); results obtained with blood taken from the left arm on day 38 (*hexagons*) (the other blood samples were taken from the right arm). Note that the abscissa for each curve is displaced relative to the others for clarity. (From Whitfield and Levy, ref. 17, with permission.)

(Fig. 1). There was an excellent linear relationship between ln APTT and heparin concentration in the 0.05- to 0.8-U/ml range that was very reproducible in any given subject (Fig. 2). The slope value for this relationship ranged from 1.51 to 3.88 ml/U (Fig. 3). Multiple linear-regression analysis revealed a linear relationship between observed slope values and slope values calculated as a function of both hematocrit and base-line APTT. Age, weight, and the concentrations of various plasma proteins did not contribute significantly to the predictability of the slope.

The results of this study gave us confidence to extend the investigation to hospitalized patients and pregnant women whose physiologic status changes with time and therefore does not allow for assessments of intraindividual variation (16,18). The blood coagulation process is so complex, involving a cascade of interrelated reactions, that the major determinants of the observed variability differ depending on the type of individuals being studied. This aspect of the variability of heparin pharmacodynamics will not be discussed here. The importance of the heparin data in the context of this overview is that they represent a definitive example of pharmacodynamic variability inasmuch as pharmacokinetic variability could be excluded by adding known concentrations of heparin to plasma *in vitro*. Heparin is a unique drug in this respect, because it is a direct anticoagulant whose effect can be measured *in vitro,* i.e., under conditions in which distribution, metabolism, and excretion of the drug are irrelevant.

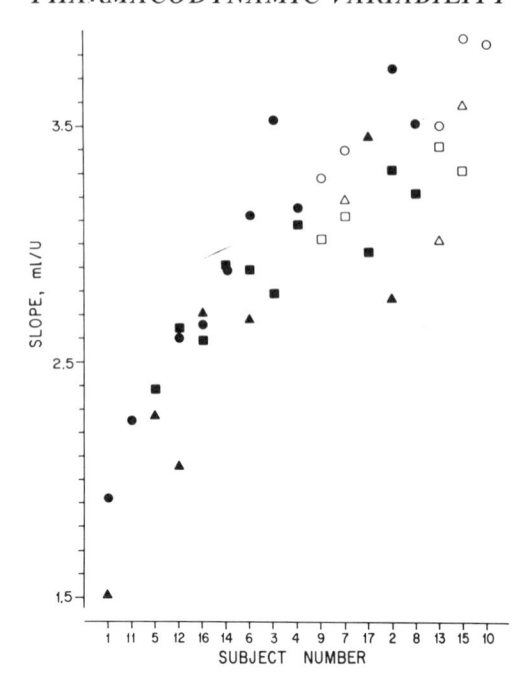

FIG. 3. Intersubject and intrasubject variability in normal subjects of the slope of the regression line relating ln APTT to concentration of added heparin in plasma. See legend to Fig. 1 for explanation of symbols. (From Whitfield and Levy, ref. 17, with permission.)

COUMARIN ANTICOAGULANTS

The indirectly acting coumarin anticoagulants can be studied only *in vivo*. They act by inhibiting the synthesis of the vitamin-K-dependent clotting factors II, VII, IX, and X. Their overall effect can be characterized in terms of the degree of inhibition of the synthesis rate of prothrombin-complex activity (10). There is an essentially linear, negative relationship between the synthesis rate of prothrombin-complex activity and the logarithm of the coumarin anticoagulant concentration in plasma, a relationship that can be characterized by its slope and intercept values. We determined these values for dicumarol in 11 normal subjects, including three separate determinations in 1 subject over 8 months (12). Eight of these subjects were restudied after they had received the microsomal enzyme inducer heptabarbital for 4 days, a treatment that increased the metabolic clearance of dicumarol but did not affect the relationship between inhibition of the synthesis rate of prothrombin-complex activity and plasma dicumarol concentration. Thus, these data could be used to assess intraindividual variability (Fig. 4). There were very large interindividual differences in slope values ($\simeq$ 10-fold), whereas the intersubject variability of the intercept values (drug concentration at zero synthesis rate) was much less pro-

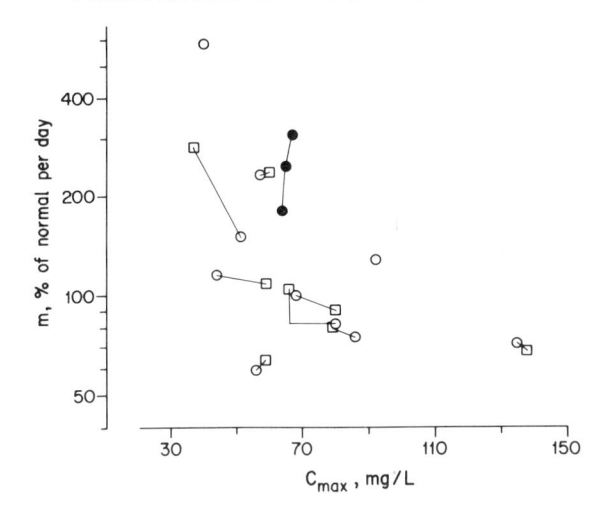

FIG. 4. Variability in the relationship between anticoagulant effect and plasma concentration of dicumarol in normal subjects. The constant $-m$ is the slope of the regression line for this relationship; C_{max} is the plasma concentration when the regression line is extrapolated to the maximum effect, i.e., when synthesis of vitamin-K-dependent clotting factors is completely inhibited: control experiments (*circles*); experiments after treatment with heptabarbital (*squares*). One subject (*filled circles*) participated in three control experiments over 8 months. The lines connect data points for a given subject. (Adapted from O'Reilly et al., ref. 12).

nounced ($\simeq$ threefold). The intraindividual differences were considerably smaller than the differences between subjects.

Interindividual variability of the slope value is of appreciable clinical significance. Individuals showing a steep slope for the relationship between drug concentration and anticoagulant effect (high slope value) will be very sensitive to small changes in drug concentration; it will be difficult to maintain their prothrombin times in the therapeutic range. The interindividual differences in the intercept values have mainly a pharmacokinetic rather than a pharmacodynamic basis, being due primarily to differences in plasma protein binding of the drug. Even the slope values are correlated with the degree of plasma protein binding (13,19), but a plot of anticoagulant effect versus the logarithm of the concentration of unbound drug has the same slope as a plot based on total concentration, because the free fractions of dicumarol and warfarin in plasma or serum are independent of concentration over the therapeutic concentration ranges of these drugs.

SUCCINYLCHOLINE

The profile of pharmacologic activity versus time for this neuromuscular blocking agent has been studied in considerable detail under various clinical conditions. One of these investigations revealed appreciable interindividual differences in duration of the effect of a 40-mg/m² dose in a group of 9 infants (15). To determine if these differences were pharmacokinetic or pharmacodynamic, the clinical data were analyzed on the basis of the following relationships (6):

$$t = \frac{2.3}{k} (\log A^0 - \log A_{min}) \quad (1)$$

$$R_e = \frac{km}{2.3} \quad (2)$$

which, when combined, rearranged, and simplified, yield

$$tR_e = m(\log A^0 - \log A_{min}) \quad (3)$$

where t is the duration of effect, R_e is the rate of decline of the effect, k is the apparent first-order elimination-rate constant of the drug, A^0 is the dose, A_{min} is the minimum effective amount of drug in the body, and m is the slope of a plot of intensity of effect versus the logarithm of the amount of drug in the body. The major assumptions underlying these equations are that the drug is administered by rapid injection, distributes instantaneously in the body, is eliminated by apparent first-order kinetics, is inactivated on biotransformation, and exhibits an essentially linear relationship between intensity of effect and the logarithm of the amount of drug in the body over the clinically relevant range. The equations based on these assumptions apply to the neuromuscular blocking effect of succinylcholine (5).

Recognizing that in these equations R_e is directly proportional to k, and t is inversely proportional to k, it is evident that the product of t and R_e is independent of k. Thus, equation (3) can be used to determine if the interindividual differences in duration of action of succinylcholine in the group of 9 infants

TABLE 3. *Pharmacokinetic analysis of neuromuscular blocking effects of succinylcholine in 9 infants*

Infant No.	Age (days)	Duration of effect (min)	Rate of decline of effect (% min⁻¹)	tR_e (%)[a]
11	28	5	40	200
10	24	6	40	240
14	37	6	40	240
15	38	6	40	240
7	10	7	20	140
4	3	9	27	243
2	1	12	27	324
5	10	14	16	224
8	20	26	9	234

[a] The average tR_e value in 20 adults was 230%.
From Levy (6), with permission, based on data of Walts and Dillon (15).

have a pharmacokinetic or pharmacodynamic basis. As shown in Table 3, all but 2 of the infants yielded tR_e values that were normal, i.e., equal to those of adults. This means that the differences in duration of effect in those 7 infants were due to corresponding differences in elimination kinetics of the drug. The 2 infants with unusual tR_e values had unusual m or A_{min} values [see equation (3)]; they differed pharmacodynamically from the other infants.

CNS-ACTIVE DRUGS

In the course of a series of studies on the effects of various diseases on relationships between drug concentration and pharmacologic activity in animal models, we have obtained data for control groups that provide some interesting information about longitudinal pharmacodynamic variability (9). Briefly, groups of adult, female, inbred Lewis rats (typically 8 animals per group) were infused intravenously with phenobarbital or ethanol until they lost their righting reflex, or with metrazol until the onset of maximal seizure. These infusions were typically between 10 and 40 min in duration, during which time the rats were on a heating pad to maintain normal body temperature. All experiments with any one drug were performed at the same time of day, and the pharmacologic endpoint was determined, with few exceptions, by the same investigator. Thus, these studies were performed under relatively ideal conditions, except that some of the control groups were subjected to sham surgery 2 days before the study (control for ureter ligation) or 5 days before the study (control for bile duct ligation), whereas other control groups received an i.v. or i.p. injection of normal saline solution or oral doses of sesame oil during the week before the pharmacologic study.

Some of the results obtained in 11 studies with phenobarbital over 15 months are summarized in Fig. 5. The average serum phenobarbital concentrations at onset of loss of righting reflex varied only slightly despite the chang-

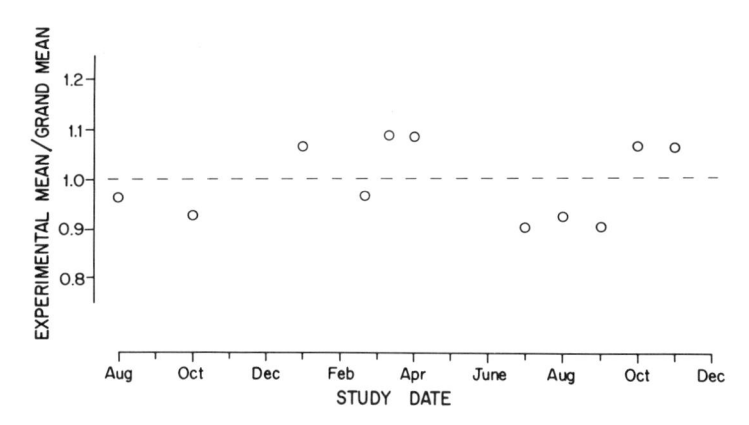

FIG. 5. Relative mean serum concentrations of phenobarbital in groups of 5 to 10 female Lewis rats at onset of loss of righting reflex, determined over 15 months.

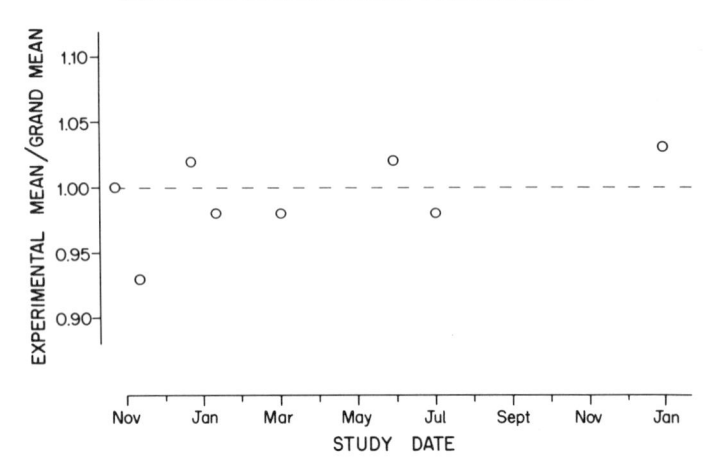

FIG. 6. Relative mean serum concentrations of ethanol in groups of 6 to 8 female Lewis rats at onset of loss of righting reflex, determined over 14 months.

ing seasons and the small number of rats per group; the individual means were within ±10% of the grand mean. These results are very encouraging in that they show good pharmacodynamic reproducibility over a long period of time. It should be noted that all animals were obtained from the same supplier, who was, however, located in another city, so that the animals had to be shipped to us. It is our practice not to use animals for research until at least 1 week after receipt.

The results of similar investigations with ethanol are summarized in Fig. 6. Eight studies performed over 14 months showed excellent reproducibility; except for one study on only 6 rats the mean serum ethanol concentrations at onset of loss of righting reflex were within ±3% of the grand mean. The very rapid distribution of ethanol to the CNS may be largely responsible for these very consistent results.

We have more limited experience with the CNS stimulant metrazol (pentylenetetrazol). This drug elicits a seizure response when administered in appropriate doses. Using a slow infusion (rather than the typical i.p. injection) to produce seizures, serum concentrations at the onset of maximal seizure were determined in seven studies over 10 months (Fig. 7). With the exception of the first experiment on only 5 animals, the mean concentrations were within ±10% of the grand mean. Thus, this drug has also shown good pharmacodynamic reproducibility in our hands. As in the other studies described in this section, some of the groups of animals were subjected to sham surgery or received saline injections during the week before the study.

CONCLUSIONS

It is at least as important to determine variability in the pharmacodynamics as in the pharmacokinetics of drugs. There is not much point in adjusting a pa-

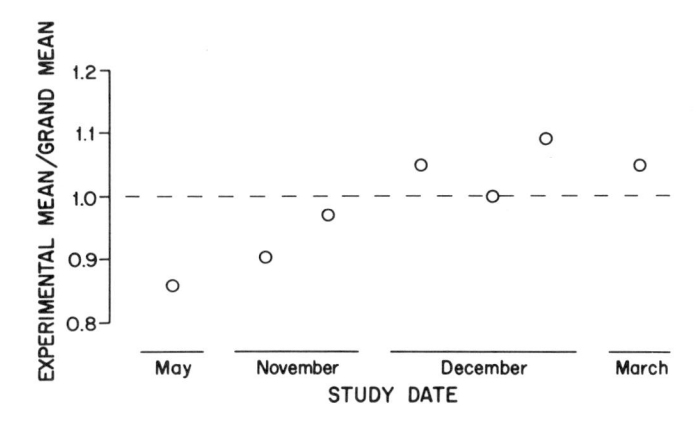

FIG. 7. Relative mean serum concentrations of metrazol in groups of 5 to 11 female Lewis rats at onset of maximal seizure, determined over 10 months.

tient's drug dosage regimen in accordance with that individual's pharmacokinetics to achieve a population-average therapeutic drug concentration if the physiologic perturbations responsible for the unusual pharmacokinetics have also altered the relationhip between drug concentration and pharmacologic activity in that patient. In the same context, experimental or clinical data thought to be indicative of interindividual pharmacodynamic variability must be supported by demonstrating intraindividual consistency. If the latter cannot be done, then a legitimate question can be raised whether the presumed interindividual variability is real or only apparent and reflective of methodologic shortcomings. Unlike chemical assays, pharmacologic measurements cannot usually be repeated under identical conditions; chemical assays can be done in duplicate or triplicate, but most pharmacologic-response measurements can be done only one after the other, and there is no way of distinguishing between methodologic variability and changes in the physiologic status of an animal or a patient with time.

Our experience in clinical and animal studies has shown that with practice and careful attention to detail, intraindividual variability in pharmacodynamics, as in pharmacokinetics, is not very pronounced in most cases. This conclusion is obviously limited to the drugs and conditions that we have investigated, but it has reinforced our view that the most important task in studies of pharmacodynamic variability is to develop effective methods for measurements of graded pharmacologic responses. This is not necessarily a matter of using sophisticated instrumentation but of recognizing and controlling incidental variables capable of affecting pharmacologic responses.

Finally, it is important to reemphasize the need to distinguish clearly between the pharmacokinetics and pharmacodynamics of a drug. A shift in the relationship between plasma drug concentration and pharmacologic activity to a lower concentration range in a cirrhotic patient is not a pharmacodynamic change if it is attributable entirely to decreased plasma protein binding! As

Sweeney (14) has stated, "pharmacodynamic deviations from 'normal' imply drug receptors which respond in an unusual fashion despite exposure to usual levels of drug." One highly regarded textbook on pharmacology contains a chapter titled "The Time Course of Drug Action" that consists entirely of pharmacokinetic material without any specific reference to the time course of pharmacologic activity! Only by keeping our semantics and our thinking clearly focused and defined will we be able to develop the appropriate protocols for the so very important assessments of pharmacodynamic variability.

ACKNOWLEDGMENT

Supported in part by grant GM-20852 from the Institute of General Medical Sciences, National Institutes of Health.

REFERENCES

1. Adam, H.K., Kay, B., and Douglas, E.J. (1982): Blood disoprofol levels in anaesthetised patients: Correlation of concentrations after single or repeated doses with hypnotic activity. *Anaesthesia*, 37:536–540.
2. Danhof, M., Hisaoka, M., and Levy, G. (1984): Kinetics of drug action in disease states. II. Effect of experimental renal dysfunction on phenobarbital concentrations in rats at onset of loss of righting reflex. *J. Pharmacol. Exp. Ther.*, 230:627–631.
3. Danhof, M., and Levy, G. (1983): Kinetics of drug action in disease states. I. Effect of infusion rate on phenobarbital concentrations in serum, brain and cerebrospinal fluid of normal rats at onset of loss of righting reflex. *J. Pharmacol. Exp. Ther.*, 229:1–7.
4. Hirsh, J., Van Aken, W.G., Gallus, A.S., Dollery, C.T., Cade, J.F., and Yung, W.L. (1975): Heparin kinetics in venous thrombosis and pulmonary embolism. *Circulation*, 53:691–695.
5. Levy, G. (1967): Kinetics of pharmacologic activity of succinylcholine in man. *J. Pharm. Sci.*, 56:1687–1688.
6. Levy, G. (1970): Pharmacokinetics of succinylcholine in newborns. *Anesthesiology*, 32:551–552.
7. Levy, G. (1974): Orientation to clinical pharmacokinetics. In: *Clinical Pharmacokinetics—A Symposium*, edited by G. Levy, pp. 1–9. American Pharmaceutical Association, Washington, D.C.
8. Levy, G. (1980): Applied pharmacokinetics—a prospectus. In: *Applied Pharmacokinetics*, edited by W.E. Evans, J.J. Schentag, and W.J. Jusko, pp. 1–3. Applied Therapeutics, San Fancisco.
9. Levy, G., Danhof, M., Hisaoka, M., and Ramzan, I. (1985): Variability in the pharmacodynamics of phenobarbital, ethanol, and pentylenetetrazol in normal rats. (*in press*).
10. Nagashima, R., O'Reilly, R.A., and Levy, G. (1969): Kinetics of pharmacologic effects in man: The anticoagulant action of warfarin. *Clin. Pharmacol. Ther.*, 10:22–35.
11. O'Reilly, R.A., Aggeler, P.M., Hoag, M.S., Leong, L.S., and Kropatkin, M.L. (1964): Hereditary transmission of exceptional resistance to coumarin anticoagulant drugs: The first reported kindred. *N. Engl. J. Med.*, 271:809–815.
12. O'Reilly, R.A., Levy, G., and Keech, G.M. (1970): Kinetics of the anticoagulant effect of bishydroxycoumarin in man. *Clin. Pharmacol. Ther.*, 11:378–384.
13. Routledge, P.A., Chapman, P.H., Davies, D.M., and Rawlins, M.D. (1979): Pharmacokinetics and pharmacodynamics of warfarin at steady state. *Br. J. Clin. Pharmacol.*, 8:243–247.
14. Sweeney, G.D. (1983): Variability in the human drug response. *Thromb. Res.* [*Suppl. IV*], pp. 3–15.

15. Walts, L.F., and Dillon, J.B. (1969): The response of newborns to succinylcholine and d-tubocurarine. *Anesthesiology,* 31:35–38.
16. Whitfield, L.R., Lele, A.S., and Levy, G. (1983): Effect of pregnancy on the relationship between concentration and anticoagulant action of heparin. *Clin. Pharmacol. Ther.,* 34:23–28.
17. Whitfield, L.R., and Levy, G. (1980): Relationship between concentration and anticoagulant effect of heparin in plasma of normal subjects: Magnitude and predictability of interindividual differences. *Clin. Pharmacol. Ther.,* 28:509–516.
18. Whitfield, L.R., Schentag, J.J., and Levy, G. (1982): Relationship between concentration and anticoagulant effect of heparin in plasma of hospitalized patients: Magnitude and predictability of interindividual differences. *Clin. Pharmacol. Ther.,* 32:503–516.
19. Yacobi, A., and Levy, G. (1977): Comparative pharmacokinetics of coumarin anticoagulants. XXVIII: Predictive identification of rats with relatively steep serum warfarin concentration–anticoagulant response characteristics. *J. Pharm. Sci.,* 66:145–146.

DISCUSSION

Discussant 1 (D1): The literature contains a number of studies that quite clearly show that for certain drugs (antiepileptics and antidepressants), a better relationship exists between plasma concentration and pharmacological effect than between the dose prescribed and ingested and the pharmacological effect. It is important to have as sharp a clinical end point as possible. I'm not sure that the awakening after anesthesia is a sharp end point. A relatively sharp end point was used by McDevitt et al. (2), who studied the effects of β-agonists during treatment with β-blockers. They found that after accounting for differences between individuals in plasma protein binding, there was only a twofold variability that remained to be explained. There have been rather few studies showing that there are marked interindividual differences in pharmacodynamic effects. Most studies done so far have not used unbound drug concentrations.

Speaker (S): The fact that there is usually a better correlation between concentration and response than between dose and response has been misinterpreted to suggest that there is little interindividual variability in pharmacodynamics. That is not true. Look at the theophylline data of Mitenko and Ogilvie (3). Look at any clinical experience with theophylline. There are some people who can be managed by 4 or 5 mg/liter whereas others need a 20-mg/liter plasma concentration. Sharpness of a pharmacologic end point is related to the rate of change of drug concentrations. If the rate of change is high, the end point is usually sharper. But then you have difficulties in determining the correct concentration; the timing of the blood sample now becomes very important.

D1: I would still like to make the point that I have not run into too many good data that can be interpreted as evidence for marked variability at the "receptor level."

S: There is a 10-fold variation in the effective blood concentrations of diisopropyl phenol (1).

D2: According to my experience with different drugs, many times the interindividual variability is 10-fold, especially with drugs that act indirectly. I mean, if you have a drug that works directly, e.g., on an alpha-receptor, you might see a smaller variability than if you are working with a drug that produces its effect indirectly, e.g., through release of transmitters.

S: To get the pharmacodynamic information is the important thing. People are staying away from pharmacodynamic measurements simply because they are too difficult to carry out. You can't argue the thing away in the absence of information, and it doesn't make any sense to emphasize pharmacokinetics and to remain ignorant of the magnitude of variability in the pharmacodynamics of a drug.

D3: What do you think about chronopharmacology as an explanation for the variability in pharmacodynamic effects?

S: Our studies on animals done over 16 months were always performed within the same 3-hr time frame. We think that this is important. In humans it depends on what type of response one is measuring.

REFERENCES

1. Adam, H.K., Kay, B., and Douglas, E.J. (1982): Blood disoprofol levels in anaesthetised patients: Correlation of concentrations after single or repeated doses with hypnotic activity. *Anaesthesia,* 37:536–540.
2. McDevitt, D.G., Frisk-Holmberg, M., Hollifield, J.W., and Shand, D.G. (1976): Plasma binding and the affinity of propranolol for a beta receptor in man. *Clin. Pharmacol. Ther.,* 20:152–157.
3. Mitenko, P.A., and Ogilvie, R.I. (1973): Rational intravenous doses of theophylline. *N. Engl. J. Med.,* 289:600–603.

Variability in Drug Therapy:
Description, Estimation, and Control,
edited by M. Rowland et al.
Raven Press, New York © 1985.

Modeling Pharmacodynamics: Parametric and Nonparametric Approaches

Lewis B. Sheiner

Department of Laboratory Medicine, School of Medicine, and Division of Clinical Pharmacology, Departments of Medicine and Pharmacy, Schools of Medicine and Pharmacy, University of California, San Francisco, California 94143

Of central interest in pharmacodynamic investigation is the equilibrium relationship between the concentration of a drug and its effect. If drug effect (E) and drug concentration at its effect site (C_e) could be measured simultaneously, then by systematically varying C_e a full description of the concentration–effect (pharmacodynamic) relationship could be obtained. However, one usually samples plasma concentration (C_p), not C_e, so that the concentration–effect relationship is obscured by equilibration delays intervening between the two concentrations. Indeed, a plot of E versus C_p measured during and after a short i.v. infusion often shows counterclockwise hysteresis (a counterclockwise loop when points are connected in time order), presumably caused by equilibration (and other) delays.

In order to suppress hysteresis and reveal the true underlying C_e–E curve, one can (a) sample the concentration at the effect site, (b) perform multiple steady-state experiments, measuring effect and C_p only when C_e is presumed to be in equilibrium with C_p, or (c) model the effect site as a new kinetic "compartment," linked to one of the pharmacokinetic compartments by a first-order process, but receiving only a negligible amount of drug. Predicted C_e can then be plotted against observed E to reveal the equilibrium concentration–effect relationship. First proposed by Segre [13], this last approach was subsequently used by Galeazzi et al. [5] for the effect of procainamide, by Dahlstrom et al. [2] to model the effect of morphine, and by Hull et al. [11] for the effect of pancuronium. The approach was subsequently elaborated by Sheiner et al. [14] and Holford and Sheiner [8–10] and used in several pharmacodynamic studies [3,7,15].

In their study, Hull et al. [11] made no assumption regarding the form of the pharmacodynamic model; they assumed only that the effect site was linked to the plasma by a single first-order process represented by a single rate constant (here called k_{eo}). Choosing two times (one time, during drug input, as C_p was rising, and one later, as C_p was falling) at which pancuronium gave 70% of its maximum effect, they estimated k_{eo} as the value producing identical concen-

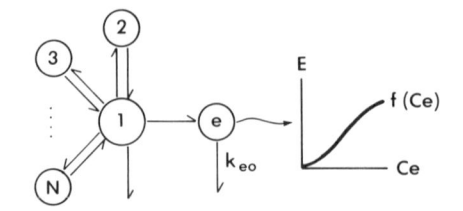

FIG. 1. The pharmacokinetic-pharmacodynamic linking model with an effect compartment. The pharmacologic effect, E, can be modeled as a parametric function, $f(C_e)$, of C_e, the concentration of drug in the hypothetical effect compartment, as in Sheiner et al. (14), or nonparametrically, as described in Fuseau and Sheiner (4). (From Fuseau and Sheiner, ref. 4, with permission.)

trations of drug in the "effect compartment" at these two times. Using the k_{eo} so estimated, they then predicted C_e for all observation times to obtain a full concentration–response curve.

A subsequent elaboration of the approach (14) used all the C_p-effect points to estimate k_{eo}, but required the analyst to postulate a particular pharmacodynamic model relating C_e to E. Recently, a new approach has returned to the more nonparametric technique of Hull et al. (11), but continues to use all the effect time points to estimate k_{eo} (4).

This chapter will briefly review some of the parametric models used to represent the C_e–E relationship and then present the nonparametric approach alluded to earlier in some detail. It is supposed in all of the discussion to follow that two models preexist: (a) a pharmacokinetic model, fully describing the time course of C_p, expressed as a sum of exponentials, the parameters of which have been determined by study of the C_p–time relationship alone, and (b) a link model, relating C_p to C_e, the parameters of which are unknown. In particular, the same link model as previously described (14) is assumed: A hypothetical effect compartment that receives only a negligible mass of drug is linked to the plasma compartment of the pharmacokinetic model by a first-order process (Fig. 1). The time course of C_e for this model is a function of k_{eo} and the pharmacokinetic parameters describing the time course of C_p. Equations predicting C_e for different drug input patterns and different pharmacokinetic models can be found elsewhere (1,8–10,14).

PARAMETRIC PHARMACODYNAMIC MODELS

Receptor theory permits the derivation of a simple mathematical form for the relationship between C_e and effect (6). The basic model has, at the receptor,

$$R + sD \rightleftharpoons RD_s$$

where R denotes the number (or concentration) of drug receptors, D is the number (or concentration) of drug molecules, and RD_s is the number (or concentration) of drug–receptor complexes (s is the number of drug molecules per receptor). Under the additional assumptions that (a) there is only one species of drug–receptor complex, (b) a negligible fraction of total drug available at the receptor is bound, (c) the effect is linearly proportional to the fraction of receptors existing as drug–receptor complex, RD_s/R_{tot}, where R_{tot} is the total number (concentration) of receptors, (d) reaction equilibrium is attained rapidly with respect to the rate of change of C_e (the concentration of D), and (e) the drug–effect relationship (in particular, drug–receptor kinetics) is time-invariant, it is not difficult to show that

$$E = E_{max} \frac{C_e^\gamma}{C_{e50}^\gamma + C_e^\gamma} \qquad (1)$$

where E_{max} is the maximum observable response, C_{e50} is the C_e yielding $E = E_{max}/2$, and γ, although theoretically equal to s, will often be found, in practice, to be noninteger. Model (1) is the sigmoid E_{max} model, often called the Hill equation, because it was first used by A. V. Hill to model the oxyhemoglobin dissociation curve. The model is illustrated in Fig. 2.

Several approximations to the sigmoid E_{max} model are in common use. The E_{max} model fixes $\gamma = 1$, but is otherwise the same as model (1):

$$E = E_{max} \frac{C_e}{C_{e50} + C_e} \qquad (2)$$

When an experiment observes E only for C_e values considerably less than C_{e50}; $C_{e50} + C_e \approx C_{e50}$, so that

$$E \approx \left(\frac{E_{max}}{C_{e50}^\gamma}\right) C_e^\gamma$$

This is often approximated by

$$E = E_0 + S \cdot C_e \qquad (3)$$

the so-called linear-effect model with constant slope (E_{max}/C_{e50}) when $\gamma = 1$. If, indeed, observations have been taken only for $C_e \ll C_{e50}$, the model is reasonable: (a) In this C_e range, the response is often fairly linear (for $\gamma < 2$), and (b) it acknowledges that the data do not provide information on C_{e50} or E_{max}.

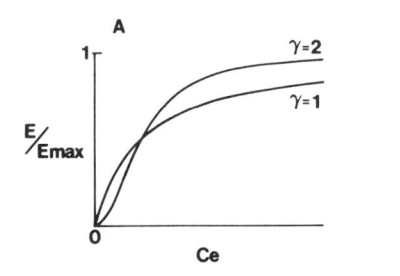

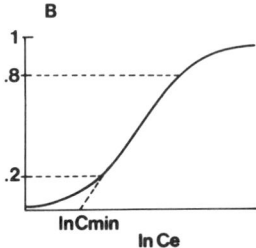

FIG. 2. Several pharmacodynamic models. **A:** the sigmoid E_{max} model [model (1)], with $\gamma = 2$, and the E_{max} model [model (2), $\gamma = 1$]. **B:** A plot of E versus ln C_e shows that between $E/E_{max} = 0.2$ and 0.8, the log-linear model [model (4)] provides a reasonable approximation, although it predicts $E = 0$ at $C_e = C_{min}$.

Naturally, the model is poor for extrapolation (prediction) outside of the observed C_e range in this circumstance, but this is a fault of the original study design, not the model. No other identifiable model would be superior. Model (3) is also sometimes used when the observed range of C_e observations is narrow, even though the range may exceed C_{e50}. In this case, the higher the range of C_e relative to C_{e50}, the smaller is S and the larger E_0. Such a use of the linear model will serve very poorly for extrapolation (prediction) outside of the observed C_e range. In this case, there is a better approach: The E_{max} model should be used instead, even though doing so involves the dual assumptions that (a) $E = 0$ when $C_e = 0$ and (b) $\gamma = 1$. The first assumption is physiologic, and the second can be regarded as a superior approximation than is use of the linear model. Reasonable predictions over a wide range of C_e should follow.

A convenient approximation to the sigmoid E_{max} model when C_e is observed only in the range causing $0.2 < E/E_{max} < 0.8$ is provided by

$$E = S(\ln C_e - \ln C_{min}) \tag{4}$$

the so-called log-linear model (see Fig. 2B). In this model C_{min} is the x intercept of the log-linear model. Although model (4) quite faithfully reproduces the sigmoid E_{max} model in the stated range, it is essentially empirical and has the added danger of suggesting that there is a threshold (C_{min}) below which the drug has no effect. Much of the controversy concerning environmental carcinogens, radiation, and other low-level toxic exposures has its roots precisely in such unwarranted extrapolations.

Some drugs produce a nonmonotonic relationship between C_e and effect, e.g., clonidine's effect on blood pressure, and this has been modeled by the difference of two sigmoid E_{max} models (12). This approach is reasonable when the drug acts to produce two opposite effects. An empirical model that describes nonmonotonicity (as well as monotonicity) can be obtained from the beta function:

$$E^* = X^r(1 - X)^s/g \tag{5}$$

where E^* is the fractional effect, E/E_{max},

$$X = C_e/(1 + C_e) + T \cdot C_e$$

$$T = 1/(C_{e_0} + C_{e_0}^2)$$

and C_{e_0} is the value (>0) at which E^* returns to zero after reaching its maximum at $C_{e_{max}} < C_{e_0}$.

$$s = \ln 0.5/z$$

$$z = [X_{max}/(1 - X_{max})] \ln(X_{50}/X_{max}) + \ln[(1 - X_{50})/(1 - X_{max})]$$

$$r = s(X_{max})/(1 - X_{max})$$

$$g = (X_{max})^r(1 - X_{max})^s$$

where X_{50} is the X value at $C_e = C_{e_{50}}$, the minimum C_e value giving 50% response ($0 < C_{e_{50}} < C_{e_{max}}$). Thus, the model is parameterized in $C_{e_{50}}$, $C_{e_{max}}$, and C_{e_0}.

When assumption (d), that drug and receptor reach equilibrium rapidly, does not hold, it is usually because RD dissociation is slow compared with the kinetics of drug in the effect compartment:

$$d\text{RD}/dt = k_{on}C_e \cdot R - k_{off}\text{RD}$$

where RD now denotes the drug–receptor complex concentration and, for simplicity, $s = \gamma = 1$ is assumed. Continuing with assumption (c), fractional effect E^* (= RD/R_{tot}) is linearly proportional to the fraction of occupied receptors:

$$dE^*/dt = k_{on}C_e(1 - E^*) - k_{off}E^* \quad (6)$$

As this equation may have no analytical solution, the fractional effect, E^*, as a function of time is often computed using numerical methods.

Assumption (e) may not hold (or may not appear to hold) if tolerance or sensitization occurs. In this case, whatever the mechanism, (apparent) fractional receptor occupancy depends on past values of C_e as well as the current one. For example, if a drug metabolite is a competitive inhibitor of the interaction of drug and receptor (but produces no effect itself), then the effect of a given concentration, C_e, will (appear to) vary with time as metabolite builds up, or wanes. It is possible to model tolerance or sensitization in a number of ways. A simple empirical model, applicable only to straightforward short-term experiments, uses the sigmoid E_{max} model but has $C_{e_{50}}$ be a function of time:

$$C_{e_{50}}(t) = C_{e_{50}}(0) + SC_e \cdot t \quad (7)$$

The slope, SC_e, will be 0 for the usual model, < 0 for sensitization, and > 0 for tolerance.

A more versatile model postulates the formation of a drug metabolite from the parent compound such that the metabolite either has a pharmacologic effect similar to that of the parent (sensitization) or is an antagonist of the parent (tolerance). This model can be adopted even for cases in which no such metabolite is known, simply to arrive at an empirical description of the observed tolerance (sensitization). The hypothetical metabolite accounting for tolerance (sensitization) can be identified with some real metabolite, if the data so indicate, by observing that the hypothetical metabolite has the same kinetics as the real one.

A minimal "metabolite" model postulates a single (infinitesimal) metabolite compartment. The hypothetical concentration of metabolite in this compartment, C_{met}, will be given by equations identical with those for C_e (1,8–10,14). However, a new kinetic parameter, k_{met} rather than k_{eo}, will be introduced to model the time lag of metabolite formation. To link the hypothetical C_{met} in the metabolite compartment to its concentration in the effect compartment, the k_{eo} as determined for the parent drug could be used, a new rate constant could be used, or, most simply, C_{met} in the metabolite compartment can be identified with C_{met} at the effect site. This last approach seems, *a priori*, most reasonable, as the equilibration rate constant for parent drug, k_{eo}, is often large relative to most other kinetic processes, and if it is also large relative to k_{met}, there will be no appreciable delay in C_{met} equilibration with the effect site. The modification of the sigmoid E_{max} model that will allow C_{met} to influence the drug effect is

$$E = E_{max} \frac{(C_e/C_{e50})^{\gamma_1} + \alpha(C_{met}/K_{met})^{\gamma_2}}{1 + (C_e/C_{e50})^{\gamma_1} + (C_{met}/K_{met})^{\gamma_2}} \qquad (8)$$

where γ_2 can be taken equal to γ_1 for simplicity. When the parameter α for C_{met} is set equal to 1, the model views C_{met} as a full agonist, or sensitizer, and when $\alpha = 0$, as a complete antagonist. The interpretation of K_{met}, the new parameter other than k_{met} associated with this model, depends on α. For $\alpha = 1$, it is exactly analogous to C_{e50}; for $\alpha = 0$, it is best understood by considering the steady state. At steady state, $C_{pss} = C_{mss}$, the steady-state concentration of the metabolite, by definition. Consequently, K_{met} must be such as to cause $(C_{pss}/K_{met})^\gamma$ to sufficiently augment the denominator of model (8) to yield E_{ss}, the fully tolerant value.

NONPARAMETRIC APPROACH TO PHARMACODYNAMIC MODELS

To return to basics, during and after a short i.v. infusion of drug, a plot of C_{p_i} versus E_i for $i = 1, \ldots, n$, the total number of (C_p, E) pairs observed, may show hysteresis; i.e., the points, when connected in time order, will show two distinct limbs, ascending (C_p rising) and descending (C_p falling). The link model (Fig. 1) predicts C_e, which lags behind C_p; the parameter k_{eo} governing the degree of lag is chosen so that the plot of C_{e_i} versus E_i shows no hysteresis. In previous work (14) this was done by fitting the observed E_i to their predictions, modeling the latter as a known function of C_e, such as in models (1)–(8).

In the nonparametric method (4), no assumptions about the pharmacodynamic model are made, but all n observation pairs, E_i plus predicted C_{e_i}, are used to estimate k_{eo}. The idea is to choose k_{eo} so that the two limbs of the C_e–E curve are superimposed. The criterion of superposition of Hull et al. (11) is the "horizontal" distance (difference) between the C_e's producing identical degrees of effect on the ascending and descending limbs (Fig. 3A). An alternative, adopted by Fuseau and Sheiner (4), is to use a function of the "vertical"-distances effect (differences at the same predicted C_e) between the two limbs of the curve as a criterion.

Formally, for a trial value of k_{eo}, the C_{e_i}, $i = 1, \ldots, n$, are first computed. Then (see Fig. 3B), for each C_{e_i}, an approximate value for the effect ($E_{int,i}$) predicted for $C_e = C_{e_i}$ on the opposite limb is obtained by linear interpolation between the nearest two observed opposite-limb effect points, renamed

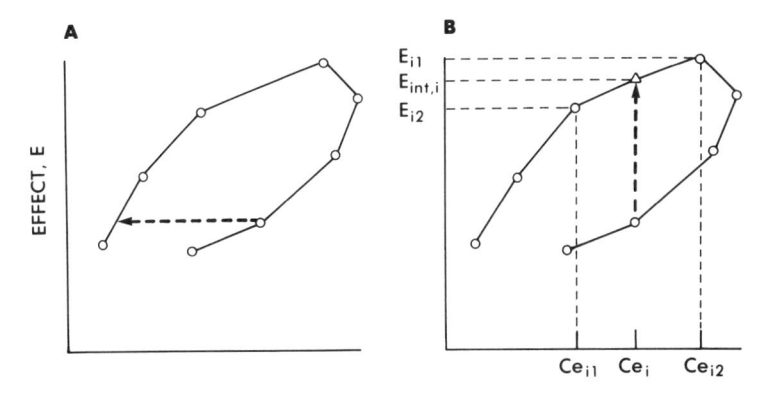

FIG. 3. Two ways to measure the degree of superposition of the two limbs of a hysteresis curve using the model of Fig. 1. **A:** In the method of Hull et al. (11), one particular effect is chosen on the ascending and descending limbs, and k_{eo} is adjusted to make C_e values at these two times be identical. **B:** In the method of Fuseau and Sheiner (4), the distance between the two limbs of the curve is evaluated by the difference of the effects between each pair of real (*circles*) and interpolated (*triangle*) points that have the same C_e; k_{eo} is chosen to minimize the mean squared effect difference. (From Fuseau and Sheiner, ref. 4, with permission.)

temporarily E_{i1} and E_{i2}. The slope, S, of the line segment connecting E_{i1} and E_{i2} is

$$S = (E_{i2} - E_{i1})/(C_{e_{i2}} - C_{e_{i1}})$$

so that

$$E_{int} = E_{i1} + (C_{e_i} - C_{e_{i1}})S$$

k_{eo} is then estimated as the value of k_{eo} minimizing the average of the n' squared differences between observed and interpolated effects:

$$O(k_{eo}) = \frac{1}{n'}\Sigma(E_k - E_{int,k})^2$$

$$O(k_{eo}) = \min_{k_{eo}} O(k_{eo})$$

The number of (interpolated) distances, n', may be less than n, depending on the value of k_{eo}, as interpolations to the opposite limb cannot be made for times less than (greater than) the first (last). As k_{eo} changes, the curve is more or less folded upon itself, and the number of points for which interpolation on the opposite limb can be made changes. This is why the average squared distance is used as a criterion, not the sum of squared distances.

No particular mechanism for the drug–effect link (e.g., drug–receptor interaction) is explicitly assumed. However, two of the previous assumptions, viz., equilibrium (d) and time invariance (e), must still hold.

Another assumption is made in the implementation that has been described (4) and is reviewed herein, but it is not intrinsic to the method, i.e., that drug input is such that a unimodal predicted C_p-time curve results.

APPLICATION TO SIMULATED DATA

Simulations can be used to evaluate the performance of the method (4). Basically, data from pharmacodynamic experiments are simulated, and the new analysis method is used to recover the (known) underlying concentration–response curves. Different choices regarding drug input, pharmacodynamic model, sampling design, and statistical model can be made.

Because primary interest focuses on recovery of the concentration–response curve, results using only one pharmacokinetic-link model are described. The pharmacokinetic model is the one-compartment open model with $k_e = 0.693$ and volume of distribution $V = 0.067$. The link model is the usual one with $k_{eo} = 7$. The equations predicting C_e for this combination of models are given elsewhere (14).

Drug input is simulated as an i.v. infusion at rate = 0.7, duration = 0.1. The maximum C_p is 1.0. Three models that obey the assumptions of the method (vide supra) are used: the E_{max} [model (2)], the sigmoid E_{max} model [model (1)], and the beta-function model [model (5)]. In order to evaluate the behavior of the approach when its assumptions are violated, models exhibiting tolerance and sensitization [model (7)] and nonequilibrium [model (6)] are also simulated.

For both the E_{max} and sigmoid E_{max} models, two C_{e50} values are used: 0.2 and 0.8. Observation times are 0.03, 0.06, 0.1, 0.2, 0.4, 0.8, 1, 2, 3, and 4. For the sigmoid E_{max} model, $\gamma = 2$. For the beta-function model, $C_{e50} = 0.2$, $C_{e_{max}} = 0.5$, and $C_{e_o} = 1$. Observation times are 0.03, 0.1, 0.15, 0.2, 0.4, 0.6, 0.8, 1, 2, and 4. For tolerance [model (7)], both $C_{e50}(0)$ and $SC_e = 0.2$, whereas for sensitization they equal 0.7 and -0.15, respectively. The $C_{e50}(t)$ so computed is used in the E_{max} model with the same observation times as specified for it earlier. For the nonequilibrium model, $k_{on} = 10$ and $k_{off} = 1$. Observation times are 0.06, 0.1, 0.14, 0.20, 0.28, 0.44, 1, 2, 3, and 4.6.

An independent random "measurement" error, ϵ_i, is added to each of the simulated effects, E_i', to yield the simulated observation, E_i:

$$E_i = E_i' + \epsilon_i$$

$$\epsilon_i = E_i' \cdot p \cdot \text{RND}$$

RND is a normal random deviate with zero mean and variance = 1; $p = 0.15$ scales the magnitude of the error and corresponds to a coefficient of variation (CV) of the error of 15%.

Figures 4, 5, and 6 show two simulations for each model, the best and the worst of 10 simulations with respect to the recovery of the true concentra-

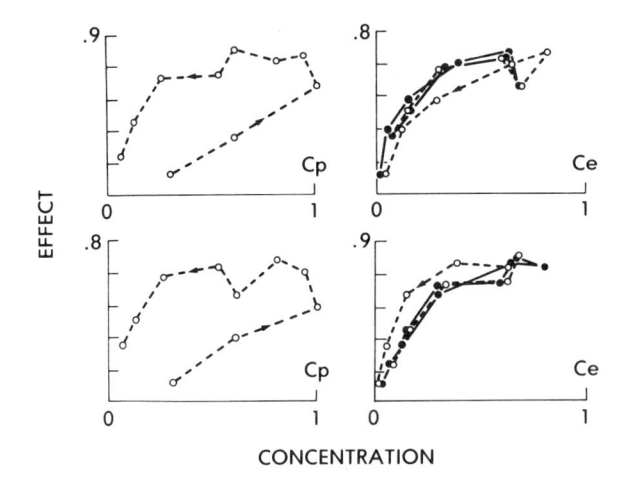

FIG. 4. Simulations of an E_{max} pharmacodynamic model with i.v. infusion, $C_{e_{50}} = 0.2$, and CV of measurement error = 15%. Dark lines and filled circles are the results of the fit; dotted lines and open circles are plots of original, simulated data. On the left is the hysteresis curve, E–C_p, and on the right the true and fitted E–C_e curve. The upper two figures are the "worst" of 10 simulations; the lower two are the "best." (From Fuseau and Sheiner, ref. 4, with permission.)

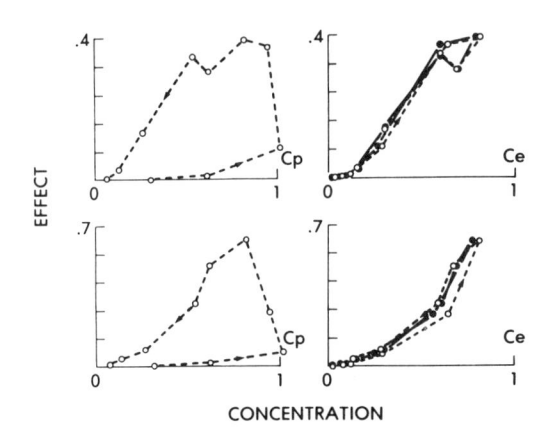

FIG. 5. Simulations of a sigmoid E_{max} pharmacodynamic model with i.v. infusion, $C_{e_{50}} = 0.8$, $\gamma = 2$, CV of measurement error = 15%. See legend to Fig. 4 for layout and symbols. (From Fuseau and Sheiner, ref. 4, with permission.)

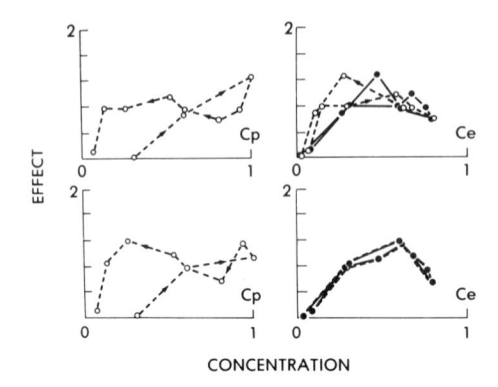

FIG. 6. Simulations of the beta-function pharmacodynamic model with i.v. infusion, $C_{e_{50}} = 0.2$, $C_{e_{max}} = 0.5$, $C_{e_o} = 1$, and CV error = 15%. See legend to Fig. 4 for layout and symbols. (From Fuseau and Sheiner, ref. 4, with permission.)

tion–effect curve. Note that even in the worst cases, the nonparametric approach recovers the shape of the original C_e–effect curve.

The simulations shown in Fig. 5, the sigmoid E_{max} model with $C_{pss_{50}} = 0.8$,[1] show a "design problem." Because C_p (and hence C_e) never exceeds $C_{pss_{50}}$ by very much, the upper part of the concentration–response curve is missing. It is therefore not possible to identify the complete E_{max} curve, and the linear model, model (3), would have to be used in a parametric approach. The nonparametric approach, however, has no problem and recovers the shape of the (incomplete) curve.

Simulations using i.v. bolus input (not shown) revealed that to estimate the concentration–response curve successfully, effect data during onset of effect as well as during offset are crucial. As a rule of thumb, at least two effect points are necessary on each side of E_{max}.

Figure 7 shows the results of simulations of the inappropriate pharmacodynamic models: tolerance, sensitization, and nonequilibrium. On the left side of each panel, dark lines show the fit of the method to data without added error. The fitted C_e–response curves even in this ideal case do not reproduce the true (broken line) curve, which actually makes a loop. The fitted curves do often show a figure-8 pattern but have far less hysteresis than the true curves.

---

[1] *Note from the editors:* The partition coefficient between the steady-state concentrations in plasma (C_{pss}) and in the effect compartment (C_{ess}) is generally unknown. Also, the plasma concentration is measured, whereas the effect compartment cannot be sampled. Accordingly, $C_{pss_{50}}$ (also denoted $C_{p_{50}}$), the plasma concentration that *at equilibrium* produces 50% of the maximum effect, is often used as a parameter of the pharmacokinetic/pharmacodynamic model instead of $C_{e_{50}}$, as if the partition coefficient were 1. In the (usual) nonsteady-state situation, the effect compartment lags behind the central (including plasma) compartment. The model-predicted effect at the time when $C_p = C_{p_{50}}$ is not equal to half E_{max}. It is lower in the ascending part of the plasma-level curve than in its declining part.

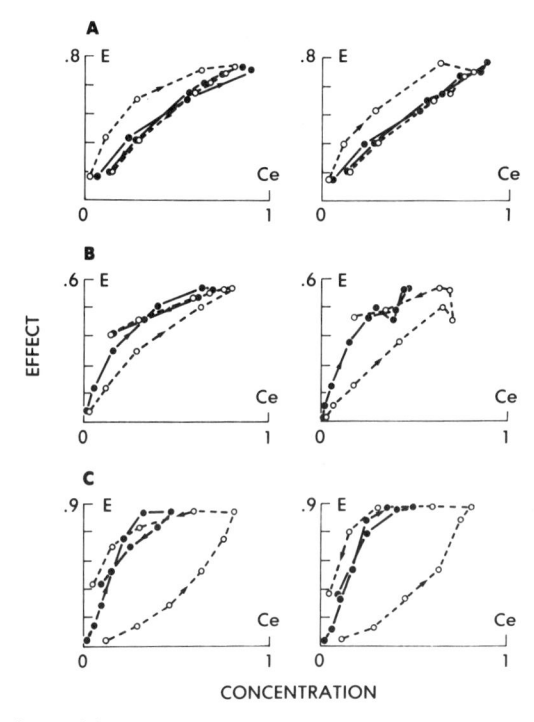

FIG. 7. Simulations of inappropriate models with i.v. infusion. **A:** Tolerance [model (7)]. **B:** Sensitization [model (7)]. **C:** Nonequilibrium [model (6)]. In all figures, the broken lines show the true curve, the solid ones the results of the fit (as in Fig. 4). The figures on the left show simulations with no added error; those on the right show simulations with added error with CV = 15%. (From Fuseau and Sheiner, ref. 4, with permission.)

DISCUSSION

A number of simple but versatile pharmacodynamic models have been suggested as structural models for the variation in drug effect correlated with variation in drug concentration at the active site. Considerable work has been done with the classic Hill model [model (1)] and approximations of it. In the future, as more attention is paid to the details of pharmacodynamics, we can expect wider use of models of sensitization or tolerance [e.g., model (7) combined with model (1)] or models that can deal with slow receptor off-rates of drugs [e.g., model (6)].

Purely pharmacodynamic models must be combined with pharmacokinetic models, and models linking C_p to C_e, in order to be useful for analysis of many non-steady-state experiments. One particular linking model (14) has been used with some success (3,7,15).

As a preliminary step to definitive structural modeling of pharmacodynamics, it is useful to view the C_e-E relationship displayed graphically. To do so for non-steady-state data, a variation of the previously described approach to simultaneous modeling of pharmacokinetics and pharmacodynamics is required. This has been described. The method recovers the underlying C_e-E relationship well when its assumptions (rapid equilibrium of C_e and effect, and a time-invariant pharmacodynamic process) hold, as revealed by simulations. However, the nonparametric method does not work when its assumptions are violated. This is not a particular fault of the nonparametric approach, as similarly distorted estimates of a parametric C_e-E model would be expected in identical circumstances. Rather, the result simply stresses the critical dependence of inferences regarding the shape of the concentration–response curve by either method on the assumption that the underlying C_e-E relationship is independent of time. When it is not, the basis for removing the hysteresis of the C_p-E curve is violated (it depends on the equilibrium and time-invariance assumptions to guarantee that C_e is the same whenever E is the same), and biased C_e-E estimates result. When the assumptions are in doubt, multiple-dose or "steady-state" experiments may reveal a time drift in the supposed (pseudo-) steady-state effect.

ACKNOWLEDGMENT

Work supported in part by NIH grants GM-26676 and GM-26691.

REFERENCES

1. Colburn, W. (1981): Simultaneous pharmacokinetic and pharmacodynamic modeling. *J. Pharmacokinet. Biopharm.*, 9:367–388.
2. Dahlstrom, B.E., Paalzow, L.K., Segre, G., and Agren, A.J. (1978): Relation between morphine pharmacokinetics and analgesia. *J. Pharmacokinet. Biopharm.*, 6:41–53.
3. Dow, J., Laquais, B., Tisne-Versailles, J., Pourrias, B., and Strolin-Benedetti, M. (1982): Pharmacokinetics and pharmacodynamics of the antiarthmic compound MD 750819 in dogs with experimentally induced arrhythmias. *J. Pharmacokinet. Biopharm.*, 10:283–296.
4. Fuseau, E., and Sheiner, L.B. (1984): Simultaneous modelling of pharmacokinetics and pharmacodynamics with a nonparametric pharmacodynamic model. *Clin. Pharmacol. Ther.*, 35:733–741.
5. Galeazzi, R.L., Benet, L.Z., and Sheiner, L.B. (1976): Relationship betwen pharmacokinetics and pharmacodynamics of procainamide. *Clin. Pharmacol. Ther.*, 20:278–289.
6. Goldstein, A., Aronow, L., and Kalman, S.M. (1968): *Principles of Drug Action*, 2, pp. 82 et seq. Wiley, New York.
7. Ham, J., Stanski, D., Newfield, P., and Miller, R.D. (1981): Pharmacokinetics and dynamics of D-tubocurarine during hypothermia in humans. *Anesthesiology*, 55:631–635.
8. Holford, N.H.G. (1981): Pharmacokinetic and pharmacodynamic modeling in vivo. *CRC Crit. Rev. Bioeng.*, 5:273–322.
9. Holford, N.H.G., and Sheiner, L.B. (1981): Understanding the dose effect relationship. *Clin. Pharmacokinet.*, 6:429–453.
10. Holford, N.H.G., and Sheiner, L.B. (1982): Kinetics of pharmacologic response. *Pharmacol. Ther.*, 16:143–165.

11. Hull, C.J., VanBeem, B.H., McLeod, K., Sibbald, A., and Watson, M.J. (1978): A pharmacokinetic model for pancuronium. *Br. J. Anaesthesia,* 50:1113–1123.
12. Paalzow, L.K., and Edlund, P.O. (1979): Multiple receptor responses: A new concept to describe the relationship between pharmacological effects and pharmacokinetics of a drug: Studies on clonidine in the rat and the cat. *J. Pharmacokinet. Biopharm.,* 7:495–510.
13. Segre, G. (1968): Kinetics of interaction between drugs and biological systems. *Il Farmaco* 23:907–918.
14. Sheiner, L.B., Stanski, D.R., Vozeh, S., Miller, R.D., and Ham, J. (1979): Simultaneous modeling of pharmacokinetics and pharmacodynamics: Application to *d*-tubocurarine. *Clin. Pharmacol. Ther.,* 25:358–371.
15. Whiting, B., Holford, N.H.G., and Sheiner, L.B. (1980): Quantitative analysis of the disopyramide concentration effect relationship. *Br. J. Clin. Pharmacol.,* 9:67–75.

DISCUSSION

Discussant 1 (D1): Do you know how to assess the precision of the estimates you obtain?

Speaker (S): First, I view the approach as a way to get a picture of the concentration–effect relationship, not to quantify it. Once you have looked at the picture, you might want to pick a functional form for the pharmacodynamic model, fit it, and get the final estimates. At that point the statistics are available. For the nonparametric approach itself, I might suggest something along the lines of a bootstrap or jackknife (1).

D2: Do you think it's possible to determine if some of the assumptions are violated by doing several experiments at different infusion rates or at different dosing levels and then trying to close all hysteresis loops simultaneously? If your assumptions were correct, this should be able to work with one k_{eo} parameter.

S: It may be possible to pursue such a course. Dr. Stanski has some experience doing experiments like that with barbiturates (3). I think the important point is this: that we need a lot of attention to be paid to experimental designs that will distinguish among models.

D3: Hysteresis may occur when the biophase of the effect is located far from the central compartment. But there is another kind of hysteresis that is due to the down- or up-regulation of receptors. In some cases receptor levels may be measured (e.g., in white cells). How can your model deal with this?

S: It's always better to model the real underlying process than to use an empirical approach such as the one I have presented. If receptors can be measured, the model should include them.

D4: The approach you have presented seems to depend on extensive data, both kinetic and dynamic. Could you comment on how to approach the problem if one either has many kinetic data in several patients, but just one or two effect measurements in each, or has a very small number of blood samples but may have extensive pharmacodynamic data.

S: The nonparametric approach cannot work with too few dynamic data points. There isn't a sufficiently specified objective function to compute. Other than using a parametric approach and simultaneous analysis, I have no suggestion. Reasonable kinetic and dynamic population-parameter estimates were obtained from such an analysis using NONMEM and only six curare blood levels and effect measurements per patient (2).

REFERENCES

1. Efron, B.E. (1979): Bootstrap methods: Another look at the jackknife. *Ann. Stat.*, 7:1–26.
2. Sheiner, L.B., Stanski, D.R., Vozeh, S., Miller, R.D., and Ham, J. (1979): Simultaneous modeling of pharmacokinetics and pharmacodynamics: Application to d-tubocurarine. *Clin. Pharmacol. Ther.*, 25:358–371.
3. Stanski, D.R., Hudson, R.J., Homer, T.D., Saidman, L.J., and Meathe, E. (1984): Pharmacodynamic modelling of thiopental anesthesia. *J. Pharmacokinet. Biopharm.*, 12:223–240.

*Variability in Drug Therapy:
Description, Estimation, and Control*,
edited by M. Rowland et al.
Raven Press, New York © 1985.

Integrating Pharmacokinetics and Dynamics: Variability in Thiopental's Dose Requirement, Pharmacokinetics, and Pharmacodynamics

Donald R. Stanski and * Jo Hermans

*Departments of Anesthesia and Medicine (Clinical Pharmacology), Stanford University Medical School, Stanford, California 94305; and Department of Anesthesia, Leiden University School of Medicine, NL-2333 AA Leiden, The Netherlands; and
* Department of Medical Statistics, Leiden University School of Medicine, NL-2333 AA Leiden, The Netherlands*

Thiopental is a barbiturate derivative used to induce anesthesia in surgical patients. It can be given as a single intravenous bolus, as multiple small intravenous boli or as a rapid intravenous infusion to induce a deep hypnotic state in a patient within 0.5 to 3 min, after which other anesthetic drugs (nitrous oxide, potent inhalational anesthetics) are used to maintain a depth of central nervous system (CNS) depression that allows the surgical procedure to be performed. Thiopental's pharmacokinetic profile is that of a large steady-state distribution volume (1.5–3.0 liters/kg), low hepatic clearance (2–4 ml/kg/min), and a terminal elimination half-life of 6 to 15 hr. It is moderately bound to plasma proteins (free fraction 0.1–0.2) (15).

The use of thiopental features rapid onset and recovery from the drug effect (anesthesia) because of its physiochemical properties. Being a thiobarbiturate it has high lipid solubility. It can readily penetrate membrane structures, including the blood-brain barrier. After a bolus intravenous injection, peak blood concentrations translate into high brain concentrations that induce CNS depression (anesthesia). Thiopental's anesthetic effect dissipates rapidly as the drug redistributes from the brain via the blood to other tissues, specifically muscle and then fat (1). Termination of thiopental's anesthetic effect is minimally dependent on its slow elimination from the body.

Recently we have developed a noninvasive, continuous measure of thiopental's drug effect on the brain using the electroencephalogram (EEG). As the dose of thiopental is progressively increased, the EEG decreases in its underlying frequency, reflecting a progressive increase in the depth of barbiturate anesthesia (10,17). Quantitating thiopental's drug effect on the brain with the EEG involves using power spectral analysis to characterize the degree of EEG slowing. We have successfully used this EEG slowing as a measure of thiopental's drug effect on the brain. Pharmacokinetic and dynamic modeling concepts have been used to relate thiopental serum concentrations to the spectral edge, a parameter that characterizes the underlying EEG frequency (10,17).

By having a sensitive, continuous measure of thiopental's drug effect on the brain, one can use a rapid intravenous infusion of the drug to precisely define the dose requirement of thiopental needed to achieve a given degree of EEG slowing. With measurements of serum concentrations and the power spectral analysis of the EEG one can quantitate both the pharmacokinetics and pharmacodynamics of the drug. These previously reported data (9) have been reanalyzed with a special focus on quantitating the degree of variability in the thiopental dose requirement relative to the two factors that determine the dose requirement: the pharmacodynamics and the pharmacokinetics. Specifically, the following issues were addressed:

1. To what extent can one identify the sources of variability in the thiopental dose requirement, the pharmacokinetics, and the pharmacodynamics using the factors of age, weight, and degree of protein binding?
2. What is the extent of unexplained variability that exists in the thiopental dose requirement, relative to the two components (pharmacokinetics and pharmacodynamics) that define the dose requirement?

METHODS

The study design, patient population, data gathering, analysis, and results have been previously reported (9). Two groups of patients were studied. In one group of 29 patients aged 19 to 88 years, thiopental was given to quantitate the dose requirement and pharmacodynamics. In a second group of 28 patients aged 23 to 88 years, thiopental pharmacokinetic data were obtained. Fourteen of the 28 patients in whom pharmacokinetic data were obtained were also in the first group of patients in whom the dose requirement and pharmacodynamics were measured.

In the first group of patients (dose requirement and pharmacodynamics), thiopental was infused at 75 to 150 mg/min until a well-defined EEG pattern of 1 to 3 sec of burst suppression was evident (within 4–10 min of starting the infusion). Clinically this represents a deep stage of thiopental anesthesia whereby ventilation is depressed, blood pressure begins to decrease, and noxious stimuli (endotracheal intubation) generally will not elicit a hemodynamic response. The amount of thiopental needed to achieve this EEG endpoint defined the dose requirement. The EEG was recorded on magnetic tape for subsequent off-line power spectral analysis. From the power spectral analysis of the EEG during the thiopental infusion and the subsequent recovery of the

EEG to an almost awake pattern (10–20 min after terminating the infusion) the spectral edge was obtained, a measure of the underlying EEG frequency. Arterial blood samples were obtained at 0.5- to 1-min intervals during the infusion and at 1- to 3-min intervals after termination of the infusion for measurements of thiopental serum concentrations. Pharmacodynamic modeling was used to estimate for each patient the following parameters: E_0, the base-line EEG frequency (Hz); E_{max}, the maximal decrease in the spectral-edge frequency (Hz) induced by thiopental; C_{p50}, the thiopental serum concentration (μg/ml) that at steady state causes one-half of the maximal EEG slowing; γ, a power function of the inhibitory sigmoid E_{max} pharmacodynamic model; $T_{1/2}k_{eo}$, the half-time (min) of equilibration for the thiopental serum concentration and EEG effect.

In the second group of 28 subjects (pharmacokinetics), thiopental was given as a rapid intravenous bolus or as a rapid intravenous infusion for the induction of anesthesia. Frequent arterial blood samples were drawn to accurately characterize the distribution–redistribution kinetics for the first 3 to 4 hr. Subsequently, venous blood samples were obtained for 24 to 48 hr to characterize the terminal elimination-phase kinetics. Thiopental serum concentrations were determined by high-performance liquid chromatography (16). Protein binding was measured with ultrafiltration (16). The data on thiopental serum concentration versus time were fitted to biexponential and triexponential equations using extended least-squares nonlinear regression (13). A proportional-error model was used. In all cases there was statistical preference for the triexponential model, based on the difference in log-likelihood value and the chi-square statistic ($p < 0.05$). Standard formulas were used to calculate the pharmacokinetic parameters. The degree of protein binding was used to express the appropriate pharmacokinetic and dynamic parameters in terms of free drug concentration.

All of the surgical patients studied were unpremedicated and without evidence of hepatic, renal, cardiovascular, or neurological dysfunction. No subjects had evidence of alcohol or drug abuse. Informed consent was obtained from each patient with the protocol reviewed by the Stanford Institutional Review Board.

DATA ANALYSIS

Descriptive linear- and nonlinear-regression analysis on the dose requirement and pharmacokinetic and pharmacodynamic parameters was performed on the BMDP Statistical Package (1982). The dose requirement and clearance and volume parameters of the pharmacokinetic analysis were first examined for a regression relationship to body weight. If a significant ($p < 0.05$) relationship existed, the parameter was divided by the body weight for the remainder of the data analysis. Simple linear regression was used to determine if an age relationship existed with the pharmacokinetic and dynamic parameters. Non-

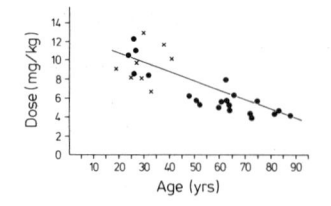

FIG. 1. Thiopental dose needed to reach burst suppression with increasing age. The *solid line* is the regression relationship indicated in Table 1. The *circles* represent surgical patients; *crosses* represent volunteer subjects. (From Homer and Stanski, ref. 9, with permission.)

TABLE 1. *Thiopental dose requirement*

No age adjustment

dose (mg/kg) mean ± SD = 7.4 ± 2.6
coefficient of variation = 36%
N = 29

Age adjustment

dose (mg/kg) = 12.39 − 0.10 × age (years) R^2 = 0.65
coefficient of variation = 21%
N = 29

linear regression was also used to characterize the relationship between the parameter versus the age relationship with an exponential equation if it was obvious that a nonlinear relationship was present. The residual sum of squares was used to distinguish between the linear and exponential models in choosing the optimal regression equation.

The degree of variability in dose requirement and pharmacokinetic and pharmacodynamic parameters was characterized with the coefficient of variation. If there was no regression relationship on age and the parameter, the coefficient of variation of the mean was calculated (standard deviation/mean × 100%). If a linear- or nonlinear-regression relationship to age existed with a parameter, the coefficient of variation was calculated from the standard error of the regression (standard error of regression/mean × 100%) (6). The standard error of the regression estimate is the square root of the residual mean square of the regression analysis. If a regression relationship does not exist, the standard error of the regression is identical with the standard deviation of the mean.

RESULTS

The total dose (mg) of thiopental needed to reach burst suppression was significantly related to body weight; therefore, the dose requirement for each subject was adjusted to body weight. Figure 1 and Table 1 indicate the dose-requirement–age relationship. There was a significant decrease in the dose requirement with increasing age. Without adjusting for age, the variability of the

TABLE 2. Thiopental pharmacodynamic parameters without an age relationship

Parameter	N	Mean	Standard deviation	Coefficient of variation
E_0 (Hz)	29	24.6	4.4	18%
E_{max} (Hz)	29	14.5	5.6	39%
Total C_{p50} (µg/ml)	29	19.4	6.8	35%
Free C_{p50} (µg/ml)	29	2.7	1.0	38%
γ [a]	28	4.9	2.9	59%
$T_{\frac{1}{2}} k_{eo}$ (min) [b]	20	1.2	0.4	37%

[a] One outlier value of 49 was excluded.
[b] Nine subjects did not exhibit hysteresis.

dose requirement (coefficient of variation) was 36%; with a linear-regression relationship to age, this index for variability decreased to 21%.

The age-related change in the dose requirement could not be explained by an age-related change in pharmacodynamics (Table 2). There was no relationship between age and the pharmacodynamic parameters indicated in Table 2. The C_{p50}, a direct measure of brain sensitivity, was derived for the total drug concentration (bound and free) and the free drug concentration. Adjustment of the C_{p50} to the free drug concentration, the therapeutically active component, did not change the relationship with age, nor did it decrease the degree of variability (35% for total drug versus 38% for free drug). The pharmacodynamic parameter that reflected the early activation of the EEG (E_0) exhibited the lowest degree of variability (18%). The power function of the inhibitory sigmoid E_{max} pharmacodynamic model had the largest degree of variability (59%). The pharmacodynamic parameters that quantitate maximal brain responsiveness (E_{max}) and the rate of blood–brain equilibration ($T_{\frac{1}{2}} k_{eo}$) had a variability between 35 and 40%.

The age-related change in the thiopental dose requirement was due to pharmacokinetic factors. The triexponential, three-compartment pharmacokinetic model used to characterize the data on thiopental serum concentration versus time can be physiologically conceptualized in terms of volumes and clearances. There are three volumes of distribution: the initial distribution volume (V_1), the rapidly equilibrating compartment (V_2), and the slowly equilibrating compartment (V_3), whose total is the volume of distribution at steady state (V_{dss}). There are also three clearances: the two distribution–redistribution clearances, rapid intercompartment clearance (QF) and slow intercompartment clearance (QS), and irreversible clearance from the body (CL) due to metabolism. Of these six parameters, the initial distribution volume, V_1, was the only pharmacokinetic parameter that was age-related (Figs. 2, 3, and 4; Tables 3 and 4). The age relationship to V_1 was best characterized with a monoexponential equation. V_2 and V_3, and therefore V_{dss}, were not age-related. None of the clearance

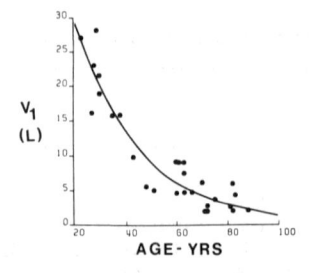

FIG. 2. Volume of the central compartment (V_1) versus age. The *solid curve* is the fitted function of the data to an exponential equation indicated in Table 3. (From Homer and Stanski, ref. 9, with permission.)

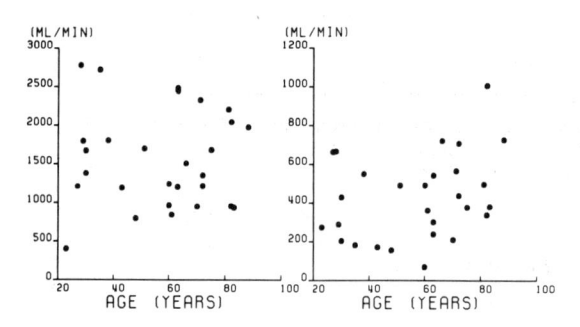

FIG. 3. Rapid **(left)** and slow **(right)** intercompartment clearances versus age. There is no age relationship to these measures of drug clearance to the peripheral tissues (compartments).

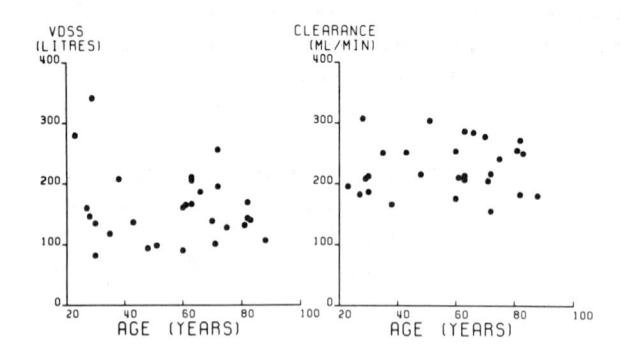

FIG. 4. Volume of distribution at steady state and total-body clearance versus age. There is no age relationship for these two pharmacokinetic measures.

TABLE 3. Thiopental pharmacokinetic parameters with an age relationship

Parameter[a]	Model	Coefficient of variation	R^2
V_1 (liters)	9.6 ± 8.0 (mean ± SD)	83%	—
V_1 (liters)	29.5 − 0.348 × age (years)	39%	0.78
V_1 (liters)	64.9 × exp[−0.039 × age (years)]	29%	0.79
Rapid-distribution half-life (min)	2.3 ± 1.5 (mean ± SD)	67%	—
Rapid-distribution half-life (min)	5.46 + 0.0548 × age (years)	48%	0.49

[a] $N = 28$ for V_1 and 27 for the rapid-distribution half-lives; one outlier value of 17.2 min was excluded from the analysis.

TABLE 4. Thiopental pharmacokinetic parameters without an age relationship

Parameter[a]	Mean	Standard deviation	Coefficient of variation
Rapid intercompartment clearance (ml/min)	1562	629	40%
Slow intercompartment clearance (ml/min)	429	219	51%
Total-body clearance (ml/min)	227	42.9	19%
V_2 (liters)	25	13	52%
V_3 (liters)	126	56	44%
V_{dss} (liters)	160	60	38%
Elimination half-life (hr)	11.9	5.4	45%
Free fraction	0.15	0.023	15%

[a] $N = 28$ for all parameters.

parameters was age-related. A composite parameter of the drug distribution process, the rapid distribution half-life, was age-related (Fig. 5) in a linear manner. Because only V_1 was age-related, the microrate constants (k_{10}, k_{12}, k_{13}) were also age-related in an exponential manner. This allows the products of V_1 and these microrate constants to result in clearance terms that were not age-related.

In Table 3 one can see that the degree of variability in V_1, as measured by the coefficient of variation, progressively decreased from 83% with no age adjustment to 39% with a linear age adjustment and then to 29% with an exponential age adjustment. The variability of the rapid distribution half-life also

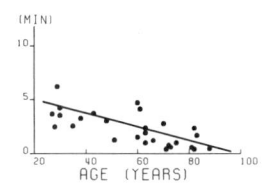

FIG. 5. Rapid-distribution half-life versus age. The solid line indicates the linear-regression relationship with age indicated in Table 3. One outlier value of 17.3 min in a 28-year-old subject was excluded from the analysis.

decreased from 67% when the mean and standard deviation were used to 48% when a linear regression with age was performed. The degrees of variability in the other primary pharmacokinetic parameters (rapid and slow intercompartment clearance, V_2, V_3) were greater than the variability found in V_1. Total-body clearance (CL) had the lowest degree of variability. None of the pharmacokinetic parameters was related to body weight. Because the degree of protein binding was not related to age, calculation of pharmacokinetic parameters based on the free drug (unbound volumes, intrinsic clearance) did not result in a decrease in the variability of the data.

DISCUSSION

Having developed a sensitive, objective, noninvasive measure of thiopental's drug effect on the brain, it has been possible to quantitate the dose–response relationship and its two component parts: the pharmacodynamics and pharmacokinetics. Other studies using clinical, quantital measures of thiopental's anesthetic effects (loss of corneal reflex, adequate hemodynamic stability) showed an age-related decrease in the thiopental dose requirement (3–5). In those studies, the age-adjusted coefficient of variation for the dose requirement based on the foregoing clinical endpoints was approximately 30 to 40%. Unfortunately, comparable regression data for age versus dose requirement were not available in those studies to compare with our results. In a very large series of 2,206 patients, Dundee et al. (8) found that in 1,907 patients aged 15 to 64 years, the (mean ± SD) dose requirement to abolish the eyelash reflex was 3.72 ± 1.22 mg/kg, CV = 33%, whereas in 246 patients older than 65 years, the dose requirement was significantly ($p < 0.05$) decreased to 3.16 ± 1.03 mg/kg, CV = 33%. The degree of variability in the data of Dundee et al. (8) was similar to that in the other studies using clinical endpoints to define the dose–response relationship.

The variability in the dose requirement obtained with the use of the EEG (age-adjusted coefficient of variation of 21%) appears to be smaller than what the other investigators cited earlier obtained with clinical measures. This may reflect the greater precision and objectivity of noninvasive, electrophysiological measures of the drug effect relative to clinical measures that are very dependent on the degree and timing of stimuli and are quantital. The degree of variability of the dose requirement was reduced with both a body-weight adjustment and age adjustment in our data.

The dose requirement of thiopental is determined by pharmacokinetics (dose–serum-concentration relationship) and pharmacodynamics (serum-concentration–drug-effect relationship). The age relationship found in the dose requirement was not seen for the pharmacodynamics. All of the measures of the brain's EEG responsiveness to thiopental (initial response E_0, maximal response E_{max}, sensitivity C_{p50}, rate of equilibration $T_{1/2}k_{eo}$) were not age-related.

The degrees of variability in the pharmacodynamics were relatively consistent at 30 to 35%, except for the power function and the initial E_0. Because the power function for the thiopental-induced EEG slowing is relatively large (values of 2-4), the concentration–response relationship begins to approach a square wave. When the concentration–response relationship is so steep, changing the value of γ may not change the shape of the curve, possibly explaining the greater degree of variability in this parameter. It is not obvious why the E_0 parameter was less variable than the other parameters of the model. Because the degrees of protein binding were relatively consistent in our subjects (Table 4), calculating the brain responsiveness based on the free $C_{p_{50}}$ did not decrease the degree of variability. A larger degree of variability in the degree of protein binding would have been needed to demonstrate that the free drug concentration is better related to the drug effect than the total drug concentration.

Thiopental's altered dose requirement in the aged was due to pharmacokinetic factors. The initial distribution volume of thiopental was related to age in a pronounced exponential manner (Fig. 2). The other distribution volumes (V_2 and V_3 and therefore V_{dss}) were not altered in the elderly. Additionally, drug clearance from the central compartment due to redistribution (rapid and slow intercompartment clearances) to the tissues or irreversible elimination from the body or total-body clearance (Fig. 3 and 4) was not related to age. Of the three clearance terms that govern drug removal from the central compartment, the rapid intercompartment clearance is the largest and therefore most important in defining the change of thiopental concentration in the central compartment during acute administration over a short period of time. Whereas drug redistribution, as measured by intercompartment clearance, is not age-related, the change in the initial distribution space causes the rapid-distribution half-life to be age-related (Fig. 5).

Thiopental's initial distribution space or central compartment is composed of the blood volume and vessel-rich tissues (lung, heart, brain, liver, kidney, endocrine organs) that have a high perfusion. This assumption is compatible with the physiological pharmacokinetic models that have been developed for thiopental (1,15). The rapidly and slowly equilibrating compartments may represent muscle and fat, respectively. The decrease in thiopental's initial distribution space may be due to the age-related decrease in cardiac output, with subsequently decreased regional blood flow, especially renal and hepatic perfusion (11,14). Thus, some of the vessel-rich tissues (liver, kidney, portal circulation) in effect would "move" from the instantaneously mixing central compartment to a more slowly equilibrating peripheral compartment. This is compatible with the fact that intercompartment clearance did not change with age.

The thiopental dose requirement is determined by the time needed to achieve a given EEG endpoint during a rapid intravenous infusion of the anesthetic. Because the infusion time needed is relatively short (4–10 min), one can collapse the triexponential pharmacokinetic model to a simple one-compartment infusion model to examine the immediate distribution and clearance terms that define the thiopental dose requirement:

$$C_{P(t)} = \frac{\text{infusion rate}}{\text{clearance}} \left[1 - \exp\left(\frac{0.693}{T_{1/2}\alpha} \cdot t\right) \right] \quad (1)$$

where $C_{P(t)}$ is a given serum concentration at time t, clearance is the global sum of rapid and slow intercompartment and metabolic clearances ($V_1 \times k_{12}, k_{13}, k_{10}$), and $T_{1/2}\alpha$ is the rapid-distribution half-life. With increasing age, the pharmacodynamics are unchanged; therefore, a given endpoint of thiopental effect (i.e., C_{P50}) will always require the same thiopental serum concentration. The global central-compartment clearance terms (rapid and slow intercompartment clearances, total clearance) did not change with age, and the infusion rate was not markedly age-adjusted. The rapid-distribution half-life ($T_{1/2}\alpha$) was age-related, becoming smaller with increasing age because of the decreasing initial distribution volume. As $T_{1/2}\alpha$ becomes smaller, the time needed to achieve a given C_p (C_{P50}) will decrease, and therefore the dose requirement will decrease (dose requirement = infusion rate × time needed to achieve a given C_p). With this model it is possible to identify which kinetic and dynamic parameters to examine for variability in defining the dose–response relationship in young and old patients. For the pharmacodynamics, C_{P50} is the most relevant parameter. For the pharmacokinetics, V_1, $T_{1/2}\alpha$, and the central-compartment clearance terms (rapid and slow intercompartment clearances, total-body clearance) define the dose requirement.

The variability found in V_1 (29%) is the smallest relative to the rapid-distribution half-life and the intercompartment clearances. Except for V_1, the degrees of variability in the pharmacokinetic parameters exceed those seen for the pharmacodynamics. It is difficult to speculate why this difference exists, or the relevance of it. As in the pharmacodynamics, protein-binding adjustments of the pharmacokinetic parameters (unbound volumes, intrinsic clearance) by the free fraction did not change any of the underlying relationships. Weight adjustments of the pharmacokinetics did not improve the degree of variability.

The degree of variability in the dose requirement (21%) is less than those for the pharmacodynamics (35%) or the pharmacokinetics (29–51%). These differences in degrees of variability may arise from the nature of the measurements. The dose requirement is determined by directly examining the EEG and defining a clear-cut EEG endpoint. There is very minimal measurement error in estimating the dose requirement; therefore, the coefficient of variation reflects mainly the interindividual variability of the patient population. The parameters of the pharmacokinetic and pharmacodynamic models involve numerous steps of sampling, measurement, data analysis, and modeling. For the pharmacodynamics, the EEG signal is first recorded on magnetic tape, digitized, and subjected to fast Fourier analysis; then the spectral edge is calculated. The spectral edge is smoothed to remove the excessive "noise." Finally, the spectral-edge data are used in the pharmacodynamic model (with nonlinear regression) to estimate the measures of drug responsiveness. In the pharmacokinetic analysis, the blood sample is first measured with an analytical technique. The serum concentration is then fitted to a pharmacokinetic model with nonlinear regression, and the model parameters are used to calculate other pharmacokinetic parameters. Although it is not possible to quantitate the degree of variability in each of these multiple steps, it is very likely that a significant portion of the variability found in the pharmacokinetics and dynamics represents global measurement error (model misspecification, data-fitting inaccuracy, etc.) that is in addition to the interindividual variability of the population.

In summary, using pharmacokinetic and dynamic modeling concepts, the thiopental dose requirement for inducing deep anesthesia has been examined. Age was found to explain a major portion of the variability in the dose requirement. Pharmacodynamics were not affected by age. The dose requirement was explained by an age-related decrease in the thiopental initial distribution space. By having a continuous measure of the drug effect, one can carefully define drug dose requirements for patients and quantitate the degree of variability due to factors that alter the dose requirement. By relating the drug effect to serum concentrations, it is possible to estimate end-organ sensitivity to the drug using pharmacodynamic modeling concepts. Finally, one can relate the given dose to the serum concentrations to characterize the drug's pharmacokinetics. The relative degrees of variability between the pharmacokinetics and dynamics can be quantitated. The key to all of the foregoing is having an accurate, sensitive measure of the drug effect in the body. By having a measure of drug effect, we can begin to improve our understanding of the clinical pharmacology of drugs in humans.

ACKNOWLEDGMENTS

We would like to thank Drs. R. J. Hudson and T. D. Homer for their contributions in collecting and analyzing the data, Dr. L. B. Sheiner for his consultations in the data analysis, and Ms. M. P. M. Toelen for preparing the manuscript. This research was supported by National Institute of Aging grant P01-AG03104, the Veterans Administration Research Service, and the Anesthesiology/Pharmacology Research Foundation of Palo Alto, California.

REFERENCES

1. Bischoff, K.B., and Dedrick, R.L. (1968): Thiopental pharmacokinetics. *J. Pharm. Sci.*, 57:1346–1351.
2. Burch, P.G., and Stanski, D.R. (1983): The role of metabolism and protein binding in thiopental anesthesia. *Anesthesiology*, 58:146–152.
3. Christensen, J.H., and Andreasen, F. (1978): Individual variation in response to thiopental. *Acta Anaesthesiol. Scand.*, 22:303–313.
4. Christensen, J.H., Andreasen, F., and Jansen, J.A. (1982): Pharmacokinetics and pharmacodynamics of thiopentone. *Anaesthesia*, 37:398–404.

5. Christensen, J.H., Andreasen, F., and Jansen, J.A. (1983): Thiopentone sensitivity in young and elderly women. *Br. J. Anaesth.,* 55:33–39.
6. Draper, N.R., and Smith, H. (1981): *Applied Regression Analysis,* p. 207. Wiley Series in Probability and Mathematical Statistics. Wiley, New York.
7. Dundee, J.W. (1954): The influence of body weight, sex and age on the dosage of thiopentone. *Br. J. Anaesth.,* 26:164–173.
8. Dundee, J.W., Hassard, T.H., McGowan, W.A.W., and Henshaw, J. (1982): The induction dose of thiopentone. *Anaesthesia,* 37:1176–1184.
9. Homer, T.D., and Stanski, D.R. (1985): The effect of increasing age on thiopental disposition and anesthetic requirement. *Anesthesiology, (in press).*
10. Hudson, R.J., Stanski, D.R., Saidman, L.J., and Meathe, E. (1983): A model for studying depth of anesthetic and acute tolerance to thiopental. *Amesthesiology,* 59:301–308.
11. Ouslander, J.G. (1981): Drug therapy in the elderly. *Ann. Intern. Med.,* 95:711–722.
12. Sheiner, L.B., Stanski, D.R., Vozeh, S., Ham, J., and Miller, R.D. (1979): Simultaneous modelling of pharmacokinetics and dynamics: Application of *d*-tubocurarine. *Clin. Pharmacol. Ther.,* 25:358–371.
13. Sheiner, L.B. (1981): ELSFIT—a program for the extended least squares fit to individual pharmacokinetic data. Technical report, Division of Clinical Pharmacology, University of California, San Francisco.
14. Shock, N.W. (1979): Systems physiology and aging. *Fed. Proc.,* 38:161.
15. Stanski, D.R., and Watkins, W.D. (1982): Intravenous anesthetics. In: *Drug Disposition in Anesthesia,* pp. 72–82. Grune & Stratton, New York.
16. Stanski, D.R., Burch, P.G., Harapat, S., and Richards, R.K. (1983): The pharmacokinetics and anesthetic potency of a thiopental contaminant isomer. *J. Pharm. Sci.,* 72:937–940.
17. Stanski, D.R., Hudson, R.J., Homer, T.D., Saidman, L.J., and Meathe, E. (1984): Pharmacodynamic modeling of thiopental anesthesia. *J. Pharmacokinet. Biopharm.,* 12:223–240.

DISCUSSION

Discussant 1 (D1): I was surprised to see that there was so little difference between the elderly and the young in the response to the same free concentration of drug, particularly as there is a drastic loss of brain neurons with age, e.g., in the monoaminergic system. Isn't there some suggestion that the effects of benzodiazepines (taking kinetic variability into consideration) are augmented with age?

Speaker (S): I am not aware of any good data in humans that demonstrate an age-related change in drug response for the benzodiazepines.

D2: Did you see if part of the variability seen with thiopental could be explained by the percentage of fat in the body, since this changes with age?

S: There was no weight relationship for any of the kinetics or dynamics, except for the dose requirement. The heavier patients required more drug to reach the EEG endpoint. We did not try to estimate lean body mass or percentage of body fat.

D3: I have a comment on the finding that the dose–effect relationship showed lower interindividual variability than the variability in C_{e50}. I think that one possible explanation for this surprising result is that you have used the standard two-stage method for estimation. It is possible that because the effect model is strongly nonlinear, the individual parameter estimates have large error, thereby inflating the interindividual variability.

S: That is a good point.

D4: The use of the coefficient of variation when comparing variability can give rise to misleading but apparently simple comparisons. My advice always is "Never use a coefficient of variation." This perhaps needs some modification if one has a logarithmic normal distribution: There is then something to be said for using a coefficient of variation, because it is effectively the standard deviation in the log distribution.

S: Your criticism is valid, but a more sophisticated statistical approach to comparing the variabilities in dose requirement, kinetics, and dynamics has not been performed on our data.

D5: It seems to me that Dr. Stanski would really like to look at the output of interest, the dose required for burst suppression, and to look at its sensitivity to the variability in the various parameters that control it. One could do this formally through a computer simulation, or one could approximate it by evaluating the (squared) partial derivatives of the output with respect to the parameters.

Variability in Drug Therapy:
Description, Estimation, and Control,
edited by M. Rowland et al.
Raven Press, New York © 1985.

Variability in Bioavailability: Concentration Versus Effect

Lennart K. Paalzow, * Gudrun H. M. Paalzow, and
† Peer Tfelt-Hansen

Department of Biopharmaceutics and Pharmacokinetics, Faculty of Pharmacy, University of Uppsala, S-751 23 Uppsala, Sweden; * Department of Pharmacology, Faculty of Pharmacy, University of Uppsala, S-751 23 Uppsala, Sweden; and † Department of Neurology, Rigshospitalet, DK-2100 Copenhagen Ø, Denmark.

Variation in the *extent* of bioavailability for a fixed dose of a drug leads to the same consequences for the pharmacological effect as would administration of variable i.v. doses. The resulting influences on the intensity and time course of the efffects depend on the characterstics of the dose–response relationship. For example, a flat dose–effect curve and a low maximal efficacy will reduce the importance of a variable bioavailability, whereas for drugs with steep dose–effect curves, small variations in bioavailability may cause dramatic changes in response, as Levy (11) has pointed out (Fig. 1).

The *rate* of bioavailability or rate of absorption can have qualitative as well as quantitative effects on drug responses, and it can also have consequences for the time course of activity. Again, the nature of the dose–response curve determines whether or not a variable rate of availability will influence the desired biological effect. We have recently become aware of the fact that several drugs interact with a variety of receptors or functional systems, depending on the administered dose or the biophase concentration attained (17–23). When a pharmacological effect is produced, we can thus observe a response from an interaction with a single type of receptor or a sum of responses elicited from various functional systems. The observed effect can therefore be regarded as a sum of l individual responses, $E = E_1 + E_2 \cdots E_l$, each of which could be of the same type or opposing to each others. Therefore, in the following, the significance of variable bioavailability will be discussed in relation to both single and composite dose–response relationships.

A SIMPLE SIGMOID DOSE–RESPONSE RELATIONSHIP

If we study the pharmacological effects of a drug using relatively large numbers of doses or establish the steady-state plasma concentrations for that partic-

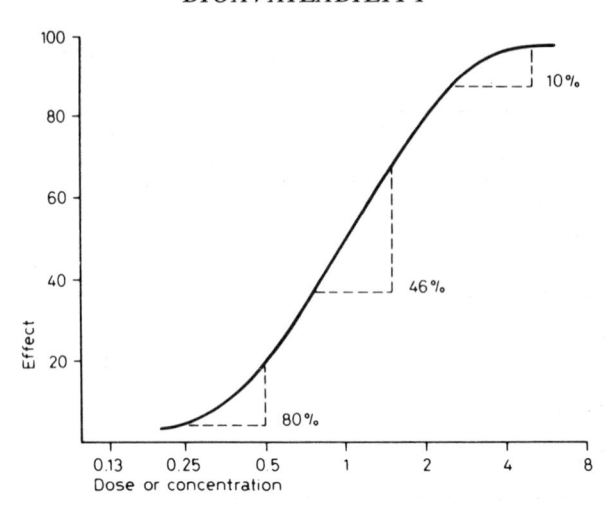

FIG. 1. Effect of a 50% decrease in bioavailability on pharmacological effect. (From Levy, ref. 11, with permission.)

ular dose range and find a typical sigmoid dose–response relationship when the effect is plotted against the logarithm of the dose, then the obtained response is most probably a consequence of activation of a single type of receptor leading to one type of effect.

A completely available dose after extravascular administration is desirable, and in such a situation the degree of variability in the amount of drug reaching the systemic blood circulation is minimized, and the variability in the effect produced should consequently be reduced. Decreased availability, on the contrary, increases the risk of greater variation in the amount taken up by the individual from time to time. However, a low extent of bioavailability does not necessarily mean that insufficient amounts of drug are reaching its site of action. The response of ergotamine on peripheral arteries can be described by a simple sigmoid E_{max} model. This is an example of a drug that has a very low bioavailability but still produces significant pharmacodynamic responses (8,28).

Ergotamine is an important agent for symptomatic relief of migraine attacks, but its use has been hampered by lack of knowledge of its clinical pharmacology. In a series of investigations we have studied the kinetics and bioavailability of ergotamine tartrate after intravenous, intramuscular, rectal, oral, sublingual, and pulmonary administration (4,5,7,8,29) using a sensitive and specific high-performance liquid chromatography (HPLC) technique for plasma analyses of ergotamine (3). Table 1 shows that an extremely low extent of availability was obtained after extravascular administration, except for the intramuscular injection; e.g., after oral administration, no ergotamine was detectable in blood samples, whereas small and very variable quantities were found after rectal administration. Therefore, regular calculations of bioavaila-

TABLE 1. *Bioavailability of ergotamine tartrate in migraine sufferers, volunteers, and patients with cluster headache*

Mode of administration and references	Dose of ergotamine tartrate (mg)	Bioavailability and maximal possible bioavailability (%) (ranges)	No. of subjects
Intramuscular (7)	0.5	46.6 ± 12.7 (SD)	5
Per os, tablet (8)	2	< (0.9–3.4)	7
Per os, tablet (4)	2–4	< 1.0	5
Per os, effervescent tablet (5)	2	< (0.6–2.6)	8
Rectal, suppository (5)	2	< (0.6–3.5)	8
Rectal, suppository (8)	2	< (0.9–10.8)	7
Rectal, solution (8)	2	<(1.6–11.1)	12
Inhalation (5)	2.2	< (0.5–2.2)	6
Sublingual (29)	2	< 1.0	4

bility could not be performed in most of the patients. An estimate of the maximal possible availability was calculated by assuming a hypothetically constant concentration of ergotamine corresponding to the limit of chemical detection (0.1 ng/ml) from time 0 up to 10 hr (five times the biological half-life). By this calculation the bioavailability ranged from 1% up to approximately 4% after oral and rectal administrations; this is, of course, an overestimation of the true values (8).

Do these findings mean that ergotamine is without any effect against migraine by the previously mentioned modes of administration? We were uncertain at first. However, after performing parallel pharmacokinetic and pharmacodynamic studies we have come to the following conclusion (30).

Ergotamine tartrate (0.5 mg) was administered intramuscularly to 10 migraine patients outside an attack. The effect on peripheral arteries was measured as a decrease in the toe systolic blood pressure and was followed for 4 days after a single dose. As can be seen in Fig. 2, ergotamine was rapidly absorbed, and the plasma concentrations reached a maximum within 30 min following administration. The levels then declined, with a half-life of approximately 2.5 hr, and reached the limit of detection after approximately 7 hr. In contrast, the effects on peripheral arteries developed slowly and reached a maximum at 4 to 6 hr after intramuscular administration of a bolus dose of 0.5 mg. The effect was well sustained for the following 2 days, as shown in Fig. 2. In order to describe the discrepancy in the temporal aspects of the pharmacodynamic effect of ergotamine in relation to its plasma concentration, we adopted the model of Sheiner et al. (26) (Fig. 2). By this approach the pronounced counterclockwise hysteresis between concentrations and effects can be resolved, and the pharmacodynamic effect (E) can be related to its steady-state plasma concentration C_{pss} according to the Hill equation:

$$E = E_{max}C_{pss}^{\gamma}/(C_{pss}^{\gamma} + C_{pss50}^{\gamma})$$

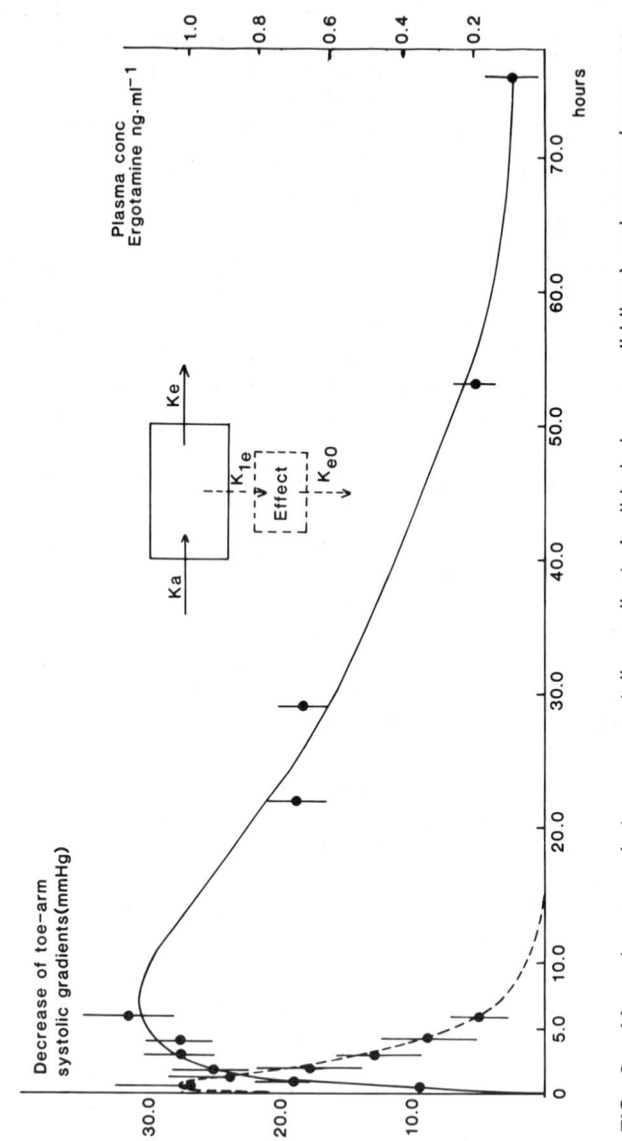

FIG. 2. Mean decreases in toe–arm systolic gradients (*solid circles on solid lines*) and mean plasma concentrations of ergotamine (*dash line*) after 0.5 mg of ergotamine tartrate i.m. to 10 patients. *Points* are actual measured values (± SE), and *lines* show the computed fit. The effect-compartment model is inserted. (From Tfelt-Hansen and Paalzow, ref. 30, with permission.)

where C_{pss50} is the steady-state plasma concentration causing 50% of the maximum response (E_{max}) and γ is a number influencing the slope of the effect–concentration relationship. The first-order rate constant characterizing the temporal aspects of equilibrium between plasma concentration and response is described by k_{eo} (Fig. 2). The equation (1) was fitted to the experimental time–effect data using the pharmacokinetic parameters of the equation for plasma concentration–time data as constants. As shown in Fig. 2, a satisfactory fit was obtained for the computed effect data to the experimental data points, and the results for the 10 patients are given in Table 2.

The rate constant k_{eo} showed a mean half-life of 9.9 hr, with a fivefold variation. The sensitivity parameter C_{pss50} showed, on the contrary, great interindividual variability that varied 40-fold from 0.044 to 1.79 ng/ml. The wide range of values obtained for the pharmacodynamic parameter (C_{pss50}) probably involves errors in measuring and modeling and in the interindividual variability in the response to ergotamine. It has been proposed that ergotamine contracts arteries by stimulation of 5-hydroxytryptamine (5-HT) receptors (15), and recently a 30-fold variability in the sensitivity of human temporal arteries to 5-HT has been reported (27). Nevertheless, 4 patients needed steady-state plasma levels for 50% of maximum effect that were less than 0.1 ng/ml, the sensitivity limit of the analytical method. Thus, a given dose of ergotamine per os or rectally can produce plasma levels between 0.05 and 0.1 ng/ml that we are unable to measure and that correspond to a systemic bioavailability less than 2%. However, such low plasma levels are still enough to produce a significant effect of ergotamine on arteries in patients sensitive to this drug (low C_{pss50} values). Obviously, ergotamine is a highly potent drug in certain individuals, and in the therapeutic situation it is desirable to titrate ergotamine responders to the optimal dose.

TABLE 2. *Effect-model parameters (k_{eo} = equilibration constant, C_{pss50} = steady-state plasma concentration causing 50% of maximal effect) for the effect of ergotamine on peripheral systolic blood pressure*

Patient	$T_{½}k_{eo}$ ± SD (hr)	C_{pss50} ± SD (ng/ml)
1	9.3 ± 0.5	0.508 ± 0.078
2	46.2 ± 0.2	0.078 ± 0.008
3	11.9 ± 3.0	1.787 ± 0.697
4	8.4 ± 0.9	0.792 ± 0.171
5	8.8 ± 0.9	0.128 ± 0.010
6	10.8 ± 2.5	0.829 ± 0.381
7	9.4 ± 2.4	0.065 ± 0.008
8	30.9 ± 2.7	0.044 ± 0.007
9	9.8 ± 1.6	0.059 ± 0.010
10	18.2 ± 5.7	1.443 ± 0.795
Mean ± SD	12.0 ± 5.0	0.573 ± 0.631
Data calculated from mean concentration ± SD	9.9 ± 0.5	0.238 ± 0.029

Consequently, low bioavailability does not necessarily mean that a drug is clinically ineffective. The *interindividual* variabilities in both pharmacodynamic responses and kinetics might be of greater importance in the therapeutic situation. For ergotamine, the variability in pharmacodynamic responses among individuals is probably more important than the obtained threefold to fivefold variability in pharmacokinetic parameters such as volume of distribution and clearance (7).

The effect of ergotamine on pheripheral arteries was characterized by a simple sigmoid E_{max} model that to our knowledge reflects an interaction with a single type of receptor. However, if a drug interacts with several types of concentration-sensitive receptor systems, producing several similar or opposing effects within a relatively small range of concentrations, another kind of complex situation will appear in establishing the pharmacodynamic response, and the relationship between drug level and effect may not always be readily apparent. This is exemplified by some of our recent studies with apomorphine (20,23), yohimbine (21), and promethazine (22), as well as by studies from the literature.

RELATIONSHIP BETWEEN PHARMACOKINETICS AND PHARMACODYNAMICS FOR DRUGS WITH MULTIPLE RESPONSE CHARACTERISTICS

In recent investigations on rats (20) we found that apomorphine induced opposing effects on pain, so that low doses (25–100 µg/kg) dose-dependently increased the sensitivity to painful stimulation. This effect then gradually declined in intensity with increasing doses, and we found that high doses, on the contrary, induced analgesia, as shown in Fig. 3. We suggested that the observed effect involved the sum of responses from at least two opposing functional systems, and we resolved the composite effect into two components, each having its particular dose–response characteristics: low doses having an ED_{50} of 36 µg/kg in producing hyperreactivity to pain, and high doses having an ED_{50} of 465 µg/kg (in the absence of hyperalgesia) for inducing antinociception.

Depending on the mode of administration, the shape of the observed dose–response curve for the effect of apomorphine on pain will have consequences for the time course of the effects. After subcutaneous administration, when drug levels are rising during the absorption phase, we are moving along the dose (concentration) axis from left to right in Fig. 3.

Figure 4 shows the temporal pattern of effects on pain for an apomorphine dose of 5 mg/kg given subcutaneously. Because apomorphine rapidly penetrates into the rat brain (23), and we did not record the effect continuously, we were not able to measure the increased reactivity to pain during the absorption phase. Therefore, after 5 min we observed analgesia that lasted 70 min and

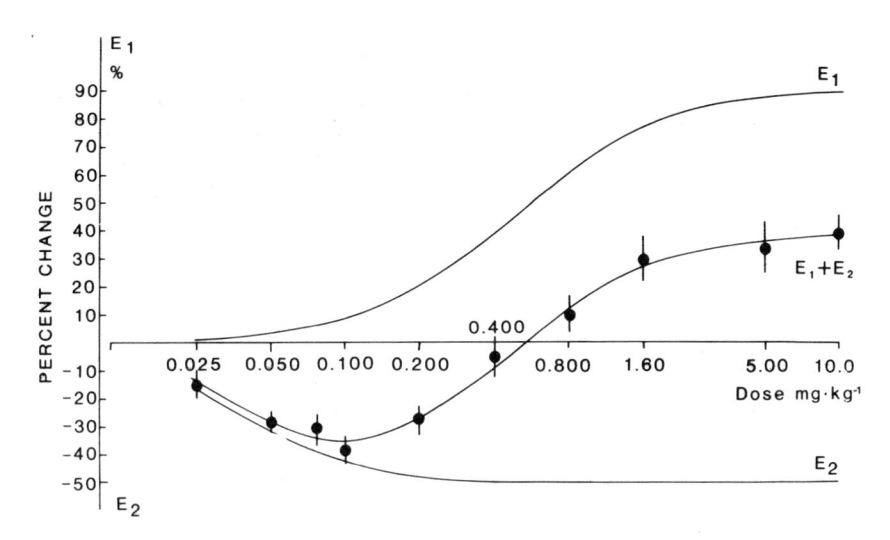

FIG. 3. Dose-response relationship for apomorphine HCl and the threshold for vocalization after s.c. administration of the drug at the time of maximum response. Each *point* represents the mean ± SE for 9 or 10 rats. The observed effect (E) is expressed as the percentage change from the pretest threshold and is dissociated into two components E_1 and E_2, representing two responses. (From Paalzow and Paalzow, ref. 20, with permission.)

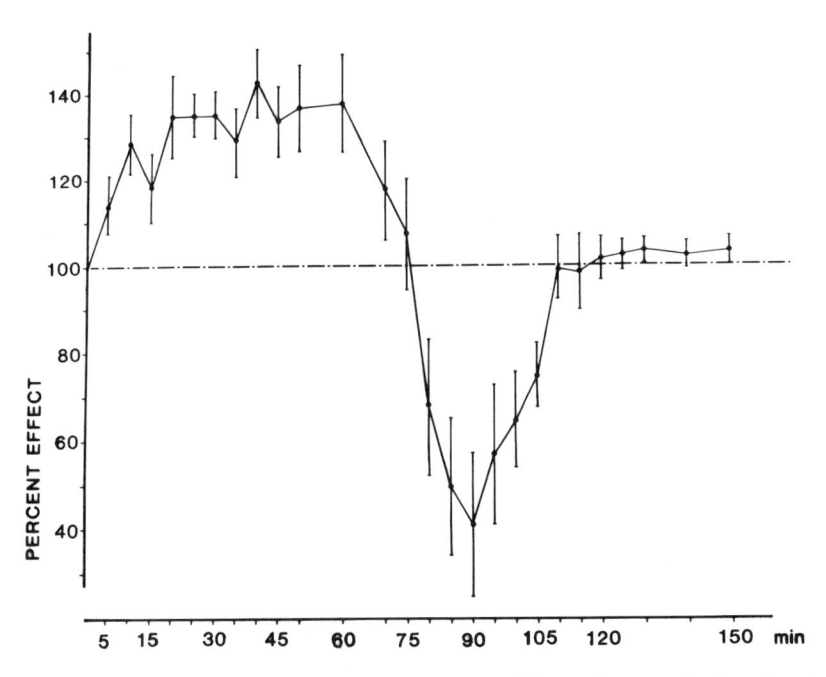

FIG. 4. Time courses of effects of apomorphine HCl on the vocalization threshold after s.c. administration of 5.0 mg/kg. The figure illustrates results from rats in which hyperalgesia was detected during the elimination phase of apomorphine. Each *point* represents the mean ± SE for 7 of 10 animals tested. (From Paalzow and Paalzow, ref. 20, with permission.)

then changed into the opposite effect, hyperalgesia, during the elimination phase, when the concentration of drug in the biophase was declining.

Another example of the same type of dose–response curve was obtained in rats after subcutaneous administration of yohimbine (21). Doses from 0.25 mg/kg to approximately 1 mg/kg produced a dose-dependent increase in sensitivity to painful stimulation that then gradually changed into analgesia with increasing doses (> 5 mg/kg s.c.) (Fig. 5). After a high dose of yohimbine (8 mg/kg s.c.) we observed a time course of opposing effects, with an initial hyperalgesia that then changed into analgesia (Fig. 6). We are presently studying the effects of yohimbine on heart rate and blood pressure in conscious rats. Analogous to the results on pain, a yohimbine dose of 8 mg/kg s.c. induces contrasting effects on heart rate during the time course of its action (Fig. 6). As yet, we have not performed any pharmacokinetic studies of yohimbine, which may, however, be expected to be a drug with a slow rate of absorption after s.c. injection.

When we used continuous recording of heart rate and blood pressure in rats, we also found opposing hemodynamic effects of apomorphine (23). Blood pressure and heart rate were studied in conscious rats at different subcutaneous doses. As shown in Fig. 7, a low dose of 50 µg/kg produced a pure bradycardia. A dose of 100 µg/kg induced an initial decrease in heart rate, followed by an increase and a decrease. When apomorphine was given at a high dose of 5 mg/kg s.c., the effect also appeared in the following sequence: bradycar-

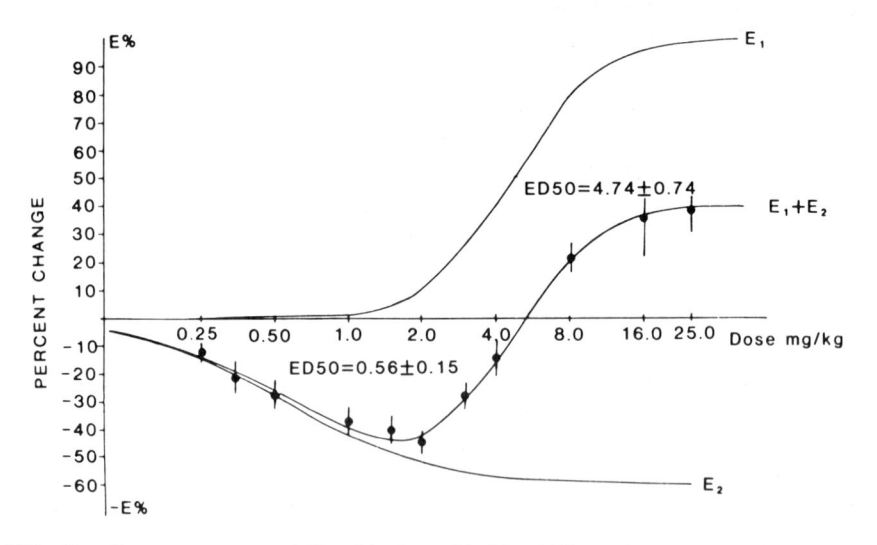

FIG. 5. Dose–response relationship for yohimbine HCl on the vocalization threshold at 30 min after s.c. injection of the alkaloid. Each *point* represents the mean ± SE for 9 to 11 rats. The observed effect (E) is expressed as the percentage change from the pretest threshold and is dissociated into two components E_1 and E_2, representing two responses from different functional systems. (From Paalzow and Paalzow, ref. 21, with permission.)

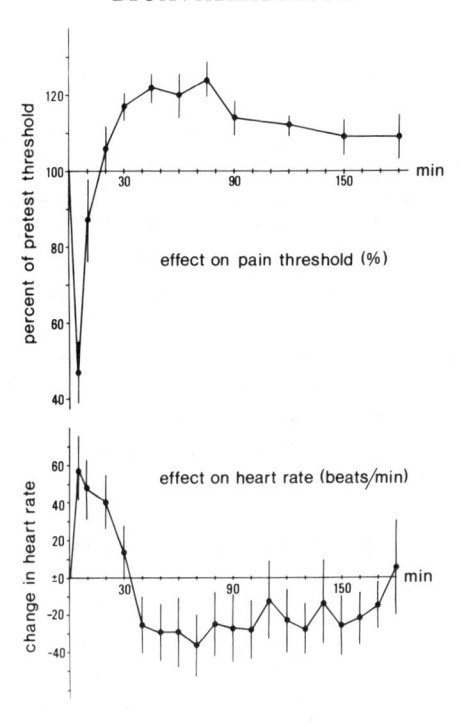

FIG. 6. Time courses of effects of yohimbine HCl on the vocalization threshold **(top)** and on heart rate **(bottom)** after s.c. administration of 8 mg/kg. Each *point* represents the mean ± SE for 8 to 10 rats.

dia-tachycardia-bradycardia. Because we have evaluated the pharmacokinetics of apomorphine in the rat (23), using an HPLC analysis, we can calculate the concentration–effect curves for apomorphine from the following equations:

$$E = \frac{E_{1max} \cdot C_p^{\gamma_1}}{C_p^{\gamma_1} + C_{pss50_1}^{\gamma_1}} + \frac{E_{2max} \cdot C_p^{\gamma_2}}{C_p^{\gamma_2} + C_{pss50_2}^{\gamma_2}} \quad (1)$$

$$C_p = A(e^{-k_e \cdot t} - e^{-k_a \cdot t}) \quad (2)$$

Apomorphine showed rapid tissue distribution after s.c. administration, and the rate of uptake and disappearance in the whole brain followed the kinetics of plasma concentrations. Therefore, the plasma levels could be used to reflect the biophase levels of apomorphine. The coefficient and rate constants of equation (2) were obtained from the kinetic studies and used as constants when fitting equations (1) and (2) to the observed effects (E) over time, and the fits are shown in Fig. 7. The calculated concentration–effect relationship can be seen in Fig. 8. The two components of the observed effects were also depicted as separate effects (bradycardia and tachycardia). As can be seen, a steady-state plasma level approximately 25 times higher is needed to produce tachycardia (C_{pss50} = 35.9 ± 2.3 ng/ml) as compared with bradycardia

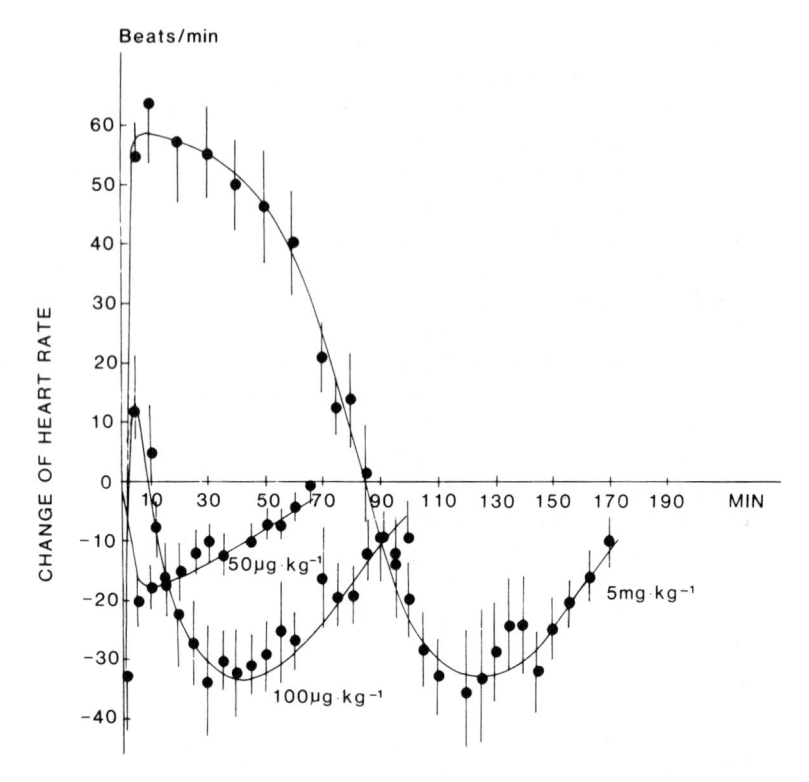

FIG. 7. Effects of apomorphine HCl on heart rate in rats after subcutaneous injection of 50 µg/kg, 100 µg/kg, and 5 mg/kg. Each *point* represents the mean ± SE for 10 to 15 rats, and the *solid line* represents the best fit of equations (1) and (2) to the observed data points.

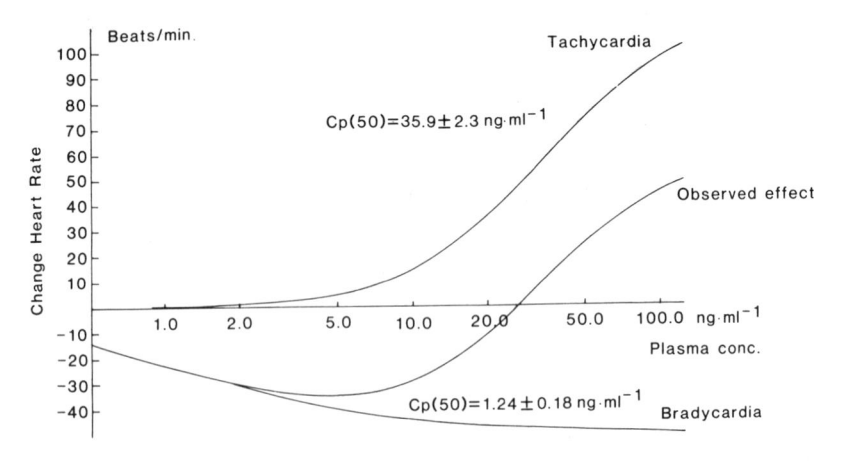

FIG. 8. Steady-state plasma-concentration–response data for the effect of apomorphine on heart rate calculated by equations (1) and (2) from the data given in Fig. 7. Cp(50) is the steady-state plasma concentration causing 50% of the maximum response (C_{pss50} in the text).

(C_{pss50} = 1.24 ± 0.18 ng/ml). We are thus moving over the observed concentration–effect curve from left to right and back again after a high s.c. dose of apomorphine of 5 mg/kg. Thus, a short-lasting bradycardia is produced during the absorption phase that rapidly turns into tachycardia at maximum load of the drug (Fig. 7). During the elimination phase, bradycardia will appear again when the concentration is continuously decreasing.

Variable bioavailability can be predicted to have a number of consequences for the pharmacodynamic effects of a drug producing multiple opposing responses, as shown for apomorphine and yohimbine. A low dose or a low bioavailability for a drug like apomorphine can produce pure bradycardia. Higher doses may, in addition to bradycardia, also produce tachycardia. Furthermore, a slow and constant rate of absorption may produce a more "pure" effect. If tachycardia is the desired effect, a rapid onset produced by a high dose and a sustained effect produced by an absorption-rate-limited disposition might be the optimal conditions to achieve therapeutic efficacy.

Problems with multiple responses during the time course after a single dose have been observed in several experimental and clinical studies, although there have not been any explanations of the findings. With a technique to continuously record the effects on motility in rats, Montanaro et al. (13) recently demonstrated that apomorphine (300 µg/kg s.c.) produced inhibition of motility for 5 to 6 min after administration and then, on the contrary, had a stimulatory effect (Fig. 9).

It should be recalled that not only during absorption but also during elimination, when drug levels decline, problems may arise after single doses of drugs with multiple response characteristics: As shown earlier, contrasting effects on

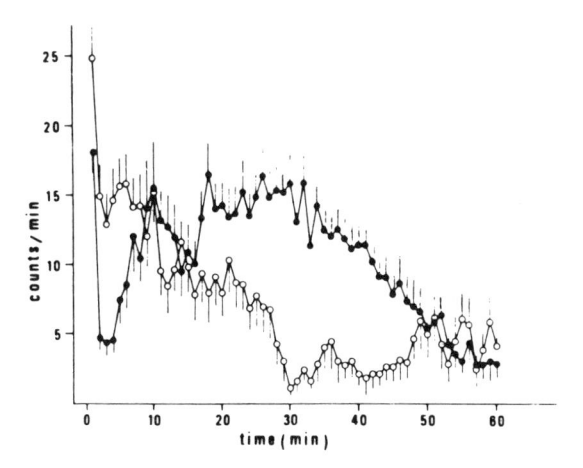

FIG. 9. Minute-by-minute time course of motility of "naive" rats treated s.c. with saline (*open circles*) or apomorphine HCl (300 µg/kg) (*filled circles*) and placed into the actometers 30 sec later. Each *point* represents the mean ± SE for 20 animals. (From Montanaro et al., ref. 13, with permission.)

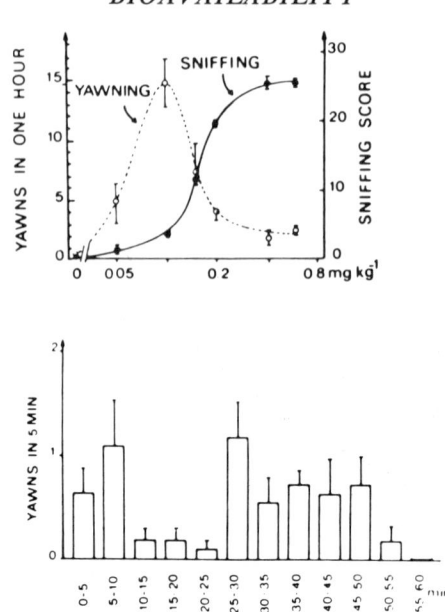

FIG. 10. Top: Effects of apomorphine on yawning and sniffing after different doses given s.c. **Bottom:** Time courses of yawning in rats treated with apomorphine 0.15 mg/kg. Yawning was observed during 12 periods of 5 min. Each point represents the mean ± SE for 6 to 14 rats. (From Protais et al., ref. 25, with permission.)

pain and heart rate were produced by a high single dose of apomorphine during the elimination phase. Accordingly, Protais et al. (25) found that the yawning effect of apomorphine in rats had a bell-shaped dose–response curve and that during the time course of 150 μg/kg s.c. the yawns appeared, disappeared, and reappeared (Fig. 10).

Thiopentone is a drug with a U-shaped dose–response curve for pain in humans (Fig. 11): Low i.v. doses induce an immediate increase in responsiveness to pain in patients, and consequently single high i.v. doses produce hyperalgesia during the elimination phase (Fig. 11) (1,2).

Concentration–response curves of many different shapes have been shown in several clinical and experimental models: A bell-shaped dose–response curve has recently been published for the effects of the mixed agonist/antagonist butorphanol on rat striatal DOPAC (3,4 dihydroxyphenylacetic acid) levels (Fig. 12). With progressively increasing doses, two types of receptors were implicated to be activated (31).

Other clinical studies have also been presented showing concentration–response curves that may be interpreted as the result of activation of at least two types of opposing or antagonizing systems by increasing concentrations. Mavroides et al. (12) showed that after haloperidol, schizophrenic patients exhibited a bell-shaped curve when improvements in symptoms were plotted against

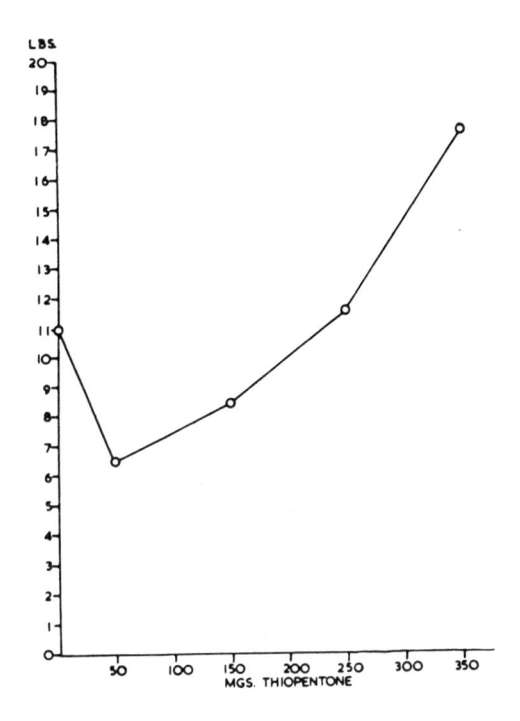

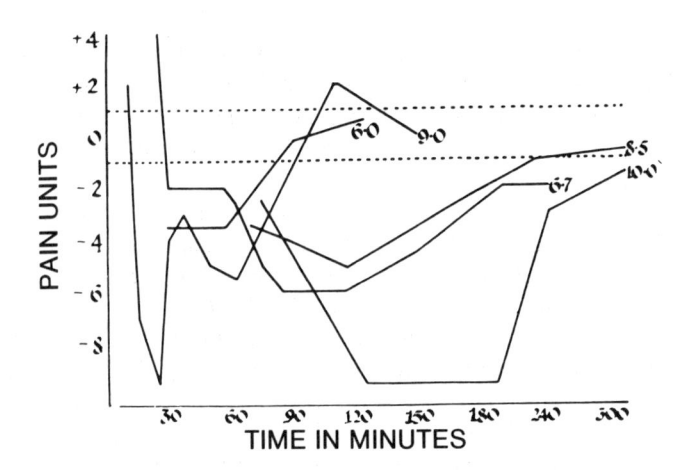

FIG. 11. Top: Effects of thiopentone at increasing i.v. doses on the pain threshold. (From Clutton-Brock, ref. 1, with permission.) **Bottom:** Postoperative pain response readings related to the control reading in patients who received large i.v. doses of thiopentone. (From Dundee, ref. 2, with permission.)

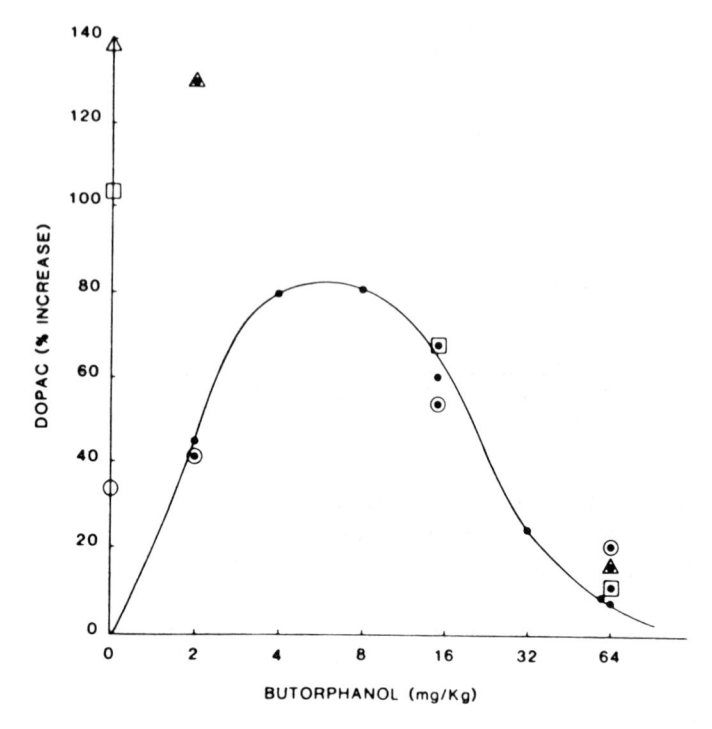

FIG. 12. Actions of morphine, butorphanol, and morphine/butorphanol combinations on rat striatal DOPAC levels. Butorphanol was administered at −6 min, and morphine at time 0, and the rats were killed at 60 min. Points are means for 7 to 10 animals, with SE less than 6%. *Solid circle,* butorphanol; *open circle,* morphine (2); *open square,* morphine (16); *open triangle,* morphine (64). (From Wood et al., ref. 31, with permission.)

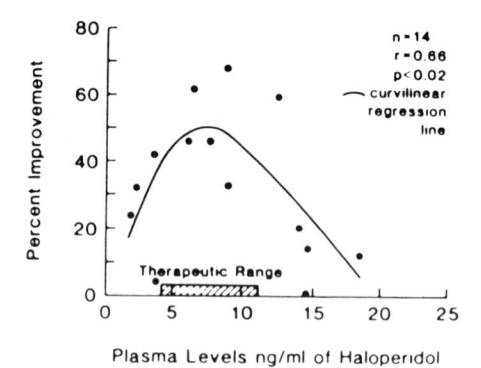

FIG. 13. Percentage clinical improvement in schizophrenia as a function of plasma level of haloperidol for the first 2 weeks of treatment. (From Mavroides et al., ref. 12, with permission.)

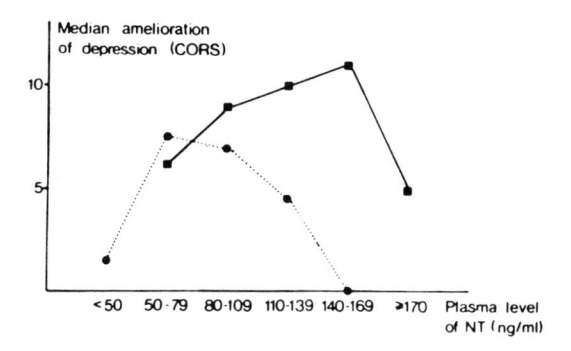

FIG. 14. Relation between plasma concentrations of nortriptyline and effect on endogenous depression after 2 weeks (Karolinska hospital; *solid circle*) and 4 weeks (Glostrup hospital; *solid square*) of treatment. (From Åsberg et al., ref. 32, and Kragh-Sørensen et al., ref. 9, with permission.)

steady-state plasma concentrations of the drug (Fig. 13). A rather narrow therapeutic window was suggested for this drug.

A similar type of window has been reported for nortriptyline (9,32) when treating patients for endogenous depression (Fig. 14). We have also found quite a narrow range of steady-state plasma concentrations of clonidine for the hypotensive effect in patients (6). A maximum decrease in mean arterial blood pressure was obtained at doses between 0.5 ng/ml and approximately 2 ng/ml. Higher levels gave no effect or a hypertensive response (Fig. 15).

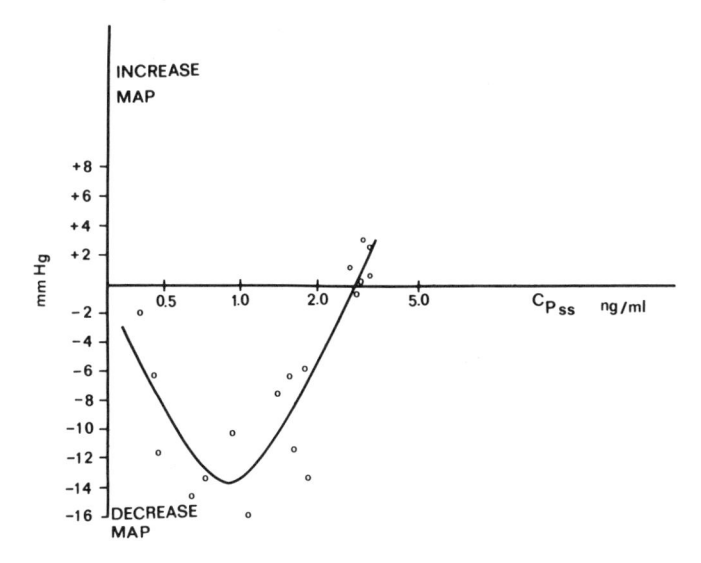

FIG. 15. Effects of clonidine on blood pressure in patients at various steady-state plasma concentrations. *Symbols* indicate individual patients. The curve is the best fit obtained from the equation $E = E_1 + E_2$, where E is the observed effect, E_1 is the calculated separate hypertensive response, and E_2 is the separate hypotensive response. (From Frisk-Holmberg et al., ref. 6, with permission.)

We have mentioned some concentration–effect relationships in which variability in bioavailability may cause not only variable degrees of responses but also variable natures of the effects. From these examples of concentration–response curves with multiple response characteristics we can predict a number of consequences for the time course of the effects dependent on the absorption and disposition characteristics of the specific drug. For example, if the low-concentration-induced effect is the desired one, a high dose given orally will produce a fluctuating effect that is on-off-on. A low dose may give a pure effect if the maximum concentration during the absorption phase does not exceed the maximum (or minimum) of the concentration–response curve. If, on the other hand, the response produced by high concentrations is desired, a high extravascular dose may give an effect pattern that is off-on-off. Variable "purity" of the effect may thus be caused by variable bioavailability.

Finally, when establishing a concentration–effect relationship, we have to consider not only factors influencing the biophase concentration but also the physiological or pathophysiological factors that may influence the biological response.

Promethazine is another example of an impure drug with dual effects on pain. Low doses produce hyperreactivity to painful stimulation in humans, rats, and mice (10,14,22), whereas higher doses produce analgesia (22). Figure 16 (22) shows the effects of different doses of promethazine on pain when we

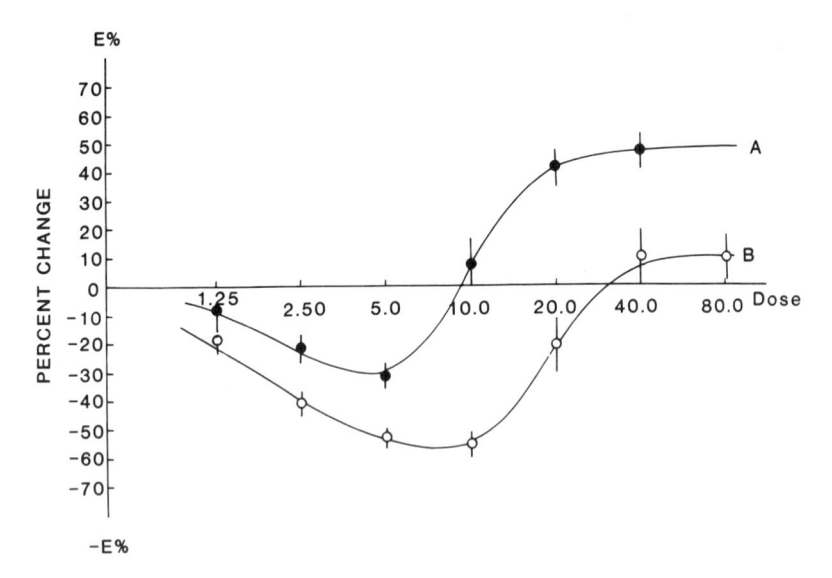

FIG. 16. Dose–response relationships for promethazine HCl and the threshold for vocalization (case A) and the threshold for vocalization when the animals were subjected to brief suprathreshold stimulation between recordings (case B). Doses of 1.25 to 80.0 mg/kg s.c. were administered, and the effects are given at the time of maximum response. Each point represents the mean ± SE for 9 or 10 rats. The observed effect is expressed as the percentage change from the pretest threshold. (From Paalzow and Paalzow, ref. 22, with permission.)

used two modes of nociceptive stimulation in rats: In case A, the stimulation was restricted to the vocalization threshold level; in case B, brief suprathreshold stimulation was applied between recordings (22). The results showed that when the intensity of the stimulation was increased, the maximal magnitude of the hyperalgesic effect was enhanced, although the potency for this effect remained unchanged. These results indicate that the net effect of promethazine on pain is balanced not only by the biophase concentration but also by the prevailing experimental situation, so that suprathreshold pain summates with the hyperalgesic properties of the drug, resulting in an increased total response to this effect, leaving the analgesic effect unchanged. Thus, with mild stimulation when the nociceptive threshold recorded is not exceeded, the potential of high composite doses to induce analgesia is more easily revealed.

We have thus exemplified how, among variables, the pharmacological testing procedure by itself may influence the response. Our guess is that also in the clinical situation there might be examples analogous to this. For example, the on-off phenomenon in the clinical response to levodopa in patients with Parkinson's disease is thought to depend both on pharmacokinetic factors and on factors influencing dopamine receptor function (16).

To summarize, the dose–response characteristics for a drug determine the consequences of variable bioavailability. In the future we should spend a great deal of effort not only on detailed evaluation of drug absorption and disposition but also on more careful characterization of the dose–effect (concentration–effect) relationships. Such studies should preferably be performed *in vivo* to enable us to detect a potential complex pharmacological effect, and a dose range as large as possible should be used.

REFERENCES

1. Clutton-Brock, J. (1961): Pain and the barbiturates. *Anaesthesia,* 16:80–88.
2. Dundee, J.W. (1960): Alterations in response to somatic pain associated with anaesthesia. II: The effect of thiopentone and pentobarbitone. *Br. J. Anaesth.,* 32:407–414.
3. Edlund, P.O. (1981): Determination of ergot alkaloids in plasma by high performance liquid chromatography and fluorescence detection. *J. Chromatogr.,* 226:107–115.
4. Ekbom, K., Paalzow, L., and Waldenlind, E. (1981): Low biological availability of ergotamine tartrate after oral dosing in cluster headache. *Cephalalgia,* 1:203–207.
5. Ekbom, K., Krabbe, A., Paalzow, G., Paalzow, L., and Tfelt-Hansen, P. (1983): Optimal routes of administration of ergotamine tartrate in cluster headache patients. A pharmacokinetic study. *Cephalalgia,* 3:15–20.
6. Frisk-Holmberg, M., Paalzow, L., and Wibell, L. (1984): Relationship between the cardiovascular effects and steady-state kinetics of clonidine in hypertension. Demonstration of a therapeutic window in man. *Eur. J. Clin. Pharmacol.,* 26:1–5.
7. Ibraheem, J., Paalzow, L., and Tfelt-Hansen, P. (1982): Kinetics of ergotamine after intravenous and intramuscular administration to migraine sufferers. *Eur. J. Clin. Pharmacol.,* 23:235–240.
8. Ibraheem, J., Paalzow, L., and Tfelt-Hansen, P. (1983): Low bioavailability of ergotamine tartrate after oral and rectal administration in migraine sufferers. *Br. J. Clin. Pharmacol.,* 16:695–699.
9. Kragh-Sørensen, P., Hansen, C.E., and Åsberg, M. (1973): Plasma levels of nortryptiline in the treatment of edogenous depression. *Acta Psychiatr. Scand.,* 49:444–456.

10. Leslie, G.B., and Nunn, B. (1968): The effect of promethazine on the antinociceptive actions of some narcotic analgesics. *J. Pharm. Pharmacol.,* 20:881–882.
11. Levy, G. (1972): Bioavailability, clinical effectiveness, and the public interest. *Pharmacology,* 8:33–43.
12. Mavroides, M.L., Kanter, D.R., Hirschowitz, J., and Garver, D.L. (1983): Clinical response and plasma haloperidol levels in schizophrenia. *Psychopharmacology,* 81:354–356.
13. Montanaro, N., Vaccheri, A., Dall'Olio, R., and Gandolfi, O. (1983): Time course of rat motility response to apomorphine: A simple model for studying preferential blockade of brain dopamine receptors mediating sedation. *Psychopharmacology,* 81:214–219.
14. Moore, J., and Dundee, J.W. (1961): Alteration in response to somatic pain associated with anaesthesia. V. The effect of promethazine. *Br. J. Anaesth.,* 33:3–8.
15. Müller-Schweinitzer, E. (1976): Evidence for stimulation of 5-HT receptors in canine saphenous arteries by ergotamine. *Naunyn Schmiedebergs Arch. Pharmacol.,* 295:41–44.
16. Nutt, J.G., Woodward, W.R., Hammerstad, J.P., Carter, J.H., and Anderson, J.L. (1984): The "on-off" phenomenon in Parkinson's disease. *N. Engl. J. Med.,* 310:483–488.
17. Paalzow, L. (1981): Pharmacokinetics and drug response. In: *Topics in Pharmaceutical Sciences,* edited by D.D. Breimer and P. Speiser, pp. 69–84. Elsevier, Amsterdam.
18. Paalzow, L., and Edlund, P.O. (1979): Multiple receptor responses. A new concept to describe the relationship between pharmacological effects and pharmacokinetics of a drug: Studies on clonidine in the rat and cat. *J. Pharmacokinet. Biopharm.,* 7:495–510.
19. Paalzow, L., and Paalzow, G. (1982): Separate noradrenergic receptors could mediate clonidine induced antinociception. *J. Pharmacol. Exp. Ther.,* 223:795–800.
20. Paalzow, G., and Paalzow, L. (1983): Opposing effects of apomorphine on pain in rats. Evaluation of the dose–response curve. *Eur. J. Pharmacol.,* 88:27–35.
21. Paalzow, G., and Paalzow, L. (1983): Yohimbine both increases and decreases nociceptive thresholds in rats: Evaluation of the dose–response relationship. *Naunyn Schmiedebergs Arch. Pharmacol.,* 322:193–197.
22. Paalzow, G., and Paalzow, L. (1985): Promethazine both facilitates and inhibits nociception in rats: Effects of the testing procedure. *Psychopharmacology,* (in press).
23. Paalzow, G., and Paalzow, L. (1985): The relationship between pharmacokinetics and cardiovascular effects of apomorphine in the conscious rats. *J. Pharm. Pharmacol.,* (in press).
24. Paalzow, L., Paalzow, G., and Tfelt-Hansen, P. (1984): Kinetics of drug action. In: *Pharmacokinetics: A Modern View,* edited by L.Z. Benet and G. Levy, pp. 327–343. Plenum Press, New York.
25. Protais, P., Dubuc, I., and Costentin, J. (1983): Pharmacological characteristics of dopamine agonists on yawning behaviour in rats. *Eur. J. Pharmacol.,* 94:271–280.
26. Sheiner, L.B., Stanski, D.R., Vozeh, S., Miller, R.D., and Ham, J. (1979): Simultaneous modeling of pharmacokinetics and pharmacodynamics: Application to *d*-tubocurarine. *Clin. Pharmacol. Ther.,* 25:358–371.
27. Skärby, T., Tfelt-Hansen, P., Gjerris, F., Edvinsson, L., and Olesen, J. (1982): Characterization of 5-hydroxytryptamine receptors in human temporal arteries: Comparison between migraine sufferers and non-sufferers. *Ann. Neurol.,* 12:272–277.
28. Tfelt-Hansen, P., Kanstrup, I.L., Christensen, N.J., and Winkler, K. (1983): General and regional haemodynamic effects of intravenous ergotamine in man. *Clin. Sci.,* 65:599–604.
29. Tfelt-Hansen, P., Paalzow, L., and Ibraheem, J.J. (1982): Bioavailability of sublingual ergotamine. *Br. J. Clin. Pharmacol.,* 13:239–240.
30. Tfelt-Hansen, P., and Paalzow, L. (1984): Plasma levels and pharmacodynamic activity of intramuscular ergotamine. *Clin. Pharmacol. Ther., (in press).*
31. Wood, P.L., McQuade, P., Richard, J.W., and Thakur, M. (1983): Agonist/antagonist analgesics and nigrostriatal dopamine metabolism in the rat: Evidence for receptor dualism. *Life Sci. [Suppl. I],* 33:759–762.
32. Åsberg, M., Cronholm, B., Sjöqvist, F., and Tuck, D. (1971): Relationship between plasma level and therapeutic effect of nortriptyline. *Br. Med. J.,* 3:331–334.

DISCUSSION

Discussant 1 (D1): You did not discuss active metabolites that might also cause some of the time dependencies in effects.

Speaker (S): When the work on ergotamine was started, there was no evidence for active metabolites. Therefore we did not consider them in the calculation.

D2: For another ergot peptide alkaloid, dihydroergotamine (DHE), several active metabolites exist *in vivo* (1,2). The main metabolite has the same activity as the parent compound, with concentrations in plasma five to seven times higher. Whereas the plasma level peaks early and falls to the detection limit within 8 hr, the venoconstriction activity remains at plateau over that period (2). There might be active metabolites of ergotamine as well.

D3: Your ergotamine data show large differences between subjects. Did you have the occasion to study the subjects a second time to see if these great differences are relatively stable within a subject?

S: No. Also of interest would be to have some biochemical measurement that would indicate which patients will be responders or nonresponders to ergotamine treatment.

D4: One point intrigues me in the case of apomorphine and yohimbine. When you cross the line from hyperalgesia to analgesia, one would expect, if this is due to the stimulation of two different types of dopaminergic receptors, as it probably is, that the variability of the results would be large, whereas your standard error was the same whatever the dose. Aren't you surprised by this?

S: If you look again at the figures, you will find that standard errors do increase for composite effects in comparison with pure effects, especially in the case of promethazine when overthreshold stimulation was used.

D5: Because of the bell-shaped response curves that you have shown, what is your feeling about controlled-release products?

S: Clonidine, for example, is marketed as a new transdermal dosage form. You have to find the right dose. If you come too much to the right on the dose–response curve, you may not get any effect.

REFERENCES

1. Aellig, W.H. (1984): Investigation of the venoconstrictor effect of 8-hydroxydihydroergotamine, the main metabolite of dihydroergotamine, in man. *Eur. J. Clin. Pharmacol.,* 26:239–242.
2. Stuermer, E. (1984): Pharmakologische und pharmakokinetische Betrachtungen über Dihydroergotamin unter besonderer Berücksichtigung neuer Aspekte. In: *Neuester Stand der Dihydergot-Forschung,* edited by P. Fitscha. Georg Thieme Verlag, Stuttgart.

*Variability in Drug Therapy:
Description, Estimation, and Control,*
edited by M. Rowland et al.
Raven Press, New York © 1985.

Optimal Design for Individual Parameter Estimation in Pharmacokinetics

Elliot M. Landaw

Department of Biomathematics, University of California at Los Angeles School of Medicine, Los Angeles, California 90024

Experiment-based model building plays an important role in pharmacokinetic analysis. Discriminating the correct structural model among several alternatives (e.g., single versus multicompartmental, linear versus nonlinear) yields valuable insights into pharmacokinetic mechanisms, and estimating model parameters is the key step for quantifying individual response and population variability. It is the purpose of this chapter to demonstrate how properly designed individual studies can significantly improve the efficiency of parameter estimation.

An individual pharmacokinetic experiment typically consists of administration of a test compound and measurement of the changing drug concentration in timed samples of blood, urine, stool, etc. Therefore, design decisions can be made at several levels:

1. which route to administer the drug (e.g., i.v., intramuscular depot, oral)
2. what dose to use (e.g., tracer versus large, single versus multiple, i.v. bolus versus continuous infusion)
3. which sites, metabolites, or "pools" to sample
4. how many samples to collect
5. what times to draw the samples

Items 4 and 5 are the most easily controlled aspects of clinical design, and we confine this exposition to optimal scheduling of sample times from a single site, such as blood. Although optimal "input" design can be quite important (8, 16), the route and dose of the drug are often determined by its pharmacological properties, particularly if the test dose is concurrent with drug therapy. Likewise, application of optimal multipool sampling (14,15) may be impractical or unnecessary for drugs that appear to follow elementary (e.g., single-compartment) pharmacokinetics.

The general goals for defining design optimality include minimization of parameter estimation errors and maximization of the ability to verify the model or discriminate against other models, coupled with constraints to minimize patient intervention and other direct and indirect costs. The full range of optimality criteria is well beyond the scope of this chapter, and several criteria may have conflicting goals (e.g., designs that are optimal for parameter estimation for a known model may be very poor for model verification). Fortunately, most of the basic principles of optimal design can be illustrated by optimizing parameter-estimate precision for the elementary one-compartment model. We refer the reader elsewhere for more complete discussions of other criteria (6,11,12,16,18), alternative pharmacokinetic models (8,9,13), and general reviews of optimal experiment design (10,20,21).

NOTATION FOR STRUCTURAL AND ERROR MODELS

We assume the following regression relation for data to be collected in a pharmacokinetic experiment:

$$y_i = f(t_i, \phi) + \epsilon_i \tag{1}$$

where t_i, $i = 1, \ldots, n$, are the sample times, y_i are the observed concentrations, f is the known structural model parameterized by a p-vector of unknown parameters $\phi = (\phi_1, \ldots, \phi_p)^T$, and ϵ_i are random "measurement errors." As usual, we assume that the errors are zero-mean and independent and that the variance of ϵ_i, $\text{Var}(\epsilon_i) = \sigma^2(t_i)$, is known at least up to a proportionality constant. It is common to use a specific model for the error variance (15). For example, one may assume that the error variance is proportional to a known power of the expected value of the observation:

$$\sigma^2(t_i) = \left[f(t_i)\right]^\zeta \sigma^2 \tag{2}$$

Here σ^2 is a proportionality constant, and $\zeta = 0, 1,$ and 2 correspond, respectively, to constant variance, counting-statistics noise, and constant coefficient-of-variation measurement error. It should be stressed that independence of the errors for different samples is assumed even for replicate samples drawn at the same time.

For the simple one-compartment model following a bolus input, we use the following structural model for f:

$$f(t_i) = Ae^{-\lambda t_i} \tag{3}$$

The unknown parameters in equation (3) are the "macroparameters" A and λ, and, more generally, for a sum of m exponentials there will be $2m$ macroparameters A_i and λ_i. Alternative parameterizations can be used in multicompartmental models (e.g., "microparameter" fractional-transfer constants). Also, a common reformulation of equation (3) is

$$f(t_i) = (D/V)e^{-CL t_i/V} \tag{4}$$

where D is the known administered dose, and the unknown parameters are the clearance CL and volume of distribution V. However, we generally find that a design that is optimal for estimation in one parameterization is optimal or near optimal for an alternative parameterization, and our examples will use equation (3).

DESIGN PROBLEM FOR PARAMETER ESTIMATION

The usual estimation problem is, given a structural model f, an error-variance model, and collected data, to find an optimal method to estimate the parameter vector ϕ. In contrast, our design problem is to specify an optimal choice of sample times t_i (the independent variable) that will produce data from which ϕ can be estimated with best precision. We use the covariance matrix for parameter estimates as the measure of precision and indicate later how this depends on the sampling design. Let $s_i(t) = \partial f/\partial \phi_i(t)$ be the "sensitivity" of the model at time t to a change in ϕ_i. Let $M(t)$ be the $p \times p$ "point information matrix" whose i,jth entry is $s_i(t)s_j(t)/\sigma^2(t)$; that is, the entries are products and cross-products of the sensitivities scaled to the measurement-error variance. If a sampling design calls for n independent samples at times $t_1, \ldots, t_n$ (repeated times indicating replication), the full information matrix for this design is

$$M = M(t_1) + \ldots + M(t_n) \tag{5}$$

and M^{-1} is the usual approximation to the covariance matrix for the estimate $\hat{\phi}$ under an optimal estimation procedure such as weighted least squares (10,15, 17). The square root of the ith diagonal entry of M^{-1} is the asymptotic standard error (SE) for $\hat{\phi}_i$, and the i,jth entry divided by the product of SE $(\hat{\phi}_i)$ and SE $(\hat{\phi}_j)$ is the asymptotic correlation coefficient between the two parameter estimates. Therefore, given a fixed value for n, the design problem can be restated as finding the set of sample times $t_1, \ldots, t_n$ that minimizes in some sense M^{-1}.

Note that if the structural model is nonlinear in some of its parameters, as is the case in equation (3), then the sensitivities are functions of the model parameters, and M^{-1} is a function of both the sample times and at least some of the values of the unknown parameters. Additionally, functional dependence of M^{-1} on model parameters can occur through error-variance models such as equation (2) when $\zeta > 0$. Therefore, one common difficulty encountered with optimal-design theory for nonlinear regression is the need to have approximate values for at least some of the parameters. For the present discussion we assume that correct or nearly correct nominal values for the parameters are being used, but we shall have more to say about this problem later.

Because optimal designs usually consist of replicate samples at a small number of distinct sample times, it is convenient to generalize the notion of design. Let t_i, $i = 1, \ldots, K$, be the distinct sample times $(t_i < t_{i+1})$, and let ρ_i be the proportion of the total sample of size n independently replicated at time t_i. For example, if $n = 4$ samples are drawn with one sample at time 0 and triplicate samples at time 10, then $K = 2$, t_1 and t_2 are 0 and 10, and ρ_1 and ρ_2 are 0.25 and 0.75. The "design measure" ξ is the set of distinct times and their proportions:

$$\xi = \{(t_1, \rho_1), \ldots, (t_K, \rho_K)\} \tag{6}$$

and the "normalized" information matrix for this design measure is

$$M(\xi) = \sum_{i=1}^{K} \rho_i M(t_i) \tag{7}$$

The advantage of this approach is that optimal sampling designs can be specified without having to refer to the sample size n. If the previous example for $n = 4$ is an optimal schedule for parameter estimation, then it can be shown that an optimal design for $n = 8$ consists of duplicate samples at time 0 and six independent replicates at time 10. This, of course, has the same design measure as the example for $n = 4$. Therefore, the optimality criteria can be redefined to find the optimal design measure to minimize a given function of $M^{-1}(\xi)$, and the usual asymptotic covariance matrix for a design consisting of n samples is $(1/n)M^{-1}(\xi)$. The disadvantage is that the optimal design measure may not result in a realizable design; in the previous example, if $n = 5$, one cannot draw 1.25 samples at time 0 and 3.75 samples at time 10. However, rounding off the $\rho_i n$ values to the nearest whole number generally produces a realizable design that is optimal or near optimal (10,13,14).

Finally, it is convenient to refer to "continuous design measures" as limiting cases for certain discrete designs. In this case the design measure becomes a continuous function of time, with total integral equal to 1, and the summation of equation (7) is replaced by an integral. For example, if a large number of samples are chosen over the interval $[T_1, T_2]$, with uniform (equal) spacing between neighboring times, the design can be approximated by the design measure

$$\xi(t) = \begin{cases} 1/(T_2 - T_1) & \text{if } T_1 \leq t \leq T_2 \\ 0 & \text{otherwise} \end{cases} \tag{8}$$

and the corresponding normalized information matrix is

$$M(\xi) = \int M(t)\xi(t)\,dt \tag{9}$$

Likewise, for geometric spacing of the sample times (constant ratio between neighboring times), the continuous design measure becomes

$$\xi(t) = \begin{cases} 1/[t \ln(T_2/T_1)] & \text{if } T_1 \leq t \leq T_2 \\ 0 & \text{otherwise} \end{cases} \tag{10}$$

OPTIMALITY CHOICES AND COMPARISON OF DESIGNS

The design problem has been stated as finding the design ξ that minimizes in some sense $M^{-1}(\xi)$. However, for $p \geq 2$ there is no unique sense of a minimum M^{-1}. For example, if the structural model is given by equation (2) and sampling is limited to times $t \geq 0$, then replicating all samples arbitrarily close to time 0 minimizes $SE(\hat{A})$, but $SE(\hat{\lambda})$ becomes arbitrarily large. Therefore, the optimal design depends on the specific function of M^{-1} to be minimized, and we focus on two main choices: D-optimality (2) and C-optimality (13). A D-optimal design is one that minimizes the determinant of $M^{-1}(\xi)$ and can be interpreted as the design that minimizes the volume of the joint asymptotic confidence region for the parameters. A C-optimal design minimizes the trace of $WM^{-1}(\xi)$, where W is a diagonal matrix with kth diagonal equal to $1/\phi_k^2$ and is interpreted as minimizing the average squared coefficient of variation of the parameter estimates.

In addition to the appeal of their interpretations, these criteria produce designs that are independent of the choice of units for the model parameters. It can be shown that a D-optimal or C-optimal design measure is "nondominated" in the sense that any other design produces an asymptotic variance for at least one parameter or function of parameters that is the same or larger than that from the optimal design. Finally, if a given model can be parameterized in two ways and either parameter set is a (locally) invertible function of the other, a D-optimal design with respect to one parameterization is also optimal with respect to the other (10,13). Thus, for example, a design that is D-optimal with respect to A and λ in equation (3) is also optimal with respect to V and CL in equation (4). D-optimal and C-optimal designs are specific examples of the broad class of L-optimal designs (10,20), and these criteria can be extended to functions or subsets of the model parameters. General properties of optimality criteria based on M^{-1} are reviewed elsewhere (10,13,20,21).

A general result is that D-optimal and C-optimal design measures for a wide class of pharmacokinetic models tend to have only as many distinct sample times as there are parameters (3,5,7,8,13). For example, if meaningful replication can be performed, the optimal design for the two-parameter model of equation (3) consists of independent replicates at just two distinct times, in contrast to the usual practice of spreading the samples over a number of different times. This result is illustrated in Table 1 for the D-optimal, C-optimal, and best uniform designs for the structural model of equation (3). If the error-variance model of equation (2) is assumed, with $\zeta = 1$, and sampling is allowed to start at time 0, then the D-optimal design consists of half of the replicates at time 0 and the remaining at time $2/\lambda$, and the C-optimal design consists of 44% of the replicates at time 0 and the remaining at time $2.26/\lambda$. The contrasting uniform design measure with the smallest determinant of M^{-1} is spread over the

TABLE 1. Comparison of sampling designs for two-parameter exponential model[a]

Design type	Design specification[b,c]	D-efficiency (percentage)	C-efficiency (percentage)	CV($\hat{A}$)[d] (percentage)	CV($\hat{\lambda}$)[d] (percentage)	r[e]
D-optimal	0 (0.50) 2/λ (0.50)	100	98	13	9	0.35
C-optimal	0 (0.44) 2.26/λ (0.56)	99	100	12	10	0.34
Uniform spacing with highest D-efficiency[c]	0–2.75/λ	62	44	16	17	0.77

[a] $y = Ae^{-\lambda t}$ + error; error variance = 0.04 $(Ae^{-\lambda t})$.
[b] D- and C-optimal designs specified as time (proportion of independent samples replicated at time).
[c] First–last times specified for uniform spacing of arbitrarily large number of sample times.
[d] CV = coefficient of variation of estimate assuming 10 total sample times.
[e] r = asymptotic correlation coefficient of $\hat{A}$, $\hat{\lambda}$.

interval from time 0 to $2.75/\lambda$. The last three columns of Table 1 show the expected asymptotic coefficients of variation for the parameter estimates and the correlation between the estimates assuming $n = 10$ samples and a proportionality constant $\sigma^2 = 0.04$ in equation (2). It is evident that the D-optimal and C-optimal designs have nearly the same performance, whereas the best uniform design has decidedly worse parameter-estimation precision and greater parameter-estimate correlation.

A useful measure for comparing the global parameter-estimation performances for designs is the design "efficiency" (1). If ξ^D and ξ^C are the D-optimal and C-optimal designs for a particular model, then the D-efficiency for a candidate design ξ is

$$e_D(\xi) = \{\det[M^{-1}(\xi^D)]/\det[M^{-1}(\xi)]\}^{1/p} \times 100\% \qquad (11)$$

and the C-efficiency is

$$e_C(\xi) = \text{trace}[WM^{-1}(\xi^C)]/\text{trace}[WM^{-1}(\xi)] \times 100\% \qquad (12)$$

where W is the diagonal matrix used in defining C-optimality. Design efficiencies are readily interpreted in terms of effective sample size and use of resources (1,9,13). For example, if a design with D-efficiency of 50% is used with total sample size n, one can achieve the same value for $\det(M^{-1})$ with a D-optimal design using only half the number of samples. Therefore, in Table 1, efficiencies for the uniform design of 62% and 44% indicate that in one sense at least 38 to 56% of the blood samples are "wasted" (vis-à-vis estimating parameters) if they are drawn using a uniform sampling schedule. Of course, one may be willing to settle for some loss in parameter-estimation efficiency if the suboptimal design has other desirable properties. Some of these issues will be discussed in a later section.

SOME GENERAL RESULTS FOR PHARMACOKINETIC MODELS

There has been some experience in applying principles of optimal experiment design for parameter estimation to standard kinetic and multicompartmental models (3,5,7–9,13–15). Some important generalizations, particularly for multiexponential models, are summarized next.

Choice of optimality criterion. For multiexponential models with sufficiently wide spacing of the rate constants λ_i (no two differ by less than a factor of 3 or 4), D-optimal and C-optimal designs are quite similar. In addition, designs that are optimal with respect to a single parameter or subset of parameters tend to have sample times close to the distinct times of the D-optimal design measure, but with different proportions of replication. D-optimal designs are highly efficient for a variety of parameter-estimation criteria.

Specification of D-optimal design. The D-optimal design for a model with p

parameters often consists of only p distinct sample times, each replicated with proportion $1/p$. For constant error variance, specification of the optimal design requires nominal values for only the λ_i, and for the general error-variance model of equation (2) easy rules of thumb can be given for specifying optimal times. For example, if sampling is limited to the interval $[T_1, T_2]$ for the single-exponential model, $t_1 = T_1$, $t_2 =$ minimum of T_2, and $t_1 + 2/[(2 - \zeta)\lambda]$. Therefore, for constant error variance ($\zeta = 0$), optimal spacing between the two samples is $1/\lambda$ or approximately 1.44 half-lives. As ζ approaches 2, t_2 approaches the maximum time T_2 [assuming that the error model of equation (2), which includes no background constant error variance, is still valid]; however, the practical limit for the spacing between the two samples is no greater than 3 half-lives. More complicated rules of thumb can be given for multiexponential models (13,15).

Sensitivity to misspecification. In multiexponential models, design specification depends primarily on nominal values for the λ_i, and when the rate constants are not closely spaced, errors as large as 20 to 30% in specifying these nominal values do not seriously degrade design efficiency. Likewise, errors of 20 to 30% in the consecutive spacing of sample times are not very serious. As noted before, the design specification under constant error variance is independent of nominal values for A_i. Under nonconstant error variance, the designs are relatively insensitive to misspecified values for A_i.

Efficiencies of standard designs. A well-chosen geometric spacing of sample times for a multiexponential model may have D-efficiencies as high as 70 to 80%. Uniform spacing is decidedly worse, efficiencies often being 50% or lower.

Ill-conditioning of multiexponential models. The use of nonoptimal sampling designs is a common and correctable cause for difficulties encountered in fitting sums of exponentials to data (15). D-optimal schedules generally reduce parameter-estimate correlations and improve the condition number of M^{-1}. Because Gauss-Newton algorithms and other modifications used in parameter estimation often use M^{-1} to guide the search, this may also result in improved numerical stability for nonlinear regression.

PRACTICAL OPTIMAL AND SUBOPTIMAL DESIGNS

The classic optimal designs are notable in the "sparseness" of the sampling (replicates at just a few distinct times), whereas conventional "intuitive" designs often spread out the sample times. This discrepancy is attributable to the critical assumptions for optimal-design theory: The structural and error-variance models are known, the errors are uncorrelated, and nominal values for at least some of the parameters are nearly correct. The greater the doubt in the validity of these assumptions, the more one may wish to deviate from the optimal design schedule. For example, sparse designs provide little or no information for checking model validity, and minor process noise or inadequacies of the structural model may lead to correlated errors for replicate or closely spaced sample times. Indeed, meaningful replicate sampling in an individual may be impractical, and subdividing one sample into a number of aliquots for assay may not represent replication of all sources of experimental error.

A number of formal alternatives to classic optimal design have been used to guard against some of these difficulties, including the use of sequential designs (7) and model-robust or error-robust designs (4,21). However, simple ad hoc modifications of classic D-optimal schedules may be sufficient for some pharmacokinetic studies. The basic idea is to use the D-optimal schedule as a guideline for the critical samples and to add a few additional samples at alternate times and/or spread out any replicate samples (9). For example, results summarized in the previous section indicate that duplicate samples may be spread $\pm 20\%$ of the spacing from the previous time without seriously affecting design performance (13). However, the nature of these modifications is determined in part by the degree to which one wishes to guard against nominal-value misspecification and correlated errors or to add a "touch" of model verification and discrimination.

The tremendous population variability that can occur for pharmacokinetic parameters means that a design based on one nominal value for ϕ may be quite inefficient for some individuals. This suggests developing a formal criterion for guarding against nominal-value misspecification. Silvey (20) has recommended developing a "maximin" design whose minimum efficiency over the range of possible parameter values is greater than that of any other design, and we discuss some representative maximin designs for the exponential model of equation (3) under the assumption of constant error variance. Maximin designs for uncertainty ranges in the error-variance parameter ζ of equation (2) are discussed by Schultz and Endrenyi (19).

If only the λ parameter is unknown in the one-exponential model, the optimal design consists of a single sample at time $1/\lambda$. We assume that the true value for an individual's λ falls in a specified "uncertainty interval" $[\lambda_{min}, \lambda_{max}]$ and search for designs that maximize the minimum D-efficiency over this interval. Notice that a maximin design is geared to doing the best for the patient who benefits the least from the design, no matter how unlikely one is to encounter that patient. Table 2 summarizes some maximin designs for $\lambda_{max} = 1$ and 2-, 4-, 10-, and 50-fold ranges in the uncertainty interval. The minimum and maximum D-efficiencies are listed for each design, and in all cases the lowest efficiency occurs at $\lambda = \lambda_{min}$ and λ_{max}.

If we restrict ourselves to one-point designs, then the maximin design is a sample at time $\ln(\lambda_{max}/\lambda_{min})/(\lambda_{max} - \lambda_{min})$. However, only when the range in the uncertainty region is greater than about fourfold can one get a better maximin design by spreading out the sample times. For very large ranges in the uncertainty interval, the one-point designs are very inefficient at the extremes,

TABLE 2. Maximin designs for one-parameter exponential model[a]

Uncertainty interval for λ	Design specification Type	Sample times[b,c]	D-efficiency (percentage) Minimum	Maximum
(0.50, 1)	One-point	1.39	89	100
(0.25, 1)	One-point	1.85	63	100
(0.10, 1)	Multipoint	1.2 (0.49) 4.6 (0.17) 7.8 (0.17) 10 (0.17)	47	54
(0.10, 1)	Geometric[c]	0.54–12.5	42	56
(0.10, 1)	One-point	2.56	29	100
(0.02, 1)	Multipoint	1.2 (0.35) 4.2 (0.15) 10 (0.15) 27 (0.15) 50 (0.20)	33	37
(0.02, 1)	Geometric[c]	0.36–82	29	34
(0.02, 1)	One-point	3.99	4	100

[a] $y = e^{-\lambda t}$ + error; constant error variance. Maximin design maximizes the minimum D-efficiency over the uncertainty interval for λ.
[b] Time (proportion of independent samples replicated at or near this time) for multipoint designs.
[c] First–last times for design with geometric spacing of arbitrarily large number of sample times.

whereas the multipoint maximin designs have nearly constant efficiencies for all values of λ. These designs are well approximated by a geometric design.

Table 3 presents maximin designs for the full two-parameter model of equation (3). For comparison, we list designs that maximize the average D-efficiency given that $\log(\lambda)$ has a uniform population distribution over the uncertainty interval (we assume that the data will dominate the prior). Preliminary studies suggest that unimodal probability distributions that are not very "wide" (i.e., have low probability tails) have sparse maximum-average-efficiency (MAE) designs and are quite similar to the D-optimal design using the population mean as nominals. Therefore, the log-uniform distribution is used as an extreme example to find "spread-out" MAE designs. The maximin designs are similar to those for the one-parameter case in Table 2 except for the addition of samples at time 0. However, spread-out nonzero times do not appear in the MAE design until the uncertainty interval is more than 10-fold wide, and the MAE design has lower efficiency at the extremes of λ than the maximin design. The efficiencies in general are larger in Table 3 than those in Table 2 because A is always estimated well. Nevertheless, it is interesting that even when the uncertainty region has a 50-fold range, the maximin design has D-efficiency no worse than 60%.

TABLE 3. Maximin and maximum average efficiency designs for two-parameter model[a]

Uncertainty interval for λ	Design specification		D-efficiency (percentage)		
	Sample time (proportion replicated)		Minimum	Maximum	Average[b]
(0.50, 1)	Maximin	0 (0.5), 1.39 (0.5)	94	100	98
(0.50, 1)	Maximum Average[b]	0 (0.5), 1.38 (0.5)	94	100	98
(0.10, 1)	Maximin	0 (0.5), 1.3 (0.3), 5.7 (0.1), 10 (0.1)	73	77	75
(0.10, 1)	Maximum Average[b]	0 (0.5), 2.52 (0.5)	53	100	81
(0.02, 1)	Maximin	0 (0.4), .8 (0.2), 1.7 (0.1), 4.3 (0.1), 12 (0.1), 50 (0.1)	60	64	62
(0.02, 1)	Maximum Average[b]	0 (0.4), 2.0 (0.3), 8.1 (0.1), 17 (0.2)	51	82	69

[a] $y = Ae^{-\lambda t}$ + error; constant error variance.
[b] Average efficiency computed assuming log-uniform distribution of λ over specified uncertainty interval.

CONCLUSION

We have seen that a well-designed pharmacokinetic study has a significant effect on the precision of parameter estimation. D-optimal designs are efficient for a variety of estimation criteria, and even when impractical to implement, they serve as useful guides for the specification of practical designs. The need to guard against misspecified nominal values or violations of the modeling assumptions leads to several formal and informal classes of suboptimal designs. If there is considerable population variability for the rate contant of a monoexponential model, sparse D-optimal designs can be quite inefficient for individuals at the extremes. In this case, maximin designs are similar to certain geometric designs and have moderate but constant efficiencies over the wide range of individuals.

The usefulness of these optimal designs for estimating population-pharmacokinetic parameters is not clear, although it should be of value in two-stage methods requiring good parameter estimates for a large number of individuals. The intriguing possibility is that efficient estimates for population variances may require a design more nearly like the maximin design in order to estimate well those individuals who deviate from the mean. In addition, patients deviating most from the mean may be the ones for whom it is most crucial to obtain the best parameter estimates for individualization of optimal treatment strategies.

ACKNOWLEDGMENTS

This work was supported primarily by National Science Foundation grant ECS 80-15965 and National Institutes of Health grant USPHS CA-16042.

REFERENCES

1. Atwood, C.L. (1969): Optimal and efficient designs of experiments. *Annals Math. Stat.*, 40:1570–1602.
2. Box, G.E.P., and Lucas, H.L. (1959): Design of experiments in nonlinear situations. *Biometrika*, 46:77–90.
3. Box, M.J. (1970): Some experiences with a nonlinear experimental design criterion. *Technometrics*, 12:569–589.
4. Cook, R.D., and Nachtsheim, C.J. (1982): Model linear-optimal designs. *Technometrics*, 24:49–54.
5. D'Argenio, D.Z. (1981): Optimal sampling times for pharmacokinetic experiments. *J. Pharmacokinet. Biopharm.*, 9:739–755.
6. D'Argenio, D.Z., and Katz, D. (1983): Sampling strategies for noncompartmental estimation of mean residence time. *J. Pharmacokinet. Biopharm.*, 11:435–446.
7. DiStefano, J.J., III (1981): Optimized blood sampling protocols and sequential design of kinetic experiments. *Am. J. Physiol.* 240(*Regulatory Integrative Comp. Physiol.* 9):R259–R265.
8. Endrenyi, L. (1981): Design of experiments for estimating enzyme and pharmacokinetic experiments. In: *Kinetic Data Analysis, Design and Analysis of Enzyme and Pharmacokinetic Experiments*, edited by L. Endrenyi, pp. 137–167. Plenum Press, New York.

9. Endrenyi, L., and Dingle, B.H. (1982): Optimal design of experiments for the precise estimation of single-exponential kinetic model parameters. In: *Pharmacokinetics During Drug Development: Data Analysis and Evaluation Techniques,* edited by G. Bozler and J.M. van Rossum, pp. 149–173. Gustav Fischer Verlag, Stuttgart.
10. Fedorov, V.V. (1972): *Theory of Optimal Experiments.* Academic Press, New York.
11. Hill, P.D.H. (1978): A review of experimental design procedures for regression model discrimination. *Technometrics,* 20:15–21.
12. Katz, D., and D'Argenio, D.Z. (1983): Experimental design for estimating integrals by numerical quadrature, with application to pharmacokinetic studies. *Biometrics,* 39:27–34.
13. Landaw, E.M. (1980): Optimal experimental design for biologic compartmental systems with applications to pharmacokinetics. Ph.D. dissertation, UCLA, University Microfilms International.
14. Landaw, E.M. (1982): Optimal multicompartmental sampling designs for parameter estimation: Practical aspects of the identification problem. *Math. Comp. Simulation,* 24:525–530.
15. Landaw, E., and DiStefano, J.J., III (1984): Multiexponential, multicompartmental and noncompartmental modeling. II. Data analysis and statistical considerations. *Am. J. Physiol.* 246(*Regulatory Integrative Comp. Physiol.* 15):R665–R677.
16. Mannervik, B. (1981): Design and analysis of kinetic experiments for discrimination between rival models. In: *Kinetic Data Analysis, Design and Analysis of Enzyme and Pharmacokinetic Experiments,* edited by L. Endrenyi, pp. 235–270. Plenum Press, New York.
17. Metzler, C.M. (1981): Statistical properties of kinetic estimates. In: *Kinetic Data Analysis, Design and Analysis of Enzyme and Pharmacokinetic Experiments,* edited by L. Endrenyi, pp. 25–37. Plenum Press, New York.
18. Pritchard, D.J., and Bacon, D.W. (1978): Prospects for reducing correlations among parameter estimates in kinetic models. *Chem. Eng. Sci.,* 33:1539–1543.
19. Schultz, M., and Endrenyi, L. (1983): Design of experiments for estimating parameters with unknown heterogeneity of the error variance. In: *Proceedings of the Statistical Computing Section,* 177–181. American Statistical Association, Washington, D.C.
20. Silvey, S.D. (1980): *Optimal Design.* Chapman & Hall, New York.
21. Steinberg, D.M., and Hunter, W.G. (1984): Experimental design: Review and comment. *Technometrics,* 26:71–97.

DISCUSSION

Discussant 1 (D1): I understand why you choose the definition of efficiency for D-optimal designs that you do. It works well in comparing designs with a fixed number of data points. However, as the number of data points increases, the relative efficiency of nonoptimal designs becomes smaller and smaller. In the limits of a uniform design with an infinite number of data points the efficiency is zero, and yet parameter estimates are perfect. Would you comment on this?

Speaker (S): Design measure efficiency is independent of the number of data points and for a uniform design is zero only if the last time is unbounded. Parameter estimates are perfect with infinite data if the spacing between times also goes to zero.

D2: I question the assumption that the covariance of successive errors is zero. This is certainly correct for 1 patient provided that the model equation itself is correct. On the other hand, if there is any model misspecification, errors from successive observations will be correlated. I wonder if your analysis can take some account of such a possibility?

S: D-optimality suggests replicating the sampling at the same time or at neighboring times. Clearly, if there is any model misspecification, the residuals will be correlated. Other design criteria do force the points to spread out and may help this problem.

D2: I have a general concern with simple definitions of optimality. If you want to estimate a straight line and you know that it is a straight line, you put all your efforts at two positions as far apart as you can. But, if things *can* go wrong, sometimes (maybe quite often) they *will* go wrong. I like to have some safeguard against that event, even though it is difficult to build it into the rather rigid concepts of optimality.

S: If you could specify a cost of missing an alternative model, then it could be incorporated into the design optimality criterion, and we would obtain a design that guards against the possibility.

D3: What happens when you use a simpler model than the data really arise from?

S: The optimality criterion assumes that the model is correct. The design will reflect this. Whether or not the design will be optimal with respect to estimation when model misspecification is present is unclear. In general, if the simpler model can be embedded in a larger model, the design can be optimized for the larger model. This result will also be good for the simpler model and yet will "protect" against poor design for any instance of the larger model.

*Variability in Drug Therapy:
Description, Estimation, and Control,*
edited by M. Rowland et al.
Raven Press, New York © 1985.

Control of Uncertain Dynamic Systems: Methods, Implementation, and Application to Drug Therapy

Darryl Katz

Department of Mathematics, California State University, Fullerton, California 92634

Pharmacokinetic models have direct applications to drug therapy with respect to determination of "appropriate" dosing regimens. Appropriate regimens are those that effectively control some performance index of interest, involving, for example, serum concentrations at specified times. We shall examine several approaches to this control problem, with emphasis on methods that employ feedback from observations, such as serum levels, made on the subject of the therapy. In addition, some of the methods to be discussed use prior information about the population from which the subject is "selected."

To provide a concrete example, we shall consider strategies for determining dosing that will minimize a specified cost function. For example, if one specifies target serum concentrations C_i^T, $i = 1, \ldots, n$, where C_i^T is the target concentration at time t_i, then an appropriate cost function might be a measure of the difference between the C_i^T and the corresponding levels, C_i, $i = 1, \ldots, n$, predicted by a suitable pharmacokinetic model. A particular example is the quadratic cost function

$$J = \sum_{i=1}^{n} (C_i^T - C_i)^2 \qquad (1)$$

Other cost functions include the maximum, over i, of $|C_i^T - C_i|$ and equation (1) with weights, w_i, in front of the individual terms to represent differential importance in minimizing the individual squared differences in the sum.

Control strategies that minimize cost functions such as equation (1) depend directly on the method used to make the predictions, C_i. For a given drug application, assuming a model of the drug kinetics, the most common methods of predicting levels of a specified dosing regimen are probably *a priori* methods, based on previous experience and measurable characteristics of the subject (1,6) and methods that estimate parameters by interpolation or nonlinear least-squares estimation (12). In order to describe some approaches to estimation, and hence control, we shall briefly look at a simple (and somewhat extreme) example that does not involve drug therapy.

Suppose that a large urn contains millions of marbles, each of which has either 1 or 3 printed on it. Based on some combination of prior experience and/or observations from this urn, we estimate that just slightly more than half of the marbles are marked 3. A marble is to be selected at random, and we are to be paid a number of dollars equal to the fourth power of the number on the marble. We wish to estimate, in advance of the draw, the size of the payoff, which will, in fact, be either $1 or $81.

Maximum-likelihood estimation would lead to $81 as the estimate, as this is the most likely value of the outcome, even though $1 is nearly as likely. (As indicated, this is an extreme example, and maximum-likelihood estimates do have important, desirable statistical properties.) A second approach might involve estimating the number on the marble to be about 2, the mean value, and hence the payoff to be $2^4 = \$16$. Finally, consider the estimate ($1 + $81)/2 = $41, which is (approximately) the mean value of the payoff. The argument in favor of the latter approach is, essentially, that it minimizes, on the average, an appropriate cost (in this case, the average squared deviation from the prediction) in terms of the quantity of interest, i.e., the payoff. The previous method, on the other hand, provides a "good" estimate of the number on the marble and then uses it to estimate a (nonlinear) function of the value. We shall return to this point later.

METHODS

In all of the methods discussed, we assume an appropriate pharmacokinetic model and, for clarity, limit the discussion to target-level control. The general arguments apply to optimization of any specified function of the model parameters and dosing regimen. The *a priori* methods (1,6) estimate the individual's parameter values from prior knowledge of the individual's population and, for example, estimate dependences of these values on measurable quantities such as body weight and renal function. Then, for some class of dosing schemes (e.g., three 1-hr infusions per 24-hr period, equally spaced), infusion rates are determined that will minimize some cost [e.g., equation (1)] for an individual with the estimated parameter values. This is, essentially, a calculus problem.

These methods are often relatively easy to implement, if sufficient useful data are available from the appropriate population. They are based on estimating parameter values and then minimizing the cost for the estimated individual. This separation of estimation and control is somewhat analogous to the $16 estimate of payoff in the marble example. In addition, *a priori* methods do not use feedback from data collected on the subject of interest.

A second class of control procedures depend entirely on feedback and use prior information only in the selection of a suitable pharmacokinetic model and, possibly, in modeling measurement error and the relationship between, for example, model parameters and measurable quantities. Drug is administered to the subject, and one or more serum levels (for example) are analyzed. These laboratory results are used, together with some estimation procedure (such as nonlinear least squares), to obtain parameter estimates. Estimation and control are again separated, and the control problem is solved as with the *a priori* methods.

It is often desirable to combine the use of prior (population) information with data collected on the current subject in the estimation of parameter values. Bayes's theorem provides a natural way to accomplish this. If ϕ represents the set of model parameters, $F(\phi)$ the prior probability density for the parameters, y_j the data collected on the subject of interest (j), and $L(y_j/\phi)$ the likelihood of the data given the parameter values ϕ, then Bayes's theorem states that

$$F(\phi/y_j) = K \cdot L(y_j/\phi) \cdot F(\phi) \qquad (2)$$

The quantity on the left is the posterior density of ϕ, given "everything" known at that point, and it provides the information necessary for estimation of ϕ.

Of course, in order to apply equation (2) to find $F(\phi/y_j)$, one must be able to calculate the quantities on the right side of the equation. The constant K can be calculated by integration, as the integral of equation (2) must be 1. $L(y_j/\phi)$ can be calculated from the pharmacokinetic model if suitable assumptions are made concerning measurement error. The prior density, $F(\phi)$, can be estimated by methods employed, for example, by NONMEM [see Sheiner et al. (8–10) for a description of this and other methods] or by direct application of equation (2), as described by Katz et al. (2,3,5). Once the posterior density is obtained, the parameters can be estimated by the maximum of the posterior density (MAP estimation) (7,11) or by the mean of the posterior density. The latter approach typically involves a much greater computational burden (we shall return to this point).

All of the methods discussed thus far separate estimation from control. The last approach to be considered, optimal stochastic control, will eliminate this separation and provide for the inclusion of prior information. Assuming that we have obtained $F(\phi/y_j)$ [equation (2)], we can now consider J [equation (1)] to be a function of the dosing regimen, as before, and of the parameters ϕ, which are random variables. We can now attempt to calculate a dosing scheme that will minimize the expected value of J, taken with respect to the density $F(\phi/y_j)$. This is analogous to the $41 estimate in the marble example in that it minimizes a quantity of direct interest, namely the expected size of an appropriate cost function. Solving for the optimal dose is no longer a "simple" opti-

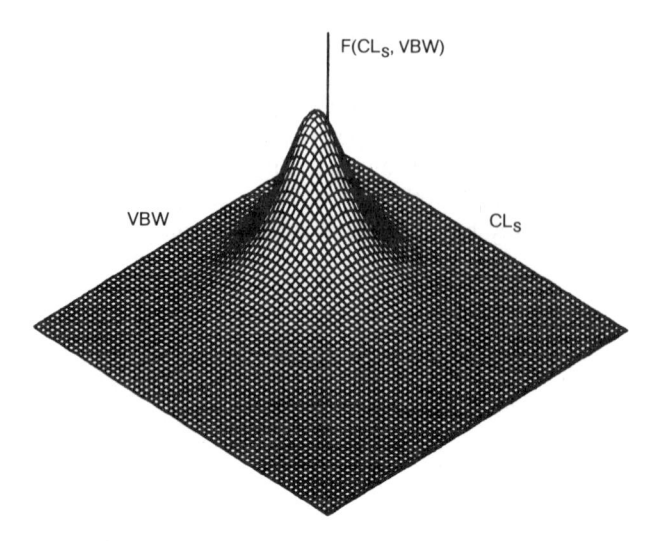

FIG. 1. Log-normal prior density for the parameters CL_s and VBW of the tobramycin kinetic model.

mization problem. Implementation and evaluation of control and estimation strategies will be discussed later.

IMPLEMENTATION PROBLEMS

Application of optimal stochastic control, as described earlier, requires calculation of the expectations of various quantities, in addition to calculations similar to those involved in the other methods. These expectations appear in the form of integrals with dimension equal to the number of parameters in the kinetic model, and generally they require numerical techniques for evaluation. The resulting computational burden is a serious problem for all but the smallest models and has hindered exploration of this approach to control. We have tried to alleviate this difficulty somewhat by a change-of-variables technique (3) that, for typical compartment models, reduces the dimension of numerical integrals by a factor of one-half, and currently we are encouraged by an alternative approach described in the following paragraph.

Let $F(\phi)$ be the prior density of the parameters ϕ obtained by some procedure, such as those described earlier. $F(\phi)$ is a continuous density function with dimension equal to the number of model parameters (Fig. 1). We shall replace $F(\phi)$ with a discrete approximation $F^*(\phi)$ (Fig. 2) that will then be used in all subsequent calculations, replacing the integral calculations by sums over relatively small numbers of terms. If $F_{cum}(\phi)$ and $F^*_{cum}(\phi)$ are the cumulative distribution functions corresponding to $F(\phi)$ and $F^*(\phi)$, respectively, we choose $F^*(\phi)$ to minimize

$$\int_\phi |F_{cum}(\phi) - F^*_{cum}(\phi)| d\phi \qquad (3)$$

where the integral is of dimension equal to the number of parameters. In other words, F^* is "L_1-optimal" with respect to the distribution functions. An algorithm has been developed to (approximately) find F^* for a given F and given number of discrete points for the approximation (4,5). The usefulness of the discrete approximations depends on their ability to yield good approximations to parameter estimates and optimal controls. The approach, as currently implemented, can probably handle models of dimension up to four or five.

PREDICTION EXAMPLE

A two-parameter model for the kinetics of i.v. tobramycin was applied to data from 42 patients to obtain the log-normal density, $F(\phi)$, shown in Fig. 1. The parameters are VBW (volume per body weight) and CL_s (the slope of the line representing the elimination-rate constant as a function of creatinine clearance). Means, variances, and covariance are in the first column of Table 1. These quantities were also calculated using a 25-point discrete approximation (Fig. 2) and an 81-point discrete approximation. As can be seen in Table 1, there is excellent agreement among the computed moments.

The probability distribution of tobramycin concentration in the serum at $t = 8$ hr following a particular infusion schedule, administered to a 70-kg subject, was calculated using $F(\phi)$ and the two discrete approximations to $F(\phi)$ described earlier. These densities were then used to calculate the expected value

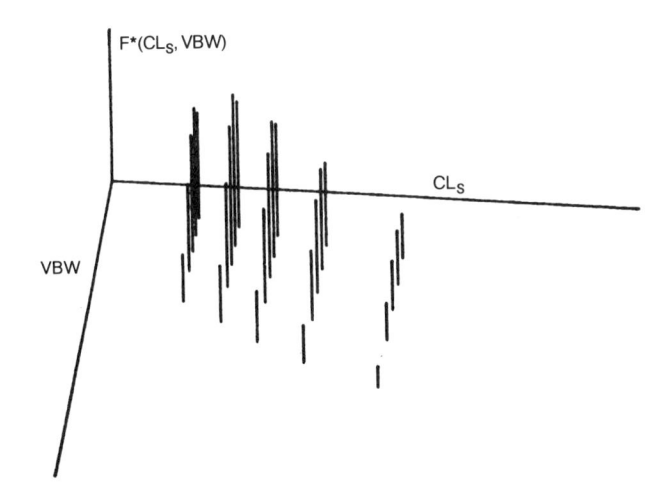

FIG. 2. Twenty-five-point discrete approximation to the log-normal prior density of Fig. 1.

TABLE 1. Parameter moments for the log-normal density in Fig. 1 and for its discrete approximations

	Log-normal	25 points	81 points
$E(VBW)$	0.318	0.311	0.313
$E(CL_s)$	0.0687	0.0676	0.0679
$Var(VBW)$	0.0154	0.0119	0.0139
$Var(CL_s)$	0.000675	0.000537	0.000615
Cov	0.00143	0.00106	0.00130

TABLE 2. Expected value and selected percentile points of the distribution of concentration at 8 hr based on the log-normal density of Fig. 1 and on its discrete approximations

	Log-normal	25 points	81 points
$E[C(t=8)]$	2.00	2.01	2.01
5%	0.845	0.878	0.881
10%	1.05	1.01	1.03
90%	3.06	3.07	2.95
95%	3.47	3.17	3.54

of the concentration as well as various percentile points of the distribution. The results, shown in Table 2, again show excellent performance by the approximate densities (although this point should be examined in the context of each new potential application). In addition to the estimates, the percentile points, and other quantities that are available as a result of having the complete density function, can be very useful in applications.

We are currently developing software to implement stochastic control using discrete approximations to facilitate computation. Once "optimal" controls are calculated, the estimation strategy of the tobramycin example can be used to obtain the probability distribution of concentrations at specified times, under the optimal regimen, together with other quantities of interest, such as expected concentrations and extreme percentile values. Solution of the control problem involves computations similar to those required by the estimation example.

We have also performed updates to $F(\phi)$, using Bayes's theorem (2) and feedback from simulated noisy measurements, in the tobramycin example (5). Again, the performance of the discrete approximations was good, and the corresponding computational burden was quite acceptable.

EVALUATION OF CONTROL STRATEGIES

In principle, optimal stochastic control will result in smaller "costs" than will alternatives that separate estimation and control. However, the magnitude of the improvement and the effects of approximations on performance, computational feasibility, and robustness with respect to assumptions must be assessed. Assuming correct models and known error structure, Monte Carlo simulation techniques can be used to compare different control strategies. Simulation can also provide insight into the sensitivity of results to violations of these assumptions. Clinical studies will, of course, be necessary to assess actual performances of promising approaches to the control of drug distribution.

ACKNOWLEDGMENTS

This work was supported in part by NIH grant RR-01629 made to the Laboratory of Applied Pharmacokinetics, University of Southern California School of Medicine. The author thanks Drs. David Z. D'Argenio and Alan Schumitzky of the University of Southern California for their helpful collaboration.

REFERENCES

1. Jelliffe, R.W., Buell, J., and Kalaba, R. (1972): Reduction of digitalis toxicity by computer-assisted glycoside dosage regimens. *Ann. Intern. Med.,* 77:891–906.
2. Katz, D. (1983): Discrete approximation to continuous density functions that are L_1 optimal. *Computational Statistics and Data Analysis,* 1:175–181.
3. Katz, D., Azen, S.P., and Schumitzky, A. (1981): Bayesian approach to the analysis of nonlinear models: Implementation and evaluation. *Biometrics,* 37:137–142.
4. Katz, D., and D'Argenio, D.Z. (1984): Discrete approximation of multivariate densities with application to Bayesian estimation. *Computational Statistics and Data Analysis,* 2:27–36.
5. Katz, D., Schumitzky, A., and Azen, S.P. (1982): Reduction of dimensionality in Bayesian nonlinear regression with a pharmacokinetic application. *Math. Biosci.,* 59:47–56.
6. Peck, C.G., Sheiner, L.B., Martin, C.M., Combs, D.T., and Melmon, K.L. (1973): Computer-assisted digoxin therapy. *N. Engl. J. Med.,* 289:441–446.
7. Sawchuk, R.J., Zaske, D.E., Cipolle, R.J., Wargin, W.A., and Strate, R.G. (1977): Kinetic model for gentamycin dosing with the use of individual patient parameters. *Clin. Pharmacol. Ther.,* 21:362–369.
8. Sheiner, L.B., and Beal, S.L. (1980): Evaluation of methods for estimating population pharmacokinetics. I. Michaelis-Menten model: Routine clinical pharmacokinetic data. *J. Pharmacokinet. Biopharm.,* 8:553–571.
9. Sheiner, L.B., and Beal, S.L. (1981): Evaluation of methods for estimating population pharmacokinetic parameters. II. Biexponential model and experimental pharmacokinetic data. *J. Pharmacokinet. Biopharm.,* 9:635–651.
10. Sheiner, L.B., Beal, S.L., Rosenberg, B., and Marathe, V.V. (1979): Forecasting individual pharmacokinetics. *Clin. Pharmacol. Ther.,* 26:294–305.
11. Sheiner, L.B., Halkin, H., Peck, C.P., Rosenberg, B., and Melmon, K.L. (1975): Improved computer-assisted digoxin therapy. *Ann. Intern. Med.,* 82:619–627.
12. Sheiner, L.B., Rosenberg, B., and Melmon, K.L. (1972): Modelling of individual pharmacokinetics for computer-aided drug dosage. *Comp. Biomed. Res.,* 5:441–459.

DISCUSSION

Discussant 1 (D1): Can you incorporate in your approach more general criteria than the quadratic cost function you mentioned?

Speaker (S): Yes. The requirements are that you have a cost function that is an expectation and a discrete approximation of the parameter distribution. If you can interchange derivatives and integrals, the expected value is just a sum of terms weighted by probabilities, and the minimization problem is standard. On the other hand, the separation idea is not optimal, because you use a method for estimating parameters that is in some sense optimal for getting parameter estimates but does not take into account the knowledge of what those estimates will be used for. Certain regimens may be real disasters if the parameters of an individual are off from what you estimate them to be, particularly for complex models.

D2: I have a simple technical question about your discretization of the distribution function and the criterion for minimizing the absolute area between the two. I would imagine this is not invariant under reparametrization: If you replace ϕ by $\log(\phi)$ or by ϕ^2, you will get a different optimal solution.

S: Yes. If we knew exactly what objective function we ultimately want to optimize, then there might be a method like maximum likelihood for choosing the right criterion. In fact, we just know that we shall be interested in various expectations. Choosing the parametrization of the model as it appears in the expectation is a possible solution. I have no reason to think that that is the best. I would, however, advocate it. Once you have an application in mind, see if it behaves reasonably well. There you have an ultimate criterion, that of getting closer attainment of target levels than if you use some alternative strategy. But I don't see a general way of getting an overall best criterion.

D3: I have some problems using cost functions as expected values of population distributions. What might happen is that you come up with a control procedure that would work for 99% of the patients; on the other hand, that 1% of the patients who would work out very poorly would not enter into the cost-function consideration because you are only looking at the expected values. Do you have any suggestions?

S: If you apply Bayes's theorem when you have almost no information on the subject, then anything can get you into trouble. That subject might be the outlier. Once you gather a reasonable amount of information on the subject of interest, that tends to start dominating the prior.

D3: I was wondering if in the initial stages of the control it might be reasonable to have a strategy that is more robust across the population.

S: Yes. An ad hoc procedure could be the following: (a) Analyze the individual data using, for example, extended least squares to get an idea of a range for the parameter values that is likely to include everybody. (b) Then go a little bit beyond that and force a little bit of density around the edges in addition to the optimal points. If there are any data at any point that would add density in the tails, at least we have a place to put that density for the computations. It's always conceivable that there is a small portion of the population that is not represented in the sample. I don't know what to do about that, except for my earlier suggestion; it is a problem with any kind of sampling.

D4: Two questions related to the goals of this meeting. The first is the following: The optimal input is of great importance for a company in order to define dose and dosage regimen. A more rational approach to this problem seems possible with your methods, one difficulty being the complexity involved. The second question is related to information for the regulatory agencies. With this approach, assuming an appropriate cost function and knowledge about outlying subjects, could various dosage regimens be compared, and could a rough indication of the probability of getting side effects in a given population of subjects be obtained?

S: Yes. If we have the right prior and the right model and so on, we can compute the distribution of whatever is important. Regarding the control of variability, this has at least two general areas of application: (a) Presumably the variability in clinical effect would be reduced without reducing the other variability just because the information was used correctly. (b) You could find the probability of something serious going wrong. However, the usual problems with modeling arise: We need to be concerned with whether or not the structural model is correct and whether or not the error model is correct.

D4: Some indications about the doses and the levels that give rise to side effects in normal subjects would be available very easily from the phase-one trials.

D5: For me, an exciting part of your work is that it allows one to examine the influence of patient variability on the outputs of interest, the cost functions, even aside from its use for individual optimization.

S: Yes. An additional way of using the approach is to compare dosing strategies, looking at what is important, e.g., the fraction of serious side effects.

D5: For this use, the prediction of probabilities of various outcomes, one only needs the prior distribution; there is no posterior, as one is not talking about individual patients.

D6: If these techniques were used for some toxic drugs that because of their small toxic margin cannot now be used clinically, we would have to have exquisite control of the input. The only place this could be done would be in an intensive-care-unit setting.

S: Quite possibly.

D1: There are two levels of application of Dr. Katz's approach. The first is to investigate dosage-regimen strategies that would be, in some sense, optimal for the *population*. Such a study has been performed for the drug lithium (1). The second is to use the approach to optimize *individual* dosage regimens. Several applications of that type have been reported (2-4). I think the first is more relevant to the drug-development process, for definition of appropriate unitary dosage and dosage regimen(s). The second is more relevant to clinical use of the drug for dosage adjustment in individual patients. Surely there is a close relationship between the two problems. Also, in both cases, a reasonable estimate of the population distribution is required.

REFERENCES

1. Gaillot, J., Steimer, J.L., Mallet, A., Thebault, J.J., and Bieder, A. (1979): A priori lithium dosage regimen using population characteristics of pharmacokinetic parameters. *J. Pharmacokinet. Biopharm.*, 7:579-628.
2. Sheiner, L.B., Beal, S., Rosenberg, B., and Marathe, V.V. (1979): Forecasting individual pharmacokinetics. *Clin. Pharmacol. Ther.*, 26:294-305.
3. Vozeh, S., Muir, K.T., Sheiner, L.B., and Follath, F. (1981): Predicting individual phenytoin dosage. *J. Pharmacokinet. Biopharm.*, 9:131-146.
4. Whiting, B., Kelman, A.W., and Struthers, A.D. (1984): Prediction of response to theophylline in chronic bronchitis. *Br. J. Clin. Pharmacol.*, 17:1-8.

*Variability in Drug Therapy:
Description, Estimation, and Control,*
edited by M. Rowland et al.
Raven Press, New York © 1985.

Clinical Application of Bayesian Feedback for Dosage Adjustment: Rationale and Experience

Samuel Vožeh, Toshihiko Uematsu, and Ferenc Follath

Division of Clinical Pharmacology, Department of Research and Internal Medicine, University Hospital, CH-4031 Basel, Switzerland

RATIONALE

Although for some drugs the use of individual-patient characteristics, e.g., body weight or renal function, significantly improves the assessment of individual dosage requirements, unpredictable interindividual variability in the dose–concentration relationship remains unacceptably large for many drugs with narrow therapeutic ranges, even after dosage adjustments for all factors known to influence their pharmacokinetics. Consider, as an example, the bronchodilating agent theophylline, whose pharmacokinetics have been carefully investigated by several groups under various clinical and laboratory conditions. Adjusting for all factors known to influence the elimination rate of theophylline still leaves an unpredictable interindividual variability in total-body clearance in a patient population with acute bronchial obstruction of more than 50% (coefficient of variation) (4). This means that the same dose that is expected to produce, on the average, a steady-state concentration of 15 mg/liter, i.e., in the middle of the recommended therapeutic range (10–20 mg/liter), may result in a subtherapeutic concentration in one patient and in toxic side effects in another (95% confidence interval: 6.0–33 mg/liter).

This large uncertainty in the dose–concentration relationship has led physicians to a cautious, and often ineffective, dosing strategy. When prescribing a drug with a narrow therapeutic range, a relatively low dose is chosen that only rarely produces potentially toxic concentrations. Although safe, such strategy results in undertreatment of many patients. Monitoring serum concentrations of phenytoin in patients treated for seizures, Koch-Weser (3) found that in more than 50% the serum phenytoin level was below the recommended therapeutic range of 10 to 20 mg/liter. We have had similar experiences in our drug-level laboratory. At least 30% of patients treated with antiarrhythmics (lidocaine, quinidine), phenytoin, aminoglycoside antibiotics, and theophylline were found to have serum concentrations below the recommended effective range.

In this situation, implementation of methods that allow the physician to accurately assess the individual dosage required to achieve a desired serum concentration is expected to result in significant improvement in treatment efficacy. These considerations and experience thus represent the theoretical basis for the development and investigation of such methods.

BAYESIAN FEEDBACK

The use of Bayesian feedback for forecasting in pharmacokinetics was first proposed by Sheiner et al. (5). In the context of control theory it can be described as a stochastic adaptive control system (10) in which the physician, aided by appropriate computer software, serves as the controller. Given the complete dosage history and one or more serum-concentration measurements, the individual pharmacokinetic parameter estimates are calculated (5). The theoretical basis of the implementation of Bayesian parameter estimation for prediction of individual pharmacokinetics has been described in detail elsewhere (6,7). Using these individual parameter estimates, the "optimal" dose is determined with the help of an interactive computer program (software developed on HP-85). The program predicts the expected serum concentration for any dosage regimen and time specified by the user. Every prediction is reported with a 68% confidence interval, indicating how well the patient's individual parameters are known or, in other words, how cautious the physician should be in changing the dose. On the basis of this information, the physician chooses the dose that appears to be effective and safe. The physician also decides whether or not additional serum-concentration measurements are necessary.

CLINICAL APPLICATION

Retrospective studies and results of computer simulations have shown that Bayesian feedback provides more accurate prediction of the individual pharmacokinetics than non-Bayesian methods (7,8). To determine the clinical usefulness of this therapeutic tool we have tested its performance in two prospective studies in patients treated with the antiarrhythmic lidocaine: (a) without intervention (group I, 10 patients) and (b) with dosage adjustment (group II, 20 patients). Results of both studies will be reported in detail elsewhere (9; S. Vožeh et al., *in preparation*).

All patients were treated with lidocaine because of acute arrhythmia, usually following a myocardial infarction. Lidocaine therapy was initiated by an intravenous bolus of 100 mg followed by a 50-mg bolus 10 min later. At the time of the first bolus, a continuous infusion was started at a rate of 60 or 120 mg/hr, depending on the presence of clinical signs of congestive heart failure. If arrhythmia persisted, the infusion rate was increased by 60 mg/hr (up to a maximum of 240 mg/hr), and an additional bolus of 50 mg was administered.

The population pharmacokinetic parameters (prior distribution) required by the Bayesian-feedback algorithm were determined in another group of 42 patients in whom more than 300 serum concentrations were collected during lidocaine therapy (9).

To estimate the individual lidocaine pharmacokinetics, a serum-concentration measurement was obtained for each patient between 2 and 4 hr after starting the infusion (at least 30 min after the last bolus dose). The serum lidocaine concentration was predicted and measured 12 and 24 hr after the commencement of treatment.

At 12 hr, serum concentrations could be predicted in both groups with excellent precision (coefficient of variation of the prediction error < 20%). The predictions of the concentration at 24 hr showed a significantly lower precision ($p < 0.01$), mainly because of the fact that in some patients the lidocaine total-body clearance decreased between 12 and 24 hr of continuous infusion. This change in lidocaine pharmacokinetics during prolonged infusion has been described by several authors, e.g., Bauer et al. (1), and is probably due to a product inhibition of lidocaine metabolism.

The individual dosage adjustments in group II resulted in all 20 patients in serum concentrations 12 hr after starting therapy within the recommended range (2–5 mg/liter). Only 2 patients did not require dosage adjustment. In 3 patients the dosage was reduced and in 15 patients it was increased on the basis of the feedback measurements. Because of the observed accumulation on prolonged infusion, in 4 of the 20 patients the 24-hr serum concentrations were above the target range of 2 to 5 mg/liter (between 5 and 6 mg/liter).

DISCUSSION

Our experience with patients treated for arrhythmias indicates that with the Bayesian-feedback method, individual dosage requirements for lidocaine can be determined within a few hours after starting therapy. Only one serum-concentration measurement obtained between 2 and 4 hr after the start of infusion (at least 30 min after the last bolus injection) is sufficient for an accurate prediction.

At the beginning of this chapter it was proposed that implementation of similar methods for drugs with narrow therapeutic ranges would be expected to result in significant improvement in treatment efficacy, the reason being the conservative dosing strategy that leads to undertreatment in a large proportion of patients. Our experience with lidocaine reported herein further supports this proposition. To achieve a serum concentration within the therapeutic range, the initially prescribed dosage had to be increased in 15 of 20 patients.

In view of these results, our own experience with other drugs (8), and the re-

TABLE 1. *Some reasons that feedback methods are not much used*

Methods
Technology
Costs
Risk of toxicity

ports of others (2,7), it is a little surprising that sophisticated computer-assisted forecasting methods are not widely used for dosage optimization for drugs with narrow therapeutic ranges. Table 1 summarizes some of the reasons that may be responsible for the fact that these methods are not used as much as one would expect. The first two factors are, of course, the lack of optimum methods and technology to employ such techniques. For many drugs, the end point, i.e., the serum concentration that is expected to produce the optimal effect, is difficult to define because of lack of controlled clinical studies investigating the concentration–effect relationship. For most drugs that could be potential candidates for Bayesian feedback we do not possess computer software that would be robust and flexible enough to be implemented under routine clinical conditions.

Another important factor is the cost involved in using sophisticated prediction methods. Every feedback problem requires the input of minimum information including a complete dosage history and patient characteristics. Even with the most user-friendly program and the modern fast personal computers, such input represents an investment of 5 to 10 min. A physician is willing to spend that amount of time for a consult, but not for a routine dosage adjustment. The situation may be different in a few years. The infrastructure in hospitals, in outpatient clinics, and in private practice may change, because computers are being more and more implemented for both administrative purposes and patient care.

The last reason that physicians are often reluctant to implement dosage-optimization methods is that their use reduces the safety margin in case of a human or technical error. With individual dosage adjustment, dosages are prescribed that, if administered to the wrong person, may cause severe toxicity. That is not the case for the presently used conservative dosage strategy, as discussed earlier, which chooses a dosage low enough not to produce severe damage even in a patient with a very low elimination rate. This increased risk of severe toxicity may require safety measures that could again considerably increase treatment costs.

In view of these considerations it appears that at the present time, Bayesian prediction methods may find implementation in the clinical routine primarily for drugs that are used under conditions requiring intensive monitoring, e.g., intensive-care unit or general anesthesia. Apart from routine therapeutic use, however, these techniques open up new possibilities for clinical trials investigating the effect–concentration relationship under controlled conditions. In this way, the development of sophisticated dosing aids helps to define the clinical situations in which routine use of serum-concentration measurements and feedback techniques is warranted.

ACKNOWLEDGMENTS

This work was supported by Swiss National Research Foundation and Prof. Max Cloëtta Foundation.

REFERENCES

1. Bauer, L.A., Brown, T., Gibaldi, M., Hudson, L., Nelson, S., Raisys, V., and Shea, J. (1982): Influence of long-term infusions on lidocaine kinetics. *Clin. Pharmacol. Ther.*, 13:433–436.
2. Beach, C.L., Lenert, L., Peck, C., Ludden, T.H., Farringer, J.A., Crawford, M.H., and Clementi, W.A. (1984): Evaluation of a two-compartment Bayesian forecasting program for lidocaine during short and long infusions. *Clin Pharmacol. Ther.*, 35:228 (abstract).
3. Koch-Weser, J. (1975): The serum level approach to individualization of drug dosage. *Eur. J. Clin. Pharmacol.*, 9:1–6.
4. Powell, J.R., Vozeh, S., Hopewell, P., Costello, J., Sheiner, L.B., and Riegelman, S. (1978): Theophylline disposition in acutely ill hospitalized patients: The effect of smoking, heart failure, severe airway obstruction, and pneumonia. *Am. Rev. Respir. Dis.*, 118:229–238.
5. Sheiner, L.B., Rosenberg, B., and Melmon, K.L. (1972): Modelling of individual pharmacokinetics for computer aided drug dosage. *Comp. Biochem. Res.*, 5:441–459.
6. Sheiner, L.B., Beal, S.B., Rosenberg, B., and Marathe, V.V. (1979): Forecasting individual pharmacokinetics. *Clin. Pharmacol. Ther.*, 26:294–305.
7. Sheiner, L.B., and Beal, S.B. (1982): Bayesian individualization of pharmacokinetics: Simple implementation and comparison with non-Bayesian methods. *J. Pharm. Sci.*, 71:1344–1348.
8. Vozeh, S., Muir, K.T., Follath, F., and Sheiner, L.B. (1981): Predicting individual phenytoin dosage. *J. Parmacokinet. Biopharm.*, 9:131.
9. Vozeh, S., Berger, M., Wenk, M., Ritz, R., and Follath, F. (1984): Rapid prediction of individual dosage requirements for liqnocaine. *Clin. Pharmacokinet.*, 9:354–363.
10. Wittenmark, B. (1975): Stochastic adaptive control methods: A survey. *Int. J. Control*, 21:705–730.

DISCUSSION

Discussant 1 (D1): The question of optimal administration of lidocaine is quite interesting in the sense that there are alternative ways of going about the problem. It is not clear whether the drug is being given to reduce arrhythmias or for prophylactic use. In the former, you could use response itself instead of plasma concentration to guide therapy. It is response that determines the size and frequency of i.v. bolus doses and response that reflects active metabolite as well as drug.

Speaker (S): In this group of patients, lidocaine was used as therapy for acute arrhythmias; so, in fact, if the patient did not respond, the clinician gave another bolus. I agree with you that it would be in the prophylactic use of lidocaine that our feedback method would be expected to result in a better treatment. And, more important, I feel that only with such methods, which allow one to adjust the serum concentration to within the desired range in every patient, can one investigate the effect–concentration relationship under routine clinical conditions.

D2: I would like to comment briefly on the use of the terminology *therapeutic range*. I think it's very important, particularly when we address ourselves to biostatisticians or mathematicians, to point out that there is no such thing as a therapeutic range without being very specific about (a) diagnosis of the patient and (b) the exclusion criteria that have been used in the few studies that have been published on the relationship between plasma concentration and effect. Moreover, we must treat the disease and the patient's symptoms, not the blood level.

S: As I mentioned in my talk, I agree that to define the therapeutic range is a difficult problem. Therefore, I advocate computer systems that do not compute the dose for the physician on the basis of a predicted target level, but give the physician the information as to what dose will result in what level, with the appropriate confidence interval. On the basis of this information the physician chooses the dose.

D3: Nobody is trying to get rid of the physician. What Dr. Vožeh has shown is that one can control something (plasma concentration) via feedback, in the real world, and that the concept can be applied to anything that one can measure, such as therapeutic response.

D4: I have partly a comment, partly a question: I don't believe the design of the experiment that you did tested the utility of the feedback method. What the design did was to test that the computer algorithm worked, which may or may not be useful. The critical question is whether or not the patients benefited by this intervention.

S: I fully agree with you. We are also interested in the therapeutic effect of adjusting the lidocaine level. A study has been started in our institution to investigate this question.

D5: There are two problems that concern me. The first, a minor one, relates to the demonstrated increase of alpha-1-acid glycoprotein post myocardial infarction, which changes the distribution of lidocaine concentrations and their meaning, because of the difference in free fraction. But more important, I see increasingly exploration, whether they be of nomograms or of control programs based on feedback, where in one group a physician gives some rigid dosing regimen predetermined or by clinical judgment, and in the other group plasma concentrations are obtained and used for feedback. There is something in between, and that is to provide the physician with plasma-concentration data and then let the physician, without the benefit of feedback programs, monitor the outcome. Failure to use this group as another control group in many studies is so incomprehensible to me that it raises questions in my mind as to whether the investigators are setting out to acquire knowledge or trying to make a self-serving point.

S: About the interpretation of drug levels by physicians, I agree completely with you when you are dealing with steady-state concentrations. If I have a patient on chronic theophylline dosing for a week, and I want to adjust the dose, then I don't have to go to a computer program. On the other hand, if you deal with a drug with clear two-compartment kinetics and if you are sampling a serum concentration 2 hr after start of the infusion, and the last bolus injection was given within 30 min, it is not very easy for a physician or even for a clinical pharmacokineticist to estimate the clearance accurately in this individual. I think it is exactly in these acute (non-steady-state) cases that these methods will probably improve our prediction abilities. But I agree with you that this must be shown in controlled studies.

D3: That was done in a study of digoxin that compared two such groups: the unaided physician versus the aided physician (1). Even for that drug, which is primarily measured in a steady-state situation, the performance was improved by the forecasting procedure, and this was for attainment of the target concentration as well as the predictions.

D6: I just wonder about the value of the so-called control group, based on the physician's judgment. Often the results entirely depend on the clinician and cannot be generalized.

D7: I seem to recall that there have been some six well-controlled trials, in three of which lidocaine was shown conclusively to be a prophylactic, and in the remaining trials not to have benefit. Now, whether or not this difference arises because the wrong dose was used or because the therapeutic range was not appropriately achieved is unknown; however, it would seem unwise to choose prophylaxis for arrhythmias with lidocaine as a test for whether or not a feedback mechanism is useful. Second, I don't believe there were any clinical endpoints, so that again the utility of plasma-concentration measurement with feedback was not assessed. Some properly designed studies are still called for.

S: I completely agree. Nonetheless, I believe that these feedback methods will help us to get to this goal.

D3: Appropriate skepticism is reasonable, but at the same time there are many of us here who have the faith, if not the proof, that by appropriately using drug levels, whether by a computer or by a physician, one can improve therapy. And if you have that faith then you have to believe that what Dr. Vožeh has shown adds something to that process, although I quite agree, and I think everyone does, that the matter needs empirical demonstration.

D8: I couldn't help reacting to the suggestion of the last discussant. Monitoring costs money, time, and effort. It behooves those people who are recommending monitoring to prove its value. Faith is not enough.

D3: No one disagrees.

REFERENCE

1. Sheiner, L.B., Halkin, H.H., Peck, C.C., Rosenberg, B., and Melmon, K.L. (1975): Improved computer-assisted digoxin therapy. *Ann. Intern. Med.,* 82:619–627.

*Variability in Drug Therapy:
Description, Estimation, and Control,*
edited by M. Rowland et al.
Raven Press, New York © 1985.

Discussion: Principles and Evaluation of Variability in Drug Therapy

Laszlo Endrenyi (Editor)

Department of Pharmacology, University of Toronto, Toronto, Ontario M5S 1A8 Canada

This edited discussion considers two main topics. The first of these deals with some principles of variability. The second main issue involves a draft proposal for conducting a pharmacokinetic screen in elderly patients, as a means of exploring variability. The proposal was contained in a discussion paper authored by Dr. Robert Temple, Acting Director of the Office of New Drug Evaluations in the U.S. Food and Drug Administration (reprinted here in its entirety as an Appendix to this chapter).

SOME QUESTIONS ABOUT VARIABILITY IN DRUG RESPONSE

What Is Variability? Definitions and Classifications

Variability in a response (beneficial or harmful) arises in drug therapy when a standard dose or dosing regimen evokes differing responses in various individuals or in a given individual at different times. In the first case, one speaks of interindividual variability, and in the latter, of intraindividual variability. Whenever it is observed, attempts should be made to explain variability if it is ultimately to be controlled.

Pharmacodynamic and Pharmacokinetic Variability

Clinically pharmacological responses are important. Generally, we would like to know, and preferably quantify, the therapeutic and toxic responses, and note their variabilities after administering a given dose of a drug.

A different, tighter definition separates the variability into pharmacokinetic and pharmacodynamic components. The pharmacodynamic component relates effect and concentration of a drug in the biophase. The pharmacokinetic component, on the other hand, relates drug concentration and dose.

Clinically, in the management of the patient, the pharmacokinetic relationship and its variability are important when the response cannot be conveniently quantified and the concentration of drug substantially predicts response.

Interindividual and Intraindividual Variabilities

Intraindividual and interindividual variabilities differ with respect to an important clinical feature: Whereas finding an optimum dose for a given individual will render the clinical problem of interindividual variation irrelevant, intraindividual variability remains a concern even if the best possible dose for this subject has been determined.

Intraindividual variability involves the change of features of a subject with time. For instance, in the case of development of tolerance or sensitization, pharmacodynamic relationships between the effect and the concentration in the biophase can change. Similarly, components of drug disposition can show changes over time, with the kinetics in the subject varying along with them. Examples include inhibition or induction of metabolic elimination, variable absorption due to pH dependence, and diurnal variation due to circadian rhythms.

Interindividual variation in the pharmacodynamic relationship can occur as evidenced by the existence of responders and nonresponders to drugs, such as observed with the antiarrhythmics. Variability in pharmacokinetics can be attributed to various factors. Some of these involve easily measurable individual characteristics (e.g., weight or sex) or disease (e.g., renal dysfunction). In other cases, the characteristics of the disease are readily identified but not easily quantified (e.g., congestive heart failure). Also, confounding factors (e.g., age and smoking) often make it difficult to identify clearly the sources of kinetic variability. The approach to drug therapy is then generally cautious and involves administering a dose low enough to yield a serum drug concentration always below the toxic range. This policy generally leads to undertreatment in a large proportion of patients. Improved therapy is possible after the major sources of variability are identified and evaluated. Then individual adjustments in drug dosage can be made.

Predictable and Unpredictable Variabilities

It is important to distinguish between variability that can be ultimately predicted and that which cannot.

The ultimately predictable components of variability involve relationships between the response and observable characteristics of the subjects. The features can be either continuous (e.g., age, weight) or discontinuous (e.g., sex, pharmacogenetic group) [see the chapter by D. J. Finney (*this volume*)].

The discrepancy between prediction and observation is the residual, unpredictable (or as yet unaccounted for) variability. Because it reflects a lack of information, it is especially important to evaluate the magnitude of the residual variability [see the chapter by J.-L. Steimer et al. (*this volume*)]. If the inexplicable variation is large, and if there is some problem with efficacy or toxicity (*vide infra*), it may be necessary to watch the patient and perhaps undertake therapeutic drug monitoring. Also, if there is a subpopulation (e.g., the elderly) with large unpredicted variability, then subjects in this group must be watched more carefully than others.

When Is Variability of Concern?

The aim of drug therapy is to achieve efficacy without toxicity. Ideally, the goal can be achieved with a single, standard dose of the drug. Thus, from the clinical point of view, variability is not a concern if a standard dose of a drug is always effective and not toxic.

Problems can arise if in some patients the drug is either ineffective or toxic at a given dose. In this case, the amount administered will have to be adjusted either on the basis of predictive relationships (*vide infra*) or empirically by titrating the patient. However, the adjustments can be difficult, often because the therapeutic or toxic effect cannot be measured accurately and early enough.

In order to deal with these concerns it is highly desirable to clarify the causes and sources of variability. Therefore, one should determine at the very earliest possible stage, preferably in a predictive animal model, the potential of a drug to do harm. One must know both the therapeutic indications and the consequences of the drug failing to be active. It is essential to have mechanistic understanding of the key processes, to help explain why a drug elicited subsequent problems. For instance, if a minor metabolite is active and is the source of variability, then clearance or bioavailability of drug should have little effect, but the formation rate of the metabolite is important, and its variability will be a cause of concern.

How Can Variability Be Either Dealt with or Reduced?

Dealing with Variability

Biological variability is an inherent feature of drug action. When considering uncontrolled variability, we can deal with it, make adjustments for it, but cannot actually change or reduce it.

The statistical methods used in dealing with variability involve establishing relationships between inputs and outputs. The inputs can be subject to control (dose, dosage pattern, route of administration) or they may be uncontrollable (e.g., the precise absorption pattern). The useful, quantifiable, desired responses represent the output (ratio of maximum and minimum responses, steady-state concentration, etc.). Models and their parameters provide the conversion, or translation, between input and output. Initially, estimates of population characteristics defining the variability in the parameters must be obtained from ad hoc data in appropriate groups of individuals. The investigator should define the objective of the given study in terms of the expected outputs (which, in turn, will determine a cost function involving a weighted combination of the outputs). The model enables calculation of the parameters, the expected values and variances of the outputs, and the distribution of the predicted responses [see the chapters by M. Rowland, J.-L. Steimer et al., and D. Katz (*this volume*)].

It depends on the main goal of the investigation whether the greatest effort should be spent on evaluating the observed responses or the model parameters. For clinical purposes, it is the predicted concentrations or pharmacodynamic responses that are important. Parameters can be useful for gaining insight, in order to understand and interpret the biological system. However, parameters are estimated with comparatively large uncertainty; they also depend on the assumed model, and their estimation is very much influenced by experimental design. Therefore, it is generally more useful to evaluate and then predict observable responses.

Reducing Kinetic Variability

Sometimes a well-defined component of drug disposition contributes substantially to the overall variability in response. Technical means of influencing this source may lead to a substantial reduction in variability. For instance, if absorption is an important source of variability, then the dosage form and the route of administration could be manipulated. If the formation of an active metabolite is highly variable, then one could consider administering the metabolite instead of the parent drug. Selecting and designing the molecular form of the active drug could modify its properties and reduce its variability. Consequently, the prospects are remarkable for being able to minimize the variability of responses during drug therapy.

PROPOSAL: A PHARMACOKINETIC SCREEN FOR DRUGS TO BE USED IN THE ELDERLY

Dr. Temple's Discussion Paper on Pharmacokinetic Screening

The report was motivated by "a perception that drugs, even drugs likely to be used in the elderly, are not studied adequately in elderly patients and that as a consequence older patients are more likely than younger patients to suffer adverse reactions to drugs." Therefore, the question of a rational approach to ascertaining drug responses in the elderly population was raised. It was noted, in addition, that in recent and current new-drug applications, substantially large numbers of older patients, over the age of 65, were included in the clinical trials. Nonetheless, the data were rarely analyzed on the basis of age.

Age-related changes in pharmacodynamics or pharmacokinetics have been observed [see the chapter entitled Modeling Pharmacodynamics: Parametric and Nonparametric Approaches (L. B. Sheiner, *this volume*)], but it is not known how common they are. In addition, it is often difficult to detect and evaluate subpopulations with different pharmacokinetic characteristics. It would therefore be desirable and useful to obtain information about therapeutic and toxic drug responses in patient populations in which the drug is likely to be used. The discussion paper makes two principal recommendations:

1. Clinical trials should be conducted in target populations, and the variability of the responses should be analyzed.

Attention should be paid to factors determining the pharmacokinetics of the drug. For instance, if a drug or an active metabolite is excreted substantially through renal mechanisms, then one should evaluate the effects of various degrees of renal impairment on the dosing requirements. Similarly, the influences of protein binding, disease states, and drug interactions ought to be assessed whenever their effects are expected to be clinically important.

Consequently, the discussion paper recommends that elderly patients should not be excluded from clinical trials of drugs to which they are expected to be exposed following approval and marketing. Also, it is expected that the analysis of the effectiveness and safety of drugs will extend to the influence of patient age and of other age-related characteristics.

2. During premarketing clinical trials of drugs, they should be subjected to a "pharmacokinetic screen." This would be a simple means of determining pharmacokinetic properties in the sampled patient population. Differences between subpopulations should be noted, including the effect of age.

The pharmacokinetic screen would require a small number of drug-level determinations to be made at steady state in many patients.

The spirit of the proposal, it was noted, was to look for unexpected phenomena and for large deviations in important features, such as side effects. Any finding could be followed up in subsequent, well-controlled trials.

It is hoped also that analysis of the trials could be pursued across the subgroups being studied. This could uncover areas in which potential problems could be anticipated without needing specific trials in the various groups.

The important questions to be asked are whether or not any of these objectives can be met and whether or not there are other goals that should be accomplished. Also, what approaches would be most suited for accomplishing their purposes?

Approaches to Assessment of Population-Kinetic Variability

Four procedures can be envisaged for obtaining information about kinetic variability. In sequence, they yield increasing information, but their investigational and analytical requirements become also higher.

Single Trough Screen

In each patient, a single blood sample would be obtained at the trough (steady-state minimum) of drug concentrations. It would be sufficient to measure drug levels close to this trough. Their relationships to characteristics of the patient (such as age, sex, disease state) could be explored by simple statistical procedures, e.g., by multiple linear regression.

This procedure is most similar to the one described in Dr. Temple's discussion paper. It would identify, essentially qualitatively, kinetically relevant factors and their differences among subgroups. The approach is quite simple and could be conducted during open, phase III trials.

However, the method would yield information only about the adjusted clearance (clearance divided by bioavailability), not about volume of distribution or half-life. The relationships to patient characteristics would be more qualitative than quantitative. Interindividual and residual variabilities could not be separated. The study would require relatively large numbers of subjects, about 20 to 40 patients for each physiological condition, altogether perhaps 400 patients with 5 to 10 conditions.

Multiple Trough Screen

Two or more blood samples would be obtained near the trough of steady-state concentrations, at least from most patients. In addition to relating blood concentrations to patient characteristics, it is possible now to separate interindividual and residual variabilities.

Because the patients are studied in greater detail, the method would require fewer subjects, and the relationships to patient characteristics could be evaluated with higher precision.

On the other hand, in order to estimate the interindividual variability of the adjusted clearance, a program designed for population-kinetic analysis (NONMEM or a similar program) should be used [see the chapter by J.-L. Steiner (*this volume*)]. This may be less familiar to the data analyst.

Full Kinetic Screen

From each subject, several blood samples (two to five samples) would be drawn at different times following the last drug administration. In addition, various drug preparations, etc., could be considered.

The approach would enable evaluating in populations not only the adjusted clearance but also the volume of distribution, adjusted for bioavailability, as well as the half-life of the drug. The three population-kinetic parameters of clearance, bioavailability, and volume of distribution could be estimated separately if i.v. administration was occasionally applied. The parameters could be assessed in various subgroups, and the effects of disease state, age, and other patient characteristics could be studied. It would also be possible to evaluate interindividual and residual variabilities of the parameters in the various subpopulations.

The method would require 10 to 20 subjects for each pathophysiological condition to be studied. The dosage history, including the timing of recent drug injections, would have to be recorded carefully. The results should be evaluated by a computer program such as NONMEM.

This method still requires only observational data that can be obtained during a clinical trial. It has been successfully tried and applied, but only retrospectively. Its potential in phase III trials, with outpatients, has yet to be tested.

Full Pharmacokinetic Study

This experimental, relatively elaborate approach could be pursued in small groups of subjects, all exhibiting potentially influential pathophysiological features. The results could be compared with those of similar studies in which the subjects had differing features.

The samples would be collected meticulously at preset, designed times. They could be evaluated in detail by standard techniques of data analysis, such as weighted nonlinear regression.

Pharmacokinetic models and parameters could be evaluated. In contrast, the clinically relevant interindividual and residual variabilities could be estimated only poorly, because sample sizes would generally be very small.

Issues of Implementation and Execution

Schedule of Pharmacokinetic Studies

The importance of understanding processes and mechanisms of drug disposition has been emphasized [see the chapters by F. Sjöqvist, M. Rowland, and G. Levy (*this volume*)]. This implies that biochemical and physiological properties of a drug should be explored early in its development.

Pharmacokinetic experiments are performed in animals and later in healthy human subjects. If exploratory studies indicate the importance and relevance of a condition or process (e.g., age, protein binding, hepatic or renal function), then its effect on the kinetics of the drug should be investigated. Such experiments could be conducted at any phase of drug development, after noting the importance of the pathophysiological factor.

Pharmacokinetic screenings would be conducted across a number of subgroups of the population. Provided that they are considered to be meaningful and useful (*vide infra*), they would be best performed during the late phase III of drug development, perhaps in the form of open-labeled trials, and involving numerous subjects.

Timing of Observations

In the simplest design relying on blood concentrations that are measured at steady state, the samples should be withdrawn near the trough, shortly before the next dose is ingested.

It is not advisable to aim at measuring peak concentrations. The time of achieving the maximum depends on the rates of all processes of drug disposition, including those of absorption, distribution, and elimination, and may vary strongly among the subjects. Consequently, the simple estimation of peak levels is subject to large uncertainty.

For the most detailed kinetic information, a number of measurements (perhaps two to five) should be obtained, in most patients, at different times relative to the last dose (*vide supra*).

Sampling of Subjects

Kinetic screening studies ought to explore features of the target populations. Consequently, the samples of subjects should be representative of patients to whom the drug will be administered.

The main purpose would be to explore the efficacy and safety of the drug in a number of assigned subpopulations (such as the elderly). Thus, it could be possible to identify subgroups at risk.

Screening investigations would not involve homogeneous samples of patients on which clinical trials often rely. In comparative trials the greater heterogeneity would undoubtedly require increased sample sizes. A stratified design could also be considered for screening trials. For instance, one could study different subgroups at different centers. However, the confounding of relevant factors should be assessed.

Methods for Data Analysis

Experimental kinetic studies could be assessed by well-known procedures, e.g., by weighted nonlinear regression. Simple observational screens, e.g., with single troughs (*vide supra*), could be evaluated by standard statistical procedures, e.g., multiple linear regression or other multivariate techniques such as cluster analysis.

More complex observational studies would probably have to be analyzed by maximum-likelihood procedures, e.g., by NONMEM, that could correct for dosage, estimate parameters of a structural model in the different subgroups, relate them to observed patient characteristics, and evaluate interindividual and residual variabilities. Analysis of the residuals could separate features of the subgroup.

Issues of Pharmacokinetic Screening

Possible Directions, Questions

In order to pursue pharmacokinetic screening trials and other population-kinetic studies, some preliminary conditions must be fulfilled. These include the availability of a specific and sensitive assay, the exploration of major metabolic pathways in humans, the demonstration of correlations between drug concentrations and clinically relevant effects, and the substantiation of a basic model for the kinetics of the drug. Other information could also be useful or even essential, e.g., whether or not the drug and/or its metabolites are active therapeutically or toxically, the possible existence of genetic influences, etc.

It could be in the common interest of all (drug industry, regulatory agencies, academic scientists, and especially patients) that subjects and their defined populations at high risk to a drug be identified. Lack of such knowledge can lead to problems. For instance, uncertainties and suspicions that poorly defined difficulties may exist could lead to substantial delays in approving the drug for marketing.

Even if some approaches to pharmacokinetic screening will ultimately be found valuable, they should not be used for regulatory purposes and should not influence the approval of the drug. Doing so would discourage innovation and encourage bad studies and ignorance. Therefore, the results of screening investigations should be used only to alert physicians to their implications and to improve therapeutic precision.

For pursuing this direction, intelligence and understanding are required from all, including the regulatory authorities. One should perceive not only what the problem is but also what its causes and solutions are.

A question remains to be answered: Whose responsibility should it be to develop population-kinetic information, and who should support it? If one considers this as research involving the development of new drugs, then these explorations would be the responsibility of drug manufacturers. If, however, the information is gained under actual conditions of use in the widespread, post-release, phase IV investigations, then it is not clear if the task should be the responsibility of the industry.

Concerns

Caution, concerns, and reservations were also expressed about the possible pharmacokinetic screening trials. Practical questions were asked about the need for taking additional blood samples and about the requirement for obtaining them near the trough. An example of a logistical problem was mentioned: the expectation of assaying numerous samples either in house or through a service.

Concerning the interpretation of trials involving the elderly, a reminder was offered: The chronological ages of patients are very different from their physiological ages. In trials, often healthy but chronologically old subjects are included. This would not be helpful for screenings. Therefore, one should look also for other factors concurrent with age, such as disease state and drugs.

Caution was advised about testing and introducing new procedures. Certainly, they should be explored and evaluated before substantial commitment is made to apply them. It should also be assessed whether or not the results are worth the time, expense, and possible delays.

Finally, anxiety was expressed about the possibility that once advisory guidelines are established, they may acquire regulatory status in the eyes of authorities who may not have a clear understanding of the fundamentals. This could occasionally lead to requiring additional time and expense during the regulatory approval process.

Consensus

Despite these concerns, participants in the workshop generally found the idea of the pharmacokinetic screening trials interesting and attractive.

The goal would be to identify (age-related) circumstances likely to require different prescribing information, or likely circumstances in which a problem would arise. Thus, subpopulations (such as the elderly) at risk could be discovered who should be excluded from having the drug, or who should be warned of possible side effects, or for whom different dosing would be recommended.

The trials could be conducted in late phase III or perhaps in phase IV of drug development, during premarketing or postmarketing of the drug, respectively. The observations would be obtained across subpopulations, either with stratified subgroups or in randomized trials with extended inclusion criteria.

Measuring a single trough level in each subject is relatively convenient. The results can be evaluated by multiple linear regression or multivariate techniques. Substantially more information can be obtained if two or more minimum trough concentrations are obtained from most subjects. However, analysis of the data will require appropriate statistical methods that, at present, require further validation. In principle, the procedure involving multiple troughs ought to be preferred.

It was generally stressed that all approaches and methods related to the principles and practice of the pharmacokinetic screening trials should be tested and evaluated before adopting them in any way. If they are found to be worthwhile and valuable, they should be used in an advisory, cautionary, and monitoring role, but not as part of the regulatory drug-approval process.

ACKNOWLEDGMENTS

What precedes is the final discussion of the workshop summarized in a substantially rearranged and edited form, plus material abstracted from manuscripts and discussion papers sent subsequently to the author by Drs. L. B. Sheiner and S. Voženh. The author would like to acknowledge all contributors.

APPENDIX: DISCUSSION PAPER ON THE TESTING OF DRUGS IN THE ELDERLY

Robert Temple

Acting Director of the Office of New Drug Evaluations in the U.S. Food and Drug Administration

There is a perception that drugs, even drugs likely to be used in the elderly, are not studied adequately in elderly patients and that as a consequence older patients are more likely than younger patients to suffer adverse reactions to drugs. It may be true that elderly patients are more likely to develop adverse reactions to drugs but, if true, the extent to which this is the result of age-related differences in drug response and insufficient clinical information about such changes, or is simply the result of an increased likelihood that the elderly will have concomitant diseases or will be using many drugs, is not really known. Most of those who have written about drugs in the elderly have found that the effect of age on the pharmacokinetics of drugs is the best-established specifically age-related problem.

A recent survey of a dozen and recently approved pending new drug applications showed that older patients (over 65) are included in reasonably large numbers in studies of most drugs. Nonetheless, it is comparatively unusual for a sponsor to direct specific attention to the elderly to determine whether there ought to be specific labeling advice for them. It is therefore worthwhile to consider whether there are specific testing and analysis requirements that should be met by anyone planning to market a drug with potential usefulness in the elderly so that the clinician will be as aware as possible of special considerations involved in using the drug in older patients.

Although specific cases of age-related changes in pharmacokinetics or pharmacodynamics are recognized, it is not clear how common such changes are, nor, except for certain obvious situations, such as the increased half-life of renal-excreted drugs in elderly patients with diminished renal function, is it clear how to predict them. This is not solely a concern related to the elderly. Subpopulations with different pharmacokinetics can exist in any age group, and detection of them has generally been difficult; a good, pharmacokinetic evaluation of a drug will therefore contribute information allowing intelligent dose adjustment in patients of all ages.

The number of documented examples of age-related pharmacodynamic differences seems too small at this time to demand formal studies comparing younger and older patients with respect to their blood-level response curves. The major impediment would be selection of an appropriate older population (well versus ill, specific decade of life, concomitant therapy or not). The approach suggested is therefore to use information collected from clinical trials that include older patients to search for possible pharmacodynamic differences.

Better information on using drugs in the elderly can be developed both from improvements in the general requirements for drug testing and from requirements related specifically to the older patient. The general requirements are:

1. For any drug that has significant renal excretion of parent drug or active metabolites, there should be formal study of the effects of altered renal status on the drug's pharmacokinetics. Dosing information in product labeling should include instructions for the dosage adjustments needed for varying degrees of renal impairment.

It would also be helpful to include in labeling for drugs needing such dosage adjustment a method for calculating the creatinine clearance from the serum creatinine, e.g.,

$$\text{male } C_{Cr} = \frac{\text{wt (kg)} \times (146 - \text{age})}{72 \times \text{Cr (mg/100 ml)}}$$

$$\text{female } C_{Cr} = 0.9 \times (\text{male } C_{Cr})$$

Such information is already commonly obtained for relatively toxic drugs; see, for example, current labeling for aminoglycoside antibiotics, a toxic group of drugs whose excretion is renal.

2. To implement a screening mechanism that will detect unanticipated pharmacokinetic problems in a setting that is reasonably comparable to clinical use.

The requirements specifically related to the elderly are:

1. To be certain elderly patients are not excluded from trials of drugs to which they will be exposed after a drug is marketed.

2. To analyze the safety and effectiveness results of clinical trials with attention specifically to the influence of patient age, as well as other characteristics that can be age-related (renal or hapatic status, muscle mass, concomitant therapy, and concomitant disease). Depending on the findings arising from screening tests and analyses, and on circumstances related to the specific drug, to carry out specific clinical trials needed to characterize the drug in the elderly.

In contemplating additional requirements related to study of drugs in the elderly, or to better evaluation of pharmacokinetics in general, the cost in time and money should be considered. It is apparent that, if planned at the outset of a drug's development, inclusion of elderly patients and analysis of results with respect to age are essentially cost-free. Exploration of pharmacokinetic questions such as the effects of renal impairment can be costly, but is plainly already a responsibility of a drug's sponsor, not a new requirement. Thus, the only significant new requirement and burden is the pharmacokinetic screening mechanism described below. Its benefits, however, appear to outweigh its costs.

Proposal

The following requirements are therefore proposed as a means of assuring that clinicians will have adequate information to use drugs appropriately in the elderly. These include general requirements, i.e., improvements in drug evaluation that are applicable to many patients but that will have particularly value with respect to the elderly, and specific requirements, i.e., requirements related solely to the older population. The new requirements would be incorporated into the existing document called "General Considerations for the Clinical Evaluation of Drugs."

I. General Requirements

A. Drugs that are excreted (parent drug or active metabolities) significantly through renal mechanisms should be studied to define the effects of altered renal function on their pharmacokinetics. Information should be developed for dosing instructions that provide appropriate adjustments for varying degrees of renal impairment. Labeling for such drugs should include a means of calculating creatinine clearance from the serum creatinine, adjusting for weight and age, because it is often difficult to obtain accurate direct measures of creatinine clearance without hospitalizing the patient for urine collections.

B. Drugs that are highly protein-bound should be studied to determine factors that might influence degree of binding, such as total blood level, pH, etc. Ordinarily, much of this study can be done using *in vitro* methods.

C. Drugs in late Phase II and Phase III should be subjected to a "pharmacokinetic screen." A pharmacokinetic screen (not previously defined) is a simple means of determining whether a drug has pharmacokinetic properties that are likely to cause it to have unanticipated problems. It consists of a small number of blood-level determinations during steady-state dosing designed to display the variability in blood levels under defined conditions of dosing.

Depending on the half-life of the drug it might be sufficient to get a trough (pre-dose) value (probably suitable if the drug has a relatively long half-life) or, alternatively, a trough and approximate peak value. If there are previous kinetic studies, the peak time can probably be estimated and one or two blood samples should be sufficient for an approximate peak level. If there are no prior studies, the peak could probably be approximated sufficiently by two or three measurements in the 1-3 hours post-dosing period. It might not be necessary to carry out these observations in every patient in Phase III but a sizeable sample, including patients in all age, race, weight, and sex groups, as well as patients with a variety of concomitant therapies and diseases, should be studied. Because a pharmacokinetic screen is relatively easy and inexpensive, at least if there is a suitable assay for the drug in body fluids, involving only 1-4 blood-level determinations per patient (a much less burdensome series of determinations than would be generated by the typical formal pharmacokinetic study) it is reasonable to cast as wide a net as possible in an effort to find atypical patients. Deviations could result from almost any factor that affected pharmacokinetics, including differences in metabolism and, of particular relevance to the elderly, differences in volume of distribution, hepatic metabolism, or renal excretion.

Studies of this kind are not intended to be similar in quality or precision to the typical formal pharmacokinetic study carried out on a new drug, and they will not be able to detect small patient-to-patient differences. Concern that such a screen is not the best possible pharmacokinetic study should not be allowed to obscure the fact that what is most important is large differences, differences likely to be clinically important.

It is inherent in the idea of a "screen" that when the screen discovers something unusual, further studies would need to be done. Thus, if a particular subpopulation (e.g., people of a certain age, or those receiving specific other drugs or with other diseases) were found to have higher (or lower) blood levels than the rest, an attempt to discover the reason for this would become necessary.

D. Drug-disease and drug-drug interactions.

1. Specific studies. Certain drug interactions are so common and so readily anticipated that it is almost always desirable to study them. These include:

a. Drugs known to have extensive protein binding can be expected to interact with specific concomitant therapies, specifically sulfonylureas, coumarin, phenytoin and certain NSAIDs, to cite a few examples. These interactions should be explored using *in vitro* or *in vivo* methods, as appropriate.

b. So many drugs affect serum levels of digoxin, which is widely used in the elderly and is potentially very toxic, that evaluation of this interaction is appropriate for virtually any drug.

c. Ophthalmic drugs (especially antiglaucoma drugs) require compatibility testing with other topical ophthalmic drugs, which are frequently used in the elderly.

d. For drugs that undergo hepatic metabolism, the pharmacokinetic effects of known hepatic enzyme inducers should be studied.

2. Interaction screen. If the drug is going to be used in conditions where specific diseases are particularly likely to be present (that is, other than the disease that is being treated with the test drug), an attempt should be made to include patients with the other diseases in the treatment population. The pharmacokinetic screen should be useful in determining whether the other diseases affect blood levels of the drug and clinical observations should permit detection of specific adverse effects associated with the other diseases. Similarly, with respect to other medications that are used concomitantly, the screen should help evaluate whether the other medications affect the kinetics of the test drug. In some cases, where a concomitant drug is used especially frequently, formal interaction studies should be carried out. For example, antianginal drugs of different pharmacologic classes (nitrate, beta-blocker, calcium antagonist) are so commonly combined that they should be subjected to formal studies of their combined effectiveness and tolerance.

It is also possible that the new drug will have an effect on the kinetics of other drugs. There is almost no limit to the number of studies that could be mounted to explore this question; therefore, a second screening mechanism would be helpful. If Phase III clinical trials include patients who are on a variety of other drug therapies (held stable during introduction of the new agent), trough blood levels of the other drugs can be obtained prior to dosing with the new agent and again after the new agent has reached steady state. It should thus be possible to detect, with relatively little effort, major effects of the new drug on many concomitant medications. The principal limit to being able to do so will be the availability of good blood-level measurements for the other agents. In general, drugs where blood levels are most critical are those for which blood-level determinations are being developed.

II. Specific Requirements Related to the Elderly

A. Determination that a Drug Is Likely to Have Significant Use in the Elderly

In many cases it is obvious that a drug will be widely used in the elderly because the diseases that it is intended to treat are characteristically diseases of aging, e.g., coronary artery disease, senile dementia, or peripheral vascular disease. In other cases it is not entirely clear what the age of ultimate population will be. A sponsor should determine through estimates of the disease prevalence by age or through examination of the age distribution for other drugs of a similar type (using the National Disease and Therapeutic Index, for example) whether his drug is likely to have significant use in the elderly.

B. Inclusion of Elderly Patients in Clinical Studies

Elderly patients should not be arbitrarily excluded from the patient population if a drug is likely to have significant use in the elderly. Sometimes, for example, patients over the age of 75 are excluded from clinical trials. There are reasons for doing this, principally, especially early in clinical studies, a desire to be sure that the patients' response to the drug will not be confounded by patients' underlying disease and fragility. Nonetheless, at least during Phase III, elderly patients should not be excluded. Ordinarily, elderly patients would be included in trials with other patients but in some cases, especially for drugs targeted to older patients or where differences in response by age are anticipated, trials could include only the elderly or, perhaps better, could specifically be designed to compare results in the older and younger patient groups.

C. Analysis of Adverse Effects and Effectiveness by Age

Adverse drug reactions and effectiveness should be analyzed taking age into account. It is possible to do a variety of analyses of effectiveness or adverse effects looking for relationship to dose, race, underlying disease, and age. This should be done both for individual studies and as an overall analysis. There would have to be a fairly substantial difference in effectiveness or adverse reaction rates by age before a difference could be detected; that is less a problem than it might seem, as unless the difference is rather large it is probably not of major importance.

This kind of analysis might need to be followed up by formal dose–response studies, or if possible, blood level response studies, specifically in the elderly; such studies might be done earlier in the drug evaluation if the drug was particularly directed at the elderly or if it was a member of a class where pharmacodynamic differences with age might be expected, such as benzodiazepines.

Alternative

There are other ways to approach the question of drugs in the elderly. Dr. Crooks of Dundee, Scotland, in a paper prepared for the Committee on Safety of Medicines, first discussed the kinds of differences that might exist between the elderly and younger people and proposed the following approach:

He identified drugs liable to produce special problems in the elderly as (1) drugs with indications for use that are commonly found in the elderly, (2) drugs with a low therapeutic ratio if associated with one or more of the following: (a) drugs primarily eliminated by renal excretion (or with biologically active metabolites excreted in the urine), (b) drugs with a high liver extraction ratio, (c) drugs that act directly on the central nervous system and (d) drugs that have an effect likely to be modified by the impairment of homeostatic mechanisms commonly found in the elderly.

He proposed that for drugs meeting those criteria a product license would require the following additional studies:

1. Single-dose pharmacokinetic studies in healthy, elderly patients (greater than 70 years old), and where the single-dose data are markedly different from the young, multiple-dose studies as well.

2. Pharmacodynamic studies in elderly patients with the condition for which the drug is indicated.

3. Safety and effectiveness of the drug must be established in the elderly under clinical trial conditions using the dosing regimen considered to be appropriate for the elderly on the basis of the pharmacokinetic and where available pharmacodynamic data.

Although this approach is in many ways similar to our proposal, I believe it has a significant problem:

The first two studies would necessarily be carried out in "healthy elderly" patients and in a rather small number of them. As the elderly are almost surely quite diverse with respect to differences from younger patients, many potential problems seem likely to be missed. Nonetheless, the recommended studies are comparatively easy to carry out and the approach is in some ways less demanding. Commentators should consider it in their responses.

*Variability in Drug Therapy:
Description, Estimation, and Control,*
edited by M. Rowland et al.
Raven Press, New York © 1985.

Concluding Remarks: Respective Roles of Pharmacokinetics and Pharmacodynamics in Drug Development

Giorgio Segre

Institute of Pharmacology, University of Siena, I-53100 Siena, Italy

Variability is a biological characteristic as well as a psychological characteristic of humans. Some of the great issues of our time, such as IQ, revolve around the question of variability. Variability in responses to drugs can often be measured and evaluated. These measurements can then be used to improve therapy by ensuring the desired effect with minimal toxicity. When dealing with variability in responses, it is good scientific practice to try to distinguish the part played by variability in pharmacokinetics from the other sources of variability, which are related to the statistical distribution in a population of the thresholds of effects and toxic signs.

To some extent, drug toxicity in patients can be anticipated from experiments in animals and from early phase II and III trials in humans. What are extremely difficult to predict are the bizarre toxicities that appear to be due to immunological and other poorly understood phenomena (1,2). Other causes of toxicity are genetic differences in drug handling, as exemplified by the existence of slow and fast acetylators of isoniazid, extensive and poor oxidizers of debrisoquine, and failure of a few subjects to rapidly hydrolyze suxamethonium. The result is sometimes a clear differentiation of patients into two or more classes.

Another factor in drug toxicity that could, in principle, be predicted is that which relates changes in excretion and biotransformation processes to disease. These changes lead to a change in some pharmacokinetic parameter, but because the distribution of the parameter in the patient population is not usually bimodal, a careful analysis is necessary to ensure appropriate stratification of the population. Such is the case of changes in renal excretion in patients with renal failure, which can lead to a dangerous accumulation of drug, e.g., aminoglycosides, unless dosage is appropriately adjusted. Here, plasma drug monitoring may be helpful in optimizing drug administration. Plasma drug monitoring is also helpful with phenytoin and theophylline, for which hepatic biotransformation is the major route of elimination and a major source of variability in clearance for these drugs.

Although animal experimentation has limited application to dosage adjustment in humans, knowing that in animals a drug is eliminated by hepatic metabolism (particularly by microsomal oxidation processes) would lead one to expect wide variations in blood levels in humans following standard doses. The use of isolated human liver cells can be of great help to examine this potential problem of variation in drug metabolism, prior to drug administration to humans.

These general considerations are of great importance, particularly in two groups of the population: the very young and the elderly. Many of the recent withdrawals from the market of medicinal products by the companies or by the registering authorities were connected with toxicity in the elderly, as exemplified by the recent case of benoxaprofen. In certain cases the toxic event is idiosyncratic, defying easy and early detection. In other cases the occurrence of severe toxicity is very low and requires a well-designed postmarketing survey in a large number of subjects to ensure detection. Many other more frequent types of toxicity can be analyzed and predicted with a high degree of confidence. Analysis of these types of toxicity requires knowledge and application of many of the statistical methods discussed in this volume.

As pointed out already, pharmacokinetic studies in humans are usually based on too few subjects. It is imperative to study the kinetics of a given drug in subgroups of the population, healthy and diseased, young and old. Also, one should study the more likely drug interactions of therapeutic importance. Both the theoretical and practical tools for doing these types of analyses are available. In addition to the presently available sophisticated instrumentation and techniques for determination of drug levels in biological fluids, there are programs for analysis of pharmacokinetic data with mainframe computers as well as microcomputers and for the study of the pharmacostatistics of a population and its stratifications: two-stage statistics and the Bayesian approach using programs for multivariate analysis or the NONMEM program.

Regarding the possible use of very early pharmacokinetic information in drug development, it should be recalled that the EEC guidelines to drug toxicity studies require an analysis of the kinetics of a drug in a few volunteers, as a preliminary step in choosing the most appropriate animal species for chronic toxicity studies (that is, the species that most resembles humans in handling the drug under study). Moreover, it is a common experience that information on the kinetics of a drug in animals can give a very early indication of its pharmacokinetic behavior in humans:

1. If a drug is well absorbed orally in rats (or in other species), it is usually well absorbed orally in humans (although the rate of absorption depends on the particular pharmaceutical preparation).
2. If a drug has a long half-life in rats, it is also likely to be long in humans (but the converse is not true).

3. If a drug rapidly enters the brain of the rat, it generally does so in humans.
4. The main route of drug handling in rats (and in other animal species) gives a good indication of what will happen in humans. For instance, if a drug undergoes extensive liver biotransformation in animals, this is likely to be so in humans, even if great quantitative differences between animals and humans exist.
5. The volume of distribution per unit body weight in humans is similar to that in animals; the same is true for protein binding.
6. Drug interactions observed in animals may well occur in humans.

One should add that a complete pharmacokinetic description of a drug requires knowledge of its metabolic profile with the attendant more complex pharmacokinetic model. In several instances in which a metabolite has been found to be active, it has subsequently been patented and introduced into the market.

The pharmacokinetics of a drug is a fundamental property that should be assessed at the earliest possible stage of development. Research into the pharmacokinetic profile of a new drug can lead to the discovery of potentially useful drugs (such as antihistaminic or opioid drugs that do not penetrate into the brain). An interesting approach that deserves more attention is to study the kinetics of drug effects. Where this approach has been adopted, useful insight into the action of a drug has been obtained. Collectively, pharmacokinetic and pharmacodynamic information will certainly improve the use of many drugs for management of the sick.

REFERENCES

1. Rawlins, M.D. (1981): Clinical pharmacology—adverse reaction to drug. *Br. Med. J.,* 282:974–976.
2. Rawlins, M.D., and Thompson, J.M. (1977): Pathogenesis of adverse drug reactions. In: *Textbook of Adverse Reactions,* edited by M.D. Davies, pp. 10–31. Oxford University Press, London.

Subject Index

A
A priori knowledge, 76,106
Absorption, 18-24
  "averaging artifact," 79-80
  and dissolution, 22
  first-order, 80,105
  and hepatic first pass, 18-19
  pharmacokinetic models, 18-24, 28
  prehepatic metabolism effect, 20-21
  zero-order, 80
Accuracy
  of assay, 76
  of estimation method, 90,103
Acetaminophen, 23
Activated partial thromboplastin time, 128-130
Active transport, 28
Acute dosage, and intrinsic clearance, 18-19
Adjusted clearance, 224
Adverse effects, 232-233
Age-dependent individuality, 2,8
Age-dependent transfer, 48-49
  and time dependence, 49
Age factors; *see also* Elderly
  benzodiazepines, 164
  and clearance, 2,8,58
  pharmacokinetic models, 116-119, 157-165
  thiopental variability, 154-165
Age-varying rate function, 42-43
Albumin, 12-13
Amiflamine, hydroxylation phenotypes, 5-7
Analgesia, 172-175,182-183,185
Animals, drug testing, 236
Antipyrine, clearance variability, 15
Apomorphine, dose-response, 172-178, 185
Approximation error, 88-89
Area under the curve, 24
Assay variability, 29-30
Assessment, pharmacokinetic variability, 223-225
AUC, 24
"Averaging artifact," 79

B
Bayes
  empirical, 103,106
Bayes's theorem, 203,206
Bayesian feedback, 85,103,211-217
Bayesian linear estimation, 85,103
Bell-shaped dose-response curve, 178, 180,185
Benzodiazepines, 164
Beta-blockers, 4-6
Beta-function model, 146,148
Bias
  assays, 29-30
  in experimental studies, 74,84
  in population studies, 76
  and two-stage estimation, 118-121
Bimodality, 96-98
Binding; *see also* Plasma binding; Receptors
  and pharmacodynamic variability, 135-137
  volume of distribution relationship, 12-13
Bioavailability, 167-185
  multiple response drugs, 172-185
  and sigmoid dose-response relationship, 167-172
Biochemical individuality, 1-2
Bioequivalence, 79
Blood levels; *see also* Concentration
  from computer simulations, 77,105-106
  from experimental studies, 72-74,84
  models of, problems, 116-118
  and pharmacodynamic variability, 127-138
  in pharmacokinetic screening, elderly, 231-232
  from population studies, 75-76
  tricyclics, and hydroxylation, 3-5
Blood pressure, 174-176
Body weight
  phenytoin variability, 116-119
  thiopental variability, 154-156
Bradycardia, 174-177
Butorphanol, 178,180

C
C-optimal designs, 191-192
Caffeine, 27

Calibration, and assay error, 29–30
Case-control study, 75
Cav, 19–20
Chlorothiazide, 77
Chronic dosage, clearance, 18–19,21
Chronopharmacology, 137–138
Clearance, 13–28
  and age, theory, 58
  and disposition, models, 11–12,15–28, 70
  pharmacogenetic variability, 6,8
  rapid intercompartment, 157–162
  slow intercompartment, 157–162
  thiopental variability, 155–165
Clonidine, 181
Closed-form solution, 87
CNS-active drugs, 133–135
Coefficient of variation, 60–61,68,84, 156–157
  interpretation, criticism, 114–116,123, 164
Compartmental systems, 31–50
Compliance, drug, 1–3
Computer generated data, 87,97
Computer generated individuals, 77,98
Computer package, 78
Computer simulation
  Bayesian feedback estimation, 211–215
  disadvantages, 214
  in drug development, 105–106
  and interpretation, 122
  nonlinear mixed-effect model, 89–91
  nonparametric maximum likelihood, 96–101
  nonparametric pharmacodynamic models, 146–149
  pharmacokinetic data, 76–78
Computer software, 65,67,89,91
Concentration; *see also* Blood levels
  Bayesian feedback prediction, 211–217
  and bioavailability, 167–185
  cost functions, 201–209
  dosage relationship, phenytoin, 116–118
  models of, problems, 118
  and drug effect, models, 139
  and drug response, 172–185
  nonparametric pharmacodynamic models, 144–152
  parametric pharmacodynamic models, 140–144
  and pharmacodynamic variability, 137
  statistical issues, 116–118
  thiopental variability, 155–165
Constant-coefficient-of-variation model, 60–61,68
Constant error variance, 194
Continuous density function, 204
"Continuous design measures," 190
Continuous solution, 96,100

Control groups, 216–217
Controlled-release products, 185
Correlation coefficients; *see also* Coefficient of variation
  interpretation, 114
Cost function, 201–208
Courmarin anticoagulants, 130–131
Covariance, 54
Covariance matrix, 83,121,189–190
Creatinine clearance, 229–230
Cross-over design, 75

D

D-optimal designs, 191–200
Data
  analysis, 102–103
  collection, 75
  naive averaging of, 78–81
  recording of, 76
  routinely-collected, 76,85,98
  transformation of, 68–69,101
Debrisoquine phenotyping, 4–7
Design optimality, 187–200
Destructive sampling, 89
Deterministic model, 32–35
Dicumarol, 130–131
Digoxin, 231
Dihydroergotamine, 27,185
3,4 Dihydroxyphenylacetic acid levels, 178,180
Diisopropylphenol, 137
Discrete solution, 100
Disoprofol, 127
Disposition, 11–12,18–28
  and clearance, 11–12,15–28
  hepatic extraction, 18–19
  intrinsic clearance relationship, 15–16
  and plasma binding, 16–17
Dissolution, and absorption, 22
Distribution, 12–13
  bimodal, 96–98,101
  bivariate, 71,94
  conditional, 92
  Dirac, 93
  discrete, 93–96,100
  empirical, 94–95,97–98
  frequency, 5,95
  gaussian, 66–67,82–84,96–98,102
  half-life, 159
  joint, 94–95
  lognormal, 90–91
  long-tailed, 101
  marginal, 93–96
  moments of, 90–91
  multivariate, 91,105
  normal, 66,96
  parametric, 66
  and pharmacokinetics, 12–13

SUBJECT INDEX 241

probability, 66–67,70,92–94
symmetric, 62,82,101
thiopental variability, and age, 157–163
two-compartment models, 34
uniform, 97
L-Dopa, 21,183
DOPAC levels, 178,180
Dosage
  form, 79
Dosage regimen
  individual adjustment of, 70,105–106
  lithium, 73,105–106
  open-loop, 106
  standard, 104
Dose-dependence, 28
Dose-response
  age and body weight factors, 156–157
  apomorphine, 172–178
  Bayesian feedback application, 211–217
  and bioavailability, 167–185
  cost functions, 201–209
  multiple response drugs, 172–185
  pharmacokinetics and pharmacodynamics, 153–165
  and receptors, 178
  yohimbine, 174
Dosing interval, 19
Drug clearance, *see* Clearance
Drug compliance, 1–3
Drug development, 103–106,235–237
Drug disease interactions, 231–232
Drug disposition, *see* Disposition
Drug distribution, *see* Distribution
Drug-drug interactions, 231–232
Drug response; *see also* Dose-response
  overview, 1–9
Drug toxicity, 223,235–236

E
Econometrics, 102
EEG measures, 153–165
Efficiency, optimal designs, 193,199
Elderly; *see also* Age factors
  pharmacokinetic screening, 222–233
  and renal status, 229–230
  special requirements, screening, 232–233
Elimination rate, succinylcholine, 132–133
EM-algorithm, 103
E_{max} model, 141–143,146–147,157
  simulations, 146–147
Empirical models, 56–59
End point determination, 29–30
Equations, and models, 117–118
Equilibrium, 139
Ergotamine, 168–172,185
Error models, notation, 188–189

Error-robust design, 195
Error variance, 194
Ethanol, 133–134
Exponential compartment model, 49
Extended least squares method, 61–62,82, 87–90,109
Extraction ratio, 12,14,16,18–19,27
Eyelash reflex, 160

F
Feedback
  control procedure, 203,206
  pharmacokinetic forecasting, 211–217
First-order absorption, 80,105
Fitting, 81
Forecasting, 88,106
Fraction of drug unbound, *see fu*
Fractional effect, 142–143
Fragmentary data, 76
fu
  and clearance, 14, 17
  and distribution, 12–13
Full kinetic screen, 224–225

G
Gamma compartment model, 41–49
Gastric emptying, 22–23
Gastrointestinal epithelium, 21
Gaussian distribution, 66–67
General error variance, 194
General heteroscedastic model, 61–62
Global two-stage method, 82–85,91,102
Glomerular filtration rate, 15
Growth curve, 102
Guanfacine, 27

H
Half-life
  in pharmacokinetic models, 12
  and variability comparisons, 27–28
Haloperidol, 178,180–181
Hazard rate, 42–43
Healthy volunteers, 72–75
Heart rate, 174–176
Heparin, 128–130
Hepatic clearance
  blood flow effect, 26–27
  and disposition, models, 18–28
  models, 14–15,18–28
Hepatic first pass, 18–19
Heteroscedastic models, 60–62
Hill model, 56–57,141–142,149
Histogram, 66–68,70–71,95–96,110
Homoscedastic model, 60
Hydroxylation phenotypes, 4–7
5-Hydroxytryptamine receptors, 171

SUBJECT INDEX

Hyperalgesia, 172–175,178,182–183,185
Hysteresis, 139,144–145,151

I

Incomplete dissolution, 22
Independent variable(s), 56–57,71
Indicator variables, 57–58
Indirect data, 69
Individual data, 70–75,79–80,87
Information matrix, 189–190
Infusion, 70,103
Initial distribution volume, 157–162
Intensity rate function, 42
Interindividual variability, 1–9
  definition, 220
  drug response, 1–9
  estimation of, pharmacokinetics, 65–111
  nonparametric maximum likelihood approach, 91–101
  pharmacodynamics, 125–138
Intestinal microflora, 20–21
Intraindividual variability, 8–9
  definition, 220
  pharmacodynamics, 125–138
  pharmacokinetics, 8–9
Intravenous infusion, 70,103
Intravenous injection, 17,70,90,96,103
Intrinsic clearance
  and disposition, 18–19
  in pharmacokinetic models, 13–14
  and plasma binding, 17
  prediction, 14
Iterated two-stage method, 83–84,102,121
Iteratively reweighted least squares, 61

K

Kernel-based methods, 96–97
Kolmogorov forward equations, 35
Kurtosis, 37,67

L

L-optimal designs, 191
Lack-of-memory property, 36
Least-squares methods, 60–62,120
Levodopa, 21,183
Lidocaine
  Bayesian feedback dosage estimation, 212–213,215–217
  hepatic clearance, disposition, 18–22, 26–27
  pharmacokinetic models, 18–22,26–27
Likelihood, population kinetics estimation, 91–96
Linear compartmental models, 31,56
Linear-effect model, 102,141,148

Linear mixed-effect models, 102
Linearity, assays, 29–30
Link model, 140,144,146,149
Lithium
  blood levels, experimental studies, 72–74
  plasma level simulations, 105–106
Liver blood flow, 26–27
Log-linear model, 56,141–142
Log-normal prior density, 204–206

M

Markov property, 36
Mathematical models, see Models
"Maximin" design, 195–198
Maximum-average-efficiency design, 196–197
Maximum likelihood estimation, 91–96, 103,120–121,202
Maximum observable response, see E_{max}
Mean
  arithmetic, 81
  empirical, 81
  geometric, 68,81
  sample, 79,100
  zero, 88,97
Mean permanence time, 41
Mean residence time, 48–50
Median, in statistical analysis, 68
MEGX, hepatic clearance, 21–22
Metabolite models, 143
Metabolites, and drug effects, 185
Method-of-moments procedure, 48
Metraxol, 133–135
Michaelis-Menten model, 56–57,83
  interpretation, statistical issues, 116–118
  nonlinear mixed-effect estimates, 90
Microcomputer, 30,83
Model-robust design, 195
Models
  criticism, 113–123
  linear with respect to the parameters, 102
  misspecification of, 98,102
  parametric and nonparametric approaches, 139–151
  pharmacokinetic/pharmacodynamic variability, 51–63
  and statistics, 69–71,116–118
  stochastic compartmental systems, 31–50
  unidentifiable, 75,85,97
  and variability, 11–28,51–63
Moment, 40–41,68,87–90,98
Monoamine oxidase inhibitors, 5–6
Monte Carlo simulations, 83–84
  and drug development, 105–106
Monitoring, 72,75

SUBJECT INDEX

Motility, drug effects, 177
Multiexponential models, 193–194
Multimodal distribution, 101
Multiple-regression analyses, 118–121
Multiple trough screen, 224,228
Multivariate approach, 54–55

N

Naive-averaging-of-data approach, 78–81
Naive-pooled-data method, 85–86, 101–102
Noise
  additive, 90,92
  multiplicative, 90
Noncompartmental approach, 39–40
Nonequilibrium model, 146,148–149
Nonlinear mixed-effect model, 84,86–91, 101–102,109
  simulations, 89–91
Nonparametric approaches, 139–151
Nonparametric maximum likelihood, 91–102
Normal subjects, 72–75
Nortriptyline
  dose-response curve, 181
  response prediction, hydroxylation, 5–7

O

Objective function, 82,87
Observational data, 75–76
Off-on-off phenomenon, 182
On-off-on phenomenon, 182–183
One-compartment models, 70,90,146, 188
One-compartment open model, 146
One exponential model, 195–196
One-point designs, 195
"Open-loop" dosage regimen, 106
Ophthalmic drugs, 231
Optimal designs, 187–200
Optimal stochastic control, 203
Optimization, 91
Ordinary least squares method, 60,64
Outliers, 101
Overdosage, 104,106

P

Pain, drug response, 172–175,178–179, 182–183,185
Pancuronium, 139–140
Parametric approaches
  optimal design, 187–200
  pharmacodynamics, modeling, 139–151
Parametric nonlinearity, 78–85

Partial thromboplastin time, 128–130
Particle location
  gamma compartment models, 44–48
  stochastic model, 33–35,44–48
Particle residence times, 35–41
Pathophysiological individuality, 1–2,8
Peak values, 231
Pentylenetetrazol, 134
Pharmacodynamics
  age factors, thiopental, 155–165
  animals and humans, 125–138
  drug development role, 235–237
  ergotamine response, bioavailability, 168–172
  individual variability, 4
  modeling, 51–63,139–151
  in multiple response drugs, 172–185
  parametric and nonparametric approaches, 139–151
  and pharmacokinetics, comparison, 132,134–135
  and pharmacokinetics, integration, 140, 144,146,149,153–165,172–185
  thiopental, 153–165
  variability in, definition, 219–220
Pharmacogenetics, 4–8
Pharmacokinetic data, 71–85
Pharmacokinetic experimental data, 72–75,78–85
Pharmacokinetic fictive data, 76–77
Pharmacokinetic-pharmacodynamic linking, 140,144,146,149
Pharmacokinetic screen, elderly, 222–228
Pharmacokinetics
  assessment, 223–225
  clinical use, controversy, 3–4
  computer simulations, 76–78
  drug development role, 235–237
  in the elderly, screening, 222–233
  ergotamine, and bioavailability, 168–172
  experimental studies, 72–75,78–85
  interindividual variability, estimation, 65–111
  comparison of methods, 101–102
  models, 11–28,51–63,69–71
  criticism, 113–123
  in multiple response drugs, 172–187
  parameter estimation in, design, 187–200
  and pharmacodynamics, comparison, 132,134–135,172–185
  and pharmacodynamics, integration, 140,144,146,149,153–165, 172–185
  population studies, 75–76,85–103
  reproducibility, 8
  stochastic compartment systems, 31–50

SUBJECT INDEX

Pharmacokinetics (contd.)
  thiopental, 153–165
    age factors, 154–165
  variability in, definition, 219–220
  variability in, reduction, 222
Pharmacostatistical model, 69–71
Phase III trials, 224–225
Phenobarbital, 133–134
Phenotyping, drug hydroxylation, 4–6
Phenytoin, 24,116,211
Pilocarpine, 1–3
Plasma binding
  and disposition variability, 16–17
  and pharmacodynamic variability, 135–137
  volume of distribution relationship, 12–13
Plasma levels, see Blood levels
Population
  approach, 54–55,59
  characteristics, 85–91
  kinetics, 75,91–103
  pharmacokinetics, 71,75–76
  variance-covariance matrix, 78,81–84
Posterior density, 203
Predictable variability, 220–221
Prediction of response, 3–4
Prehepatic metabolism, 20–22
Prevost's algorithm, 83
Prior density, 203–205
Probability
  density, 71,92,99
  density-function, 71,98
  distribution, 35,66–67,70,92–94,101
Promethazine, 182–183
Proportional flows, 34–35
Propranolol, 18
Protein binding, 135–137,153–165
Prothrombin-complex activity, 130–131
"Pseudocompartments," 44–45
Psychological individuality, 1–2

Q
Quadratic cost function, 201
Quinidine, 104

R
Random
  effect, 88,90,104
  number generator, 76–77,97
  sampling, 75,97
  variable, 66,70
Rapidly equilibrating compartment, 157–162
Rats, drug testing, 236

Rebound, 79
Receptors; see also Binding
  and bioavailability, 171
  concentration-effect models, 140–144, 151
  dosage effects, 178,180
  and drug variability, 136–137
Reference-individual, 86,101
Regression models, 51–55
  criticism, 118–123
Renal clearance, models, 15
Renal status, 229–230
Reproducibility, drug kinetics, 8
Residence time, 36–41,48–50
Retention time, 36–37,43–45,48
Righting reflex, 133–134
Robustness, 102

S
Salicylamide, 24
Sampling, and assay error, 29
Sampling in experimental studies, 72–75
Sampling in pharmacokinetic screening, 226
Saturable elimination, 23–24
Secondary peak, 79–80
Sensitivity, assays, 29–30
Sensitization, models, 143,146
  simulations, 148–149
Sequential designs, 195
Serotonin receptors, 171
Serum concentration, see Concentration
Sex factors, 116–119
Side effects, 232–233
Sigmoid dose-response, 167–172
Sigmoid E_{max} model, 140–143,146–147, 157
  simulations, 146–148
Simulations, see Computer simulation
Single trough screen, 224,228
Skewness
  nonparametric maximum likelihood use, 101
  and statistics, 68
Slowly equilibrating compartment, 157–162
Smoothing, 79–80,96–100
Sojourn time, 48
Sparteine phenotyping, 4,6
Stability, drug kinetics, 8
Standard deviation, 68
Standard two-stage method, 68,81–85, 102
Standardized design, 79,102
Statistical approach
  and models, criticism, 113–123

SUBJECT INDEX

pharmacokinetic variability, 66–69
population kinetics analysis, 102–103
Statistical moments, usefulness, 40–41
Steady-state concentration
  apomorphine, and heart rate, 175–176
  clonidine, hypotensive effect, 181
  and computer simulated prediction, 216
  models, statistical interpretation, 116–118
  and pharmacodynamic effect, ergotamine, 169–171
  and saturable elimination, 24
Stochastic compartmental systems, 31–50
  age-varying transfer rates, 41–47
  particle location, 33–35
  particle residence times, 35–41
  pharmacokinetic variability modeling, 31–50
"Stochastic parameter regression," 102
Stochastic prediction, 100
Structural models
  notation, 188–189
  parameter estimation, design problem, 189–190
  pharmacokinetics/pharmacodynamics, 52,55–57
Succinylcholine, 131–133
Sum of exponentials model, 56
Symmetric distribution, 101

T

Tachycardia, 175–177
Target concentration, 75,106
Temporal aspects, see Time factors/time course
Theophylline
  interindividual variability, 211
  pharmacodynamic variability, 137
  pharmacokinetic models, 15,19,26–27
Therapeutic index, 75,103
Therapeutic range, 216
Therapeutic window, 181
Thiopental, 153–165
Thiopentone, 178–179
Three compartment model, 157–165
Time-average concentration, 19–20
Time dependence, 49
Time factors/time course
  "averaging artifact," 79–80
  and individual pharmacokinetic data, 56
  multiple response drugs, 177
  pharmacodynamics, 137–138
  and plasma concentration, 169–171
Time lag, 79–80

Time series, 69,102
Tobramycin kinetic model, 204–206
Tolerance, models, 143,146,148–149
Total body clearance, 157–163
Toxicity, 223,235
Transport, 28
Tricyclic antidepressants
  hydroxylation phenotypes, 4–5
  individual differences, response, 3–5
Triexponential model, 155,157
Trough values, 224,228,231–232
Two-compartment model
  and computer simulated prediction, 216–217
  nonlinear mixed-effect estimates, 90
  pharmacokinetics, 31–50
  population approach, 110–111
Two-parameter exponential model, 192
Two-parameter model, 196–197,205–206
Two-stage methods, 81–85,109–110
  criticism, 118–122

U

U-shaped dose-response curve, 178
Unbalanced data, 75–76
Unbound fraction, see f_u
Unbound volume of distribution, 12–13, 16
Uncertain dynamic systems, 201–207
"Uncertainty interval," 195–197
Unchanged drug, 72
Underdosage, 104,106
Unimodal distribution, 101
Unpredictable variability, 220–221
Unweighted least squares, 30,60,64
Urine levels, experimental studies, 72–74

V

V, see Volume of distribution
Variability, definition and assessment, 219–221
Variance, 67–68
Variance-covariance matrix, 82–83,88–89, 121
Variance models, 52–53,59–64
Visitations, 36–37
Vocalization threshold, 173–175,182–183
Volume of distribution
  pharmacokinetic models, 11–12
  and plasma binding, 12–13
  thiopental variability, 155–165
Volunteers, experimental studies, 72–75

W

Weighted least squares method, 30, 60–61, 120
Workup, and assay error, 29

Y

Yawning, drug effect, 178
Yohimbine, dose-response, 173, 185